VOLUME NINETY TWO

VITAMINS AND HORMONES

Anorexia

VOLUME NINETY TWO

VITAMINS AND HORMONES

Anorexia

Editor-in-Chief

GERALD LITWACK, PhD

Toluca Lake, North Hollywood, California

ELSEVIER

AMSTERDAM • BOSTON • HEIDELBERG • LONDON
NEW YORK • OXFORD • PARIS • SAN DIEGO
SAN FRANCISCO • SINGAPORE • SYDNEY • TOKYO

Academic Press is an imprint of Elsevier

Cover photo credit:
Yosten, G.L.C.
Novel Neuropeptides in the Control of Food Intake:
Neuronostatin and Nesfatin-1
Vitamins and Hormones (2013) 92, pp. 1–26.

Academic Press is an imprint of Elsevier
32 Jamestown Road, London, NW1 7BY, UK
The Boulevard, Langford Lane, Kidlington, Oxford, OX5 1GB, UK
Linacre House, Jordan Hill, Oxford OX2 8DP, UK
225 Wyman Street, Waltham, MA 02451, USA
525 B Street, Suite 1800, San Diego, CA 92101-4495, USA

First edition 2013

ISBN: 978-0-12-410473-0
ISSN: 0083-6729

Printed and bound in USA
13 14 15 16 11 10 9 8 7 6 5 4 3 2 1

CONTENTS

Contributors *xiii*
Preface *xvii*

1. Novel Neuropeptides in the Control of Food Intake: Neuronostatin and Nesfatin-1 **1**

Gina L. C. Yosten

1. Introduction 2
2. Neuronostatin 8
3. Nesfatin-1 11
4. Conclusions 16

References 19

2. Anorexia and Hypothalamic Degeneration **27**

Ida A. K. Nilsson, Charlotte Lindfors, Martin Schalling, Tomas Hökfelt, and Jeanette E. Johansen

1. Introduction 28
2. The *anx/anx* Mouse 30
3. General Aspects of Mechanisms Underlying Weight Disturbances 42
4. Neurodegeneration and Mitochondrial Dysfunction Related to Eating Disorders in Humans 48
5. Conclusions and Future Directions 49

Acknowledgments 49
References 50

3. The Role of Ghrelin in Anorexia–Cachexia Syndromes **61**

Bobby Guillory, Andres Splenser, and Jose Garcia

1. Introduction 62
2. Discovery of Ghrelin 63
3. Ghrelin, GHS-R1a, and GOAT 64
4. Mechanisms of Action of Ghrelin 66
5. Ghrelin and Sarcopenia of Aging 72
6. Ghrelin and Cancer Cachexia 73
7. Ghrelin and COPD-Induced Cachexia 83
8. Ghrelin and Anorexia Nervosa 85
9. Ghrelin and CHF-Induced Cachexia 87

10. Ghrelin and ESRD 89
11. AIDS-Associated Cachexia 90
12. RA-Associated Cachexia 91
13. Conclusions 93
Acknowledgments 93
References 93

4. Ghrelin Gene Variants and Eating Disorders **107**

Tetsuya Ando

1. Introduction 108
2. Ghrelin Signaling System 108
3. Physiological Functions of Ghrelin 110
4. Ghrelin and Eating Disorders 110
5. Ghrelin Gene Variants and Eating Disorders 111
6. Association of Ghrelin Polymorphisms with Anthropometry and Eating Pathology in Young Women 116
7. Association of Ghrelin Polymorphisms with Changes in Eating Disorder Phenotypes 117
8. Conclusions 117
References 118

5. Steroid Metabolism and Excretion in Anorexia Nervosa **125**

Wassif Samuel Wassif and Andrew Rashad Ross

1. Introduction 125
2. Steroid Metabolism in Health 126
3. Steroid Metabolism in AN 129
4. Steroid Excretion in AN 130
5. Effects of Refeeding 136
6. Conclusions 137
Acknowledgments 138
References 138

6. Anorexia Nervosa and Estrogen Receptors **141**

Nicolas Ramoz, Audrey Versini, and Philip Gorwood

1. Introduction 142
2. Anorexia Nervosa 142
3. Estrogens and Estrogen Receptors and Pathways 145
4. Estrogen and Anorexia 147
5. Human Genetics of Estrogen Pathway in Anorexia Nervosa 151

6. Conclusions 155
References 156

7. Cannabinoid Receptors and Cholecystokinin in Feeding Inhibition 165

Francisco Alén, M. Teresa Ramírez-López, Raquel Gómez de Heras, Fernando Rodríguez de Fonseca, and Laura Orio

1. Introduction: Peripheral Regulation of Food Intake: A Place for Endocannabinoids and Cholecystokinin 166
2. The Endocannabinoids and Feeding Regulation 168
3. CCK and Feeding Regulation 175
4. Interactions Between CCK and Endocannabinoid Receptors in the Regulation of Feeding 181
5. Conclusions and Clinical Relevance 183

Acknowledgments 184
References 184

8. Treatment of Cachexia: Melanocortin and Ghrelin Interventions 197

Jeremy Steinman and Mark Daniel DeBoer

1. Introduction 198
2. Molecular Mediators of Cachexia 199
3. Peripheral and Central Appetite Regulation 201
4. Cancer Cachexia 209
5. Cardiac Cachexia 215
6. Renal Cachexia 219
7. Other Cachexia 220
8. Summary of Treatment Effects 225
9. Future Directions 226

References 227

9. The Influence of Estrogen Therapies on Bone Mineral Density in Premenopausal Women with Anorexia Nervosa and Amenorrhea 243

Jocelyn Lebow and Leslie Sim

1. Introduction 244
2. Estrogen Therapy and Bone Mass 245
3. Potential Clinical Drawbacks of Estrogen Therapy for Patients with AN 246
4. Influence of Oral Contraceptives on Bone Mineral Density 247
5. Influence of Hormone Replacement Therapy on Bone Mineral Density 248

6. The Role of Insulin-Like Growth Factor 1 and Estrogen on Bone Mineral Density 251
7. Implications 252
References 256

10. Clinical and Hormonal Variables Related to Bone Mass Loss in Anorexia Nervosa Patients 259

María Luisa Fernández-Soto, Amalia González-Jiménez, Marta Chamorro-Fernández, and Socorro Leyva-Martínez

1. Introduction 260
2. Materials and Methods 261
3. Results 263
4. Discussion 265
Acknowledgments 267
References 267

11. Mechanism-Based Therapeutic Approaches to Cachexia 271

Fabio Penna, Gabriella Bonelli, Francesco M. Baccino, and Paola Costelli

1. Introduction 272
2. Body and Tissue Wasting 273
3. Anorexia 274
4. Inflammation 275
5. Tissue Wasting in Cachexia: Hypoanabolism or Hypercatabolism? 279
6. From Mechanistic Alterations to Therapeutic Strategies 281
7. Nutritional Interventions 281
8. Anti-Inflammatory Strategies 283
9. Inhibition of Cytokine Production 284
10. Interference with Cytokine-Receptor Interaction 285
11. Strategies to Correct Metabolic Alterations 286
12. Conclusions 290
References 290

12. Cisplatin-Induced Anorexia and Ghrelin 301

Tomohisa Hattori, Koji Yakabi, and Hiroshi Takeda

1. Introduction 302
2. Cisplatin-Induced Overproduction of 5-HT 303
3. Cisplatin, 5-HT-Induced Ghrelin Regulation 307
4. Treatment of Ghrelin- and Ghrelin Enhancer-Based, Cisplatin-Caused Dyspepsia 311

5. Conclusion 315
References 315

13. Anorexia of Aging **319**

Zbigniew Kmieć, Erika Pétervári, Márta Balaskó, and Miklós Székely

1. Introduction 320
2. Animal Studies 322
3. Human Studies 335
4. Anorexia of Aging May Result from the Imbalance of Catabolism and Anabolism: Convergence of Animal and Human Studies 341
5. Therapeutic Approaches to Overcome the Anorexia of Aging and Its Deleterious Effects on Body Functions 345
6. Conclusions and Perspectives 346

Acknowledgments 347
References 347

Index *357*

CONTRIBUTORS

Francisco Alén
Departamento de Psicobiología, Facultad de Psicología, Universidad Complutense, Madrid, Spain

Tetsuya Ando
Section of Stress Research, Department of Psychosomatic Research, National Institute of Mental Health, National Center of Neurology and Psychiatry, Ogawahigashi-cho, Kodaira, Tokyo, Japan

Francesco M. Baccino
Department of Clinical and Biological Sciences, University of Torino, Turin, Italy

Márta Balaskó
Department of Pathophysiology and Gerontology, Medical School, University of Pécs, Pécs, Hungary

Gabriella Bonelli
Department of Clinical and Biological Sciences, University of Torino, Turin, Italy

Marta Chamorro-Fernández
Department of Psychiatry, University Hospital Carlos Haya, Málaga, Spain

Paola Costelli
Department of Clinical and Biological Sciences, University of Torino, Turin, Italy

Mark Daniel DeBoer
Division of Pediatric Endocrinology, Department of Pediatrics, P.O. Box 800386, University of Virginia, Charlottesville, Virginia, USA

María Luisa Fernández-Soto
Eating Disorders Unit, Department of Endocrinology and Clinical Nutrition, University Hospital San Cecilio, Granada, Spain

Jose Garcia
Division of Diabetes, Endocrinology and Metabolism, Michael E DeBakey Veterans Affairs Medical Center, and Department of Molecular and Cell Biology, Huffington Center on Aging, Baylor College of Medicine, Houston, Texas, USA

Raquel Gómez de Heras
Departamento de Psicobiología, Facultad de Psicología, Universidad Complutense, Madrid, Spain

Amalia González-Jiménez
Department of Medicine, University of Granada, Granada, Spain

Philip Gorwood
INSERM UMR894, Centre de Psychiatrie et Neurosciences, and CMME, Sainte-Anne Hospital, Paris Descartes University, Paris, France

Bobby Guillory
Division of Diabetes, Endocrinology and Metabolism, Michael E DeBakey Veterans Affairs Medical Center, Baylor College of Medicine, Houston, Texas, USA

Tomohisa Hattori
Tsumura Research Laboratories, Tsumura & Co., Yoshiwara, Ami-machi, Inashiki-gun, Ibaraki, Japan

Tomas Hökfelt
Department of Neuroscience, Karolinska Institutet, Stockholm, Sweden

Jeanette E. Johansen
Department of Molecular Medicine & Surgery, Karolinska Institutet, and Center for Molecular Medicine, Karolinska University Hospital, Stockholm, Sweden

Zbigniew Kmieć
Department of Histology, Medical University of Gdansk, Gdansk, Poland

Jocelyn Lebow
Department of Psychiatry and Psychology, Mayo Clinic, Rochester, Minnesota, USA

Socorro Leyva-Martínez
Eating Disorders Unit, Department of Endocrinology and Clinical Nutrition, University Hospital San Cecilio, Granada, Spain

Charlotte Lindfors
Department of Molecular Medicine & Surgery, Karolinska Institutet, and Center for Molecular Medicine, Karolinska University Hospital, Stockholm, Sweden

Ida A.K. Nilsson
Department of Molecular Medicine & Surgery; Center for Molecular Medicine, Karolinska University Hospital, and Department of Neuroscience, Karolinska Institutet, Stockholm, Sweden

Laura Orio
Departamento de Psicobiología, Facultad de Psicología, Universidad Complutense, Madrid, Spain

Fabio Penna
Department of Clinical and Biological Sciences, University of Torino, Turin, Italy

Erika Pétervári
Department of Pathophysiology and Gerontology, Medical School, University of Pécs, Pécs, Hungary

Nicolas Ramoz
INSERM UMR894, Centre de Psychiatrie et Neurosciences, Paris, France

M. Teresa Ramírez-López
Departamento de Psicobiología, Facultad de Psicología, Universidad Complutense, Madrid, Spain

Fernando Rodríguez de Fonseca
Departamento de Psicobiología, Facultad de Psicología, Universidad Complutense; Fundación IMABIS, Hospital Universitario Carlos Haya, Málaga, and CIBEROBN, Instituto Salud Carlos III, Madrid, Spain

Andrew Rashad Ross
Department of Ophthalmology, University Hospital, Assiut, Egypt

Martin Schalling
Department of Molecular Medicine & Surgery, Karolinska Institutet, and Center for Molecular Medicine, Karolinska University Hospital, Stockholm, Sweden

Leslie Sim
Department of Psychiatry and Psychology, Mayo Clinic, Rochester, Minnesota, USA

Andres Splenser
Division of Diabetes, Endocrinology and Metabolism, Michael E DeBakey Veterans Affairs Medical Center, Baylor College of Medicine, Houston, Texas, USA

Jeremy Steinman
Division of Pediatric Endocrinology, Department of Pediatrics, P.O. Box 800386, University of Virginia, Charlottesville, Virginia, USA

Miklós Székely
Department of Pathophysiology and Gerontology, Medical School, University of Pécs, Pécs, Hungary

Hiroshi Takeda
Pathophysiology and Therapeutics, Hokkaido University, Faculty of Pharmaceutical Sciences, and Department of Gastroenterology and Hematology, Graduate School of Medicine, Hokkaido University, Kita-ku, Sapporo, Japan

Audrey Versini
INSERM UMR894, Centre de Psychiatrie et Neurosciences, Paris, France

Wassif Samuel Wassif
Department of Clinical Biochemistry, Bedford Hospital NHS Trust, Kempston Road, MK42 9DJ Bedford, United Kingdom

Koji Yakabi
Department of Gastroenterology and Hepatology, Saitama Medical Center, Saitama Medical University, Tsujido-machi, Kamoda, Kawagoe, Saitama, Japan

Gina L.C. Yosten
Department of Pharmacological and Physiological Science, Saint Louis University School of Medicine, Saint Louis, Missouri, USA

PREFACE

Anorexia nervosa is a syndrome in which a young person limits food consumption to the point where he/she is seriously underweight, a condition that can become life threatening. Young females, more than young males, seem to be the most representative. An anorexic can have the view that his/her body is always overweight, when, in fact, it can be seriously underweight. Until recently, rather little by way of basic science was understood about this condition. Newer research indicates the involvement of many factors, nervous and hormonal. This volume focuses on the newer scientific bases for this disease, and clinical observations and treatments generated through scientific knowledge.

Chapter 1 on "Novel neuropeptides in the control of food intake: neuronostatin and nesfatin-1" is contributed by G.L.C. Yosten. "Anorexia and hypothalamic degeneration" is the topic of I.A.K. Nilsson, C. Lindfors, M. Schalling, T. Hökfelt, and J.E. Johansen (Chapter 2). B. Guillory, A. Splenser, and J. Garcia discuss "The role of ghrelin in anorexia-cachexia syndromes" in Chapter 3. T. Ando, in Chapter 4, reports on "Ghrelin gene variants and eating disorders." The topic of W.S. Wassif and A.R. Ross is "Steroid metabolism and excretion in anorexia nervosa" (Chapter 5). In a related theme, N. Ramoz, A. Versini, and P. Gorwood review "Anorexia nervosa and estrogen receptors" in Chapter 6. "Cannabinoid receptors and cholecystokinin in feeding inhibition" is the subject of F.A. Fariñas, M.T. Ramírez-López, R. Gomez de Heras, F. Rodríguez de Fonseca, and L. Orio (Chapter 7).

Trending toward the clinical observations and treatments, J. Steinman and M.D. DeBoer contribute "Treatment of cachexia: melanocortin and ghrelin interventions" (Chapter 8). "The influence of estrogen therapies on bone mineral density in premenopausal women with anorexia nervosa and amenorrhea" is the topic of J. Lebow and L. Sim (Chapter 9). "Clinical and hormonal variables related to bone mass loss in anorexia nervosa patients" is reviewed by M.L. Fernández-Soto, A. González-Jiménez, M. Chamorro-Fernández, and S. Leyva-Martínez in Chapter 10. F. Penna, G. Bonelli, F.M. Baccino, and P. Costelli present "Mechanism-based therapeutic approaches to cachexia" in Chapter 11. "Cisplatin-induced anorexia and ghrelin" is discussed in Chapter 12 by T. Hattori, K. Yakabi, and H. Takeda. The final chapter is a treatise on "Anorexia of aging" by Z. Kmieć, E. Pétervári, M. Balaskó, and M. Székely (Chapter 13).

The figure on the cover of the book is Fig. 1.1 from Chapter 1.

Mary Ann Zimmerman and Helene Kabes of Elsevier, Oxford, UK, were instrumental in the assembly of this volume.

Gerald Litwack, PhD
November 13, 2012

CHAPTER ONE

Novel Neuropeptides in the Control of Food Intake: Neuronostatin and Nesfatin-1

Gina L.C. Yosten[1]

Department of Pharmacological and Physiological Science, Saint Louis University School of Medicine, Saint Louis, Missouri, USA

[1]Corresponding author: e-mail address: gyosten@slu.edu; glcyosten@yahoo.com

Contents

1. Introduction 2
   1.1 Anatomic basis for the neural control of appetite 2
   1.2 The central melanocortin system 4
   1.3 The central oxytocin system 6
2. Neuronostatin 8
   2.1 Introduction 8
   2.2 Neuronostatin-induced anorexia 9
3. Nesfatin-1 11
   3.1 Introduction 11
   3.2 Nesfatin-1-induced anorexia 12
4. Conclusions 16
   4.1 The proposed central POMC–CRH–OT feeding circuit 16
   4.2 Oxytocinergic and nonoxytocinergic-mediated anorexia 18
References 19

Abstract

Food intake is a complex, multifaceted process that involves the integration of numerous nutritional signals and behavioral outputs. Dozens of centrally acting peptide hormones that contribute to the control of appetite and food intake have been identified. Two recently described peptide hormones, neuronostatin and nesfatin-1, both act in the brain to induce anorexia, albeit through potentially different mechanisms. In this chapter, the central circuits mediating the anorexigenic effect of these two hormones, their interaction with the central melanocortin and oxytocin systems, and the physiological relevance of these hormones in appetite control are described and an integrated model of hypothalamic control of energy intake is presented.

Vitamins and Hormones, Volume 92
ISSN 0083-6729
http://dx.doi.org/10.1016/B978-0-12-410473-0.00001-5

1. INTRODUCTION

Food intake is a complex, multifaceted process that is regulated by a combination of centrally derived hormonal signals and hormonal and neural signals originating in the periphery. Numerous hormones that alter food intake have been identified and the number is continually increasing. Slight infarctions/perturbations in the delicate hormonal control of food intake have disastrous effects, as evidenced by the severe obesity exhibited by leptin- or leptin receptor-deficient animals (Brunner et al., 1997; Ingalls, Dickie, & Snell, 1950) and humans (Ozata, Ozdemir, & Licinio, 1999), and anorexia observed in humans with reduced ghrelin production (Neary et al., 2004). Dozens of neuropeptides have been identified over the past few decades, which act in the brain, particularly in the hypothalamus, to alter food intake and energy expenditure. The production and actions of these peptides have been shown to be altered in obese states and several have been shown to be physiologically relevant regulators of appetite and glucose metabolism. One example is leptin, which is produced by adipocytes and acts in the brain to decrease food intake (Bray & York, 1997). The amount of leptin produced by the body is proportional to the number of adipocytes, so obese patients have higher circulating levels of leptin than normal weight individuals (Sinha et al., 1996). Several theories exist as to how the brain integrates and responds to nutritional status information, such as adipostatic leptin signaling, and clearly that the hypothalamus and brainstem are intimately involved in this process.

1.1. Anatomic basis for the neural control of appetite

Studies on the neural control of appetite have historically focused on the hypothalamus and certain areas of the brainstem, such as the nucleus of the solitary tract (Berthoud, 2002). The hypothalamus is a highly complex brain region forming the walls of the third cerebroventricle below the thalamus. It extends roughly from the area of the anterior commissure (at the midline)/optic chiasm rostrally to the posterior limits of the mammillary nuclei caudally (Daniel, 1976). The hypothalamus comprises over 40 distinct nuclei (Berthoud, 2002) that have been linked to important homeostatic functions, in addition to food intake, including cardiovascular function, fluid homeostasis, thermoregulation, and the endocrine control of the function of both the anterior and posterior lobes of the pituitary (Toni, Malaguti, Benfenati, & Martini, 2004). The hypothalamus is functionally and physically connected to the anterior and posterior pituitary, respectively. Releasing and inhibiting factors (such as growth hormone-releasing hormone, somatostatin, dopamine, corticotropin-releasing hormone (CRH), gonadotropin-releasing hormone, and thyroid-stimulating hormone) are produced in the neurons of various hypothalamic nuclei. These catecholaminergic or peptidergic neurons project to the median eminence, where, upon depolarization, they release their synaptic contents into the intracellular space adjacent to the fenestrated capillary endothelium that begins the hypophyseal portal system. The long portal veins then deliver these peptides/catecholamines to the anterior pituitary, or adenohypophysis, where they stimulate (or inhibit) the release of pituitary hormones such as growth hormone, prolactin, thyroid-stimulating hormone, luteinizing hormone, follicle-stimulating hormone, and adrenocorticotrophic hormone. The posterior pituitary, or neurohypophysis, is physically connected to the hypothalamus. Neurons originating in the hypothalamus, particularly in the paraventricular and supraoptic nuclei, send axons to the posterior pituitary, where they terminate. These neurons predominantly produce oxytocin and/or vasopressin, which are released directly into the peripheral bloodstream (Melmed, 1995).

Several hypothalamic nuclei have been implicated in appetite control. The arcuate nucleus is situated medially below and surrounding the ventral aspect of the third ventricle, dorsal to the median eminence. Because of its location, neurons in this nucleus are thought by many to be in a prime location for sensing metabolic signals, such as glucose, leptin, or insulin (Cone et al., 2001); however, there remains controversy concerning how peripherally derived factors reach neurons in the arcuate, since, as reviewed by Ferguson, Latchford, and Samson (2008), no direct evidence for the absence of the blood brain barrier in the arcuate has been convincingly presented. The arcuate nucleus contains one of only two populations of pro-opiomelanocortin (POMC)-producing neurons (the other population is located in the nucleus of the solitary tract). POMC neurons from both brain nuclei form an important metabolic and autonomic regulatory circuit (Cone, 2005). The arcuate nucleus communicates extensively with the paraventricular nuclei, which are a pair of bilaterally located nuclei positioned adjacent to the dorsal aspect of the third ventricle (Berthoud, 2002). The paraventricular nuclei contain basically three types of neurons. Magnocellular neurons are large cells that produce vasopressin and/or oxytocin and project either to the posterior pituitary or to other brain sites. Preautonomic parvocellular neurons are smaller cells that project to brainstem autonomic centers, such as the nucleus of the solitary tract and the rostral ventral lateral medulla. Neuroendocrine parvocellular neurons send their axons to the median eminence, where they deliver releasing hormones to the hypophyseal portal system (Ferguson et al., 2008).

Brainstem nuclei are also important in the control of appetite. The nucleus of the solitary tract, in addition to the arcuate nucleus of the hypothalamus, contains one of only two major populations of POMC-producing neurons and also is a major site of melanocortin receptor expression (Berthoud, 2002). The nucleus of the solitary tract receives direct vagal inputs, which signal changes in appetitive state (Berthoud, 2002). The nucleus of the solitary tract has direct reciprocal connections with the hypothalamus and may modulate sympathetic preganglionic neurons through its interconnections with the rostroventrolateral medulla (Berthoud, 2002).

Neurons within these important brain structures form neural circuits that control appetite. These circuits communicate by means of peptide neurotransmitters, such as alpha-MSH and oxytocin, which may act synchronously or in series to exert their effects. Two of these circuits are the central melanocortin system and the central oxytocin system.

1.2. The central melanocortin system

The central melanocortin system is defined anatomically as neurons arising in the arcuate nucleus of the hypothalamus and in the nucleus of the solitary tract in the brainstem, which produce either alpha-melanocyte-stimulating hormone alpha-MSH, a product of the POMC preprohormone, or neuropeptide Y (NPY) and agouti-related peptide (AgRP) (Cone, 2005; Fig. 1.1). These neurons project to target neurons that produce the melanocortin 3/4 receptors, located throughout the brain, but especially in other hypothalamic nuclei, including the preoptic nucleus, paraventricular nucleus, periventricular area, and the dorsal hypothalamic area, as well as in the nucleus of the solitary tract, dorsal motor nucleus of the vagus, the parabrachial nucleus, the caudate, and the putamen (Kishi et al., 2003). Activation of the melanocortin 3/4 receptors by alpha-MSH leads to a potent inhibition of food intake, and antagonism of the melanocortin 3/4 receptors by AgRP, which is a natural antagonist of these receptors, results in a stimulation of food intake (Cone, 2005). In addition to the antagonist activity of AgRP, NPY/AgRP neurons can directly inhibit POMC neurons by releasing GABA (Cone, 2005).

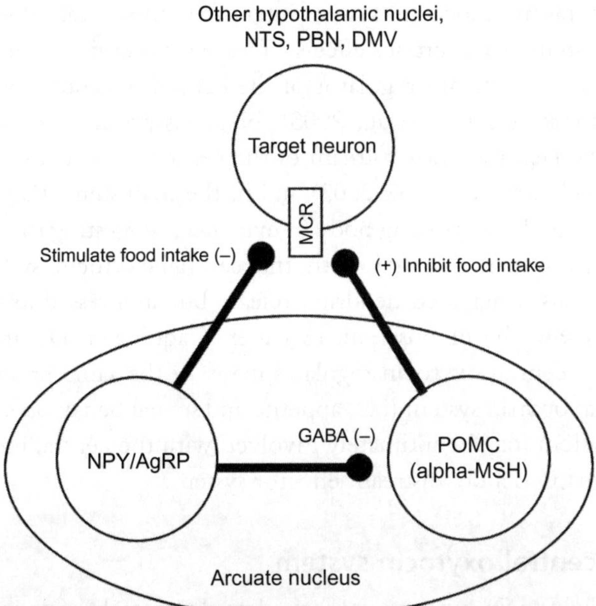

Figure 1.1 The central melanocortin system. Neuropeptide Y (NPY)/agouti-related peptide (AgRP) and proopiomelanocortin (POMC, precursor of alpha-melanocyte-stimulating hormone (alpha-MSH)) neurons originating in the arcuate nucleus project to melanocortin receptor (MCR)—producing neurons to either inhibit or stimulate food intake. NTS, nucleus of the solitary tract; PBN, parabrachial nucleus; DMV, dorsal motor nucleus of the vagus.

The importance of the central melanocortin system in the central control of appetite has been demonstrated in numerous animal and human studies. Melanocortin 4 receptor knockout mice are hyperphagic and obese (Huszar et al., 1997) and also have altered cardiovascular parameters (Tallam, da Silva, & Hall, 2006). Ectopic overexpression of the agouti protein, which, like AgRP, is a natural antagonist of melanocortin receptors, in the brain results in Agouti Obesity Syndrome (Fan, Boston, Kesterson, Hruby, & Cone, 1997), in which affected mice are profoundly obese. Additionally, melanocortin agonists, when injected centrally, decrease food intake (Cone, 2005) and increase sympathetic nervous system activity (Matsumura, Tsuchihashi, Abe, & Mitsuo, 2002). Human genetic analyses also indicate that mutations in components of the central melanocortin system, particularly in the melanocortin 4 receptor, may account for as many as 1 in 16 cases of human obesity (Loos et al., 2008).

The central melanocortin system interacts with several other identified neuronal systems to exert its effects. The serotonergic system has been shown to be an upstream regulator of the central melanocortin system to alter food intake (Heisler et al., 2003). Neurons producing brain-derived neurotrophic factor act downstream of the central melanocortin system in both the forebrain (Xu et al., 2003) and in the brainstem (Bariohay et al., 2009). There is also a growing body of evidence, suggesting that the central melanocortin system interacts with the central oxytocin system. Melanocortin agonists increased dendritic release but suppressed axonal release of oxytocin into the bloodstream (Sabatier, Caquineau, Dayanithi, et al., 2003). Since central oxytocin regulates many of the same processes as the central melanocortin system (i.e., appetite and sexual behaviors), the central oxytocin system may be intimately involved with the central melanocortin system, perhaps as a downstream effector system.

1.3. The central oxytocin system

The central oxytocin system is comprised predominately of neurons located in the paraventricular nucleus and the supraoptic nucleus of the hypothalamus (Fig. 1.2). There are two types of oxytocin-producing neurons.

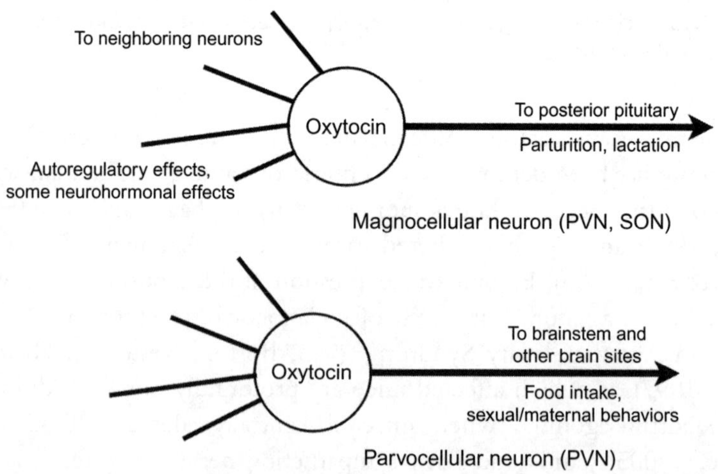

Figure 1.2 The central oxytocin system. Magnocellular oxytocin neurons originating in the paraventricular (PVN) and supraoptic (SON) nuclei of the hypothalamus release oxytocin dendritically to exert autoregulatory effects and project an axon to the posterior pituitary, where oxytocin is released into the general circulation. Parvocellular oxytocin neurons originating in the PVN project to the brainstem and other brain sites to affect food intake and other behaviors.

Magnocellular oxytocin neurons (in both the paraventricular and supraoptic nuclei) project to the posterior pituitary where oxytocin is released into the general circulation (Sabatier, Caquineau, Douglas, & Leng, 2003). Magnocellular oxytocin neurons can also release oxytocin dendritically to affect neighboring neurons. Dendritically released oxytocin has been shown to have some neurohormonal effects as well as some autoregulatory actions (Sabatier, Caquineau, Douglas, et al., 2003). For example, dendritically released oxytocin may be important in the positive feedback loop during parturition and may also modulate the hypothalamic–pituitary–adrenal axis during stress (Neumann, 2007). Parvocellular oxytocin neurons are located predominantly in the paraventricular nucleus and project to the brainstem and other brain sites to affect appetite and a wide variety of behaviors and homeostatic mechanisms. Oxytocin neurons play a physiologically relevant role in the hypothalamic regulation of sodium appetite, feeding, affiliative and maternal behaviors, central cardiovascular control, and reproduction (Michelini, Marcelo, Amico, & Morris, 2003; Puryear, Rigatto, Amico, & Morris, 2001; Sabatier, Caquineau, Douglas, et al., 2003).

Like the central melanocortin system, the central oxytocin system has been shown to be important in appetite control. Centrally injected oxytocin dose-dependently decreased food intake in male rats (Arletti, Benelli, & Bertolini, 1989; Olson, Drutarosky, Chow, et al., 1991; Olson, Drutarosky, Stricker, & Verbalis, 1991), and oxytocin-deficient mice ingested significantly more sucrose (Miedlar, Rinaman, Vollmer, & Amico, 2007) and sodium (Amico, Morris, & Vollmer, 2001; Puryear et al., 2001). Oxytocin-deficient mice also developed late-onset obesity (Takayanagi et al., 2008).

Several lines of evidence support the hypothesis that oxytocin is a downstream mediator of the central melanocortin system. Intracerebroventricular administration of the melanocortin 3/4 receptor agonist, alpha-MSH led to c-Fos accumulation in oxytocin-producing neurons (Caquineau et al., 2006). Pretreatment with the oxytocin receptor antagonist, OVT reversed the anorexigenic effect of leptin (Blevins, Schwartz, & Baskin, 2004), a peptide that is dependent on the central melanocortin system to exert its activities (Dunbar & Lu, 1999). As mentioned previously, alpha-MSH was shown also to modulate the dendritic and axonal release of oxytocin (Sabatier, Caquineau, Dayanithi, et al., 2003, Sabatier, Caquineau, Douglas, et al., 2003).

Understanding the way in which neuronal circuits, like the central melanocortin system and the central oxytocin system, interact may provide insight into how the brain controls appetite and food consumption. With that knowledge, we can better understand the pathogenesis of diseases like obesity and anorexia, and perhaps design novel therapeutic strategies to prevent or ameliorate the impact of these conditions. This chapter focuses on the neuronal networks activated by two recently described neuropeptides, nesfatin-1 (Oh-I et al., 2006) and neuronostatin (Samson et al., 2008) and describes the involvement of the central melanocortin and oxytocin systems in the expression of their anorexigenic action.

2. NEURONOSTATIN

2.1. Introduction

Somatostatin is a neuroendocrine and gut hormone that was originally described in 1972, on the basis of its ability to inhibit growth hormone release from the anterior pituitary (Vale et al., 1972). It is now known that somatostatin exerts broad, inhibitory actions in a variety of biological systems through an interaction with five related G protein-coupled receptors (GPCR) (SSTR1-5) (Reisine & Bell, 1995). The preprohormone of somatostatin is a 116-amino acid precursor, consisting of a 24-amino acid signal peptide at the N-terminus, and the two forms of somatostatin, somatostatin-14 and the N-terminally extended somatostatin-28, at the C terminus (Funckes et al., 1983; Samson et al., 2008). For many years, there was speculation that the somatostatin preprohormone encoded another biologically active peptide, although this potential peptide remained elusive for 30 years.

On the basis of bioinformatic analyses of conserved sequences and potential dibasic cleavage sites, an additional peptide hormone was identified and named neuronostatin (Samson et al., 2008). Neuronostatin was found to be highly conserved across species, from human to goldfish, with only one amino acid difference between human and rodent (mouse and rat) sequences (Samson et al., 2008). Using an antibody directed against synthetic neuronostatin, the endogenous peptide was purified from porcine pancreas and spleen and was found to be a 13-amino acid peptide that was C-terminally amidated (Samson et al., 2008). As expected, neuronostatin was produced in the same tissues as somatostatin, including the pancreas, hypothalamus, heart, cerebrum, spleen, and stomach (Samson et al., 2008). Although neuronostatin and somatostatin were detected in the same tissues, they were present in differing amounts (Samson et al., 2008), likely due to differential posttranslational processing required for the two peptides (neuronostatin is C-terminally amidated, while somatostatin is cyclized by a disulfide bond).

Despite sharing a common preprohormone and expression pattern, neuronostatin and somatostatin possess biological activities that are distinct from each other. While somatostatin is known to inhibit growth hormone release from the anterior pituitary, neuronostatin failed to alter basal, growth hormone-releasing hormone- or ghrelin-stimulated, or somatostatin-inhibited growth hormone secretion in primary anterior pituitary cell cultures (Samson et al., 2008). As detailed below, neuronostatin inhibited food intake and increased mean arterial pressure when injected centrally (Samson et al., 2008), while central somatostatin did not consistently alter either appetite or cardiovascular function (Brown, 1988; Carretta et al., 1989; Lotter et al., 1981; Stengel et al., 2010). Furthermore, somatostatin exerts its primarily inhibitory effects via five related GPCRs coupled to Gi proteins. Although the neuronostatin receptor, postulated to be an orphan GPCR, remains unconfirmed, neuronostatin does not activate any of the SSTRs (Samson et al., 2008).

2.2. Neuronostatin-induced anorexia

2.2.1 Central circuits involved in neuronostatin-induced anorexia

Because of the relatively high expression of neuronostatin in the hypothalamus, a region of the brain that is known to be important in the control of food intake, it was hypothesized that neuronostatin would play a role in the control of appetite and metabolism. Indeed, central administration of neuronostatin significantly reduced food and water intake in adult male rats (Samson et al., 2008). Although neuronostatin was detected in various brain regions in addition to hypothalamus, including hippocampus, cortex, amygdala, and cerebellum (Dun et al., 2010), the site of neuronostatin's anorectic action may be primarily forebrain/hypothalamus, since injection into either lateral (Samson et al., 2008; Yosten & Samson, 2010a, 2010b) or third (Carlini et al., 2011) ventricles reduced food intake. However, parenchymal injection of neuronostatin into the hippocampus had no effect on food intake (Carlini et al., 2011). Furthermore, neuronostatin-induced anorexia was abolished by pretreatment with the melanocortin 3/4 receptor antagonist, SHU9119 (Yosten & Samson, 2010a, 2010b), indicating that neuronostatin exerts its central activities via the central melanocortin system, suggesting either a hypothalamic or brainstem site of action. Although centrally projecting oxytocin fibers have been implicated as downstream mediators of melanocortin action (Sabatier, Caquineau, Dayanithi, et al., 2003, Sabatier, Caquineau, Douglas, et al., 2003), pretreatment with an oxytocin receptor antagonist failed to alter neuronostatin-induced anorexia (Yosten & Samson, 2010a).

2.2.2 Relationship between neuronostatin-induced anorexia and autonomic function

In addition to its effect on appetite, neuronostatin also elevated mean arterial pressure when injected into the lateral cerebroventricle of conscious male rats (Samson et al., 2008; Yosten, Pate, & Samson, 2011). This effect was found to be at least partially dependent upon the central melanocortin system (Yosten et al., 2011) and involved activation of the sympathetic nervous system and release of vasopressin from the posterior pituitary gland (Yosten et al., 2011). Most neuropeptides that alter food intake also influence autonomic activity (e.g., orexin (Ferguson & Samson, 2003), alpha-MSH (Cone, 2005), adrenomedullin (Taylor & Samson, 2001)), although it is unclear which of these effects is the primary action of these multifunctional peptides. The effect of neuronostatin on food intake potentially could be secondary to autonomic activation, since central administration of neuronostatin reduced gastric emptying and gastrointestinal transit in rats (Su et al., 2012). Like the effects of neuronostatin on food intake and mean arterial pressure, this action of neuronostatin was reversed by pretreatment with a melanocortin receptor antagonist (Su et al., 2012). Inhibition of gastric emptying and transit, which can lead to a decrease in food intake (Clegg & Shafat, 2010), is often due to a increase in sympathetic nervous system activity (Czimmer, Million, & Tache, 2006; Nagase, Nakajima, Sekihara, York, & Bray, 2002; Nakade, Tsukamoto, Pappas, & Takahashi, 2006), indicating that the primary action of neuronostatin may be modulation of autonomics.

2.2.3 Physiological relevance of neuronostatin-induced anorexia

Because neuronostatin is derived from the somatostatin preprohormone (Samson et al., 2008), studies into the physiological relevance of the peptide in regulating food intake are limited, since any attempt to compromise the production of neuronostatin would compromise somatostatin as well. Preliminary studies utilizing passive immunoneutralization revealed that inhibition of endogenous neuronostatin action led to a decrease in food intake (Yosten & Samson, 2011). This finding was surprising; however, antiserum-treated animals were also hypotensive and exhibited an impairment in baroreflex function (Yosten & Samson, 2011), indicating again that the effect of neuronostatin on food intake indeed may be secondary to its role in regulating autonomic activity. Because the technique of passive immunoneutralization has many inherent challenges associated with implementation and interpretation of data (Culler & Negro-Vilar, 1989), these results must be corroborated with knockdown experiments in which the neuronostatin receptor has been compromised.

3. NESFATIN-1

3.1. Introduction

Nesfatin-1 is an 82-amino acid hormone that is derived from the nucleobindin 2 (NUCB2)/NEFA precursor protein (Oh-I et al., 2006). Nesfatin-1 is highly conserved across species (Oh-I et al., 2006), and its production has been verified in goldfish (Kerbel & Unniappan, 2012), mouse (Oh-I et al., 2006), rat (Oh-I et al., 2006), and human (Tan, Hallschmid, Kern, Lehnert, & Randeva, 2011; Zhang et al., 2012) tissues. In humans, nesfatin-1 has been mapped to chromosome 11, and to chromosomes 1 and 7 in rats and mice, respectively (NCBI Gene). The localization of nesfatin-1 has been extensively studied in rodents and humans, and these studies have revealed the production of the protein by numerous structures in the brain (Brailoiu et al., 2007; Foo, Brismar, & Broberger, 2008; Goebel-Stengel, Wang, Stengel, & Tache, 2011) as well as by many peripheral tissues (Foo, Brauner, Ostenson, & Broberger, 2010; Gonzalez, Tiwari, & Unniappan, 2009; Ramanjaneya et al., 2010; Tagaya, Miura, Okada, Ohshima, & Mori, 2012; Tagaya, Osaki, et al., 2012). In the brain, nesfatin-1/NUCB2 mRNA or immunoreactivity has been detected in various hypothalamic nuclei, including feeding centers such as the arcuate nucleus, paraventricular nucleus, lateral hypothalamic area, dorsomedial hypothalamus, and ventromedial hypothalamus (Brailoiu et al., 2007; Foo et al., 2008; Goebel-Stengel et al., 2011). Additionally, nesfatin-1 has been detected in the nucleus of the solitary tract, locus coeruleus, Edinger–Westphal nucleus, raphe pallidus, parabrachial nucleus, and the dorsal vagal complex (Foo et al., 2008; Goebel-Stengel et al., 2011). In the periphery, nesfatin-1 is produced by white adipose tissue (Ramanjaneya et al., 2010; Tagaya, Miura, et al., 2012; Tagaya, Osaki, et al., 2012), particularly by subcutaneous fat depots (Ramanjaneya et al., 2010), and by pancreatic beta cells (Foo et al., 2010; Gonzalez et al., 2009; Mohan & Unniappan, 2012; Zhang et al., 2010). Additionally, nesfatin-1 has been detected in endocrine cells of the gastric mucosa (Mohan & Unniappan, 2012; Stengel, Goebel, Yakubov, et al., 2009;

Zhang et al., 2010), particularly the ghrelin-producing X/A-like cells (Stengel, Goebel, Yakubov, et al., 2009), in Brunner's glands of the duodenum (Mohan & Unniappan, 2012; Zhang et al., 2010), colon (Zhang et al., 2010), small intestine, liver, esophagus, and adrenal glands (Konczol et al., 2010). Given the central and peripheral expression pattern of the peptide, nesfatin-1 is perfectly positioned to influence energy intake and metabolic homeostasis.

3.2. Nesfatin-1-induced anorexia

3.2.1 Central circuits mediating nesfatin-1-induced anorexia

Nesfatin-1 was originally described on the basis of its ability to potently inhibit food intake in adult male rats when injected intracerebroventricularly (Oh-I et al., 2006). This effect was found to be independent of the action of the adipocyte-derived adipokine, leptin, since nesfatin-1 exerted an anorexigenic action in Zucker fa/fa rats (Oh-I et al., 2006), which lack functional leptin receptors (Brunner et al., 1997). However, central injection of alpha-MSH elevated expression of the *NUCB2* gene (Oh-I et al., 2006). Furthermore, the inhibitory effect of nesfatin-1 on food intake was reversed by central pretreatment with the melanocortin 3/4 receptor antagonist, SHU9119, indicating that nesfatin-1 requires the presence of functional brain melanocortin receptors to exert its anorexigenic activity (Oh-I et al., 2006; Yosten & Samson, 2009).

Several neurotransmitters and peptides have been proposed to act as downstream mediators of the central melanocortin system, and consequently nesfatin-1, including CRH (Kawashima, Sakihara, Kageyama, Nigawara, & Suda, 2008) and oxytocin (Sabatier, Caquineau, Dayanithi, et al., 2003; Sabatier, Caquineau, Douglas, et al., 2003). Nesfatin-1 colocalized with CRH in the hypothalamus (Foo et al., 2008; Kohno et al., 2008; Noetzel et al., 2009) and incubated with nesfatin-1 increased calcium mobilization in isolated neurons that were immunoreactive for CRH (Yoshida et al., 2010). CRH signals via two related GPCR, CRH1R and CRH2R (Grammatopoulos & Chrousos, 2002). Pretreatment with the CRH1R/CRH2R antagonist, astressin-B, or the CRH2R-specific antagonist, astressin2-B, abolished nesfatin-1-induced anorexia when nesfatin-1 was administered into the forebrain but not the hindbrain (Stengel, Goebel, Wang, et al., 2009), suggesting that the anorexigenic effect of nesfatin-1 is dependent upon the activation of CRH2 receptors in the hypothalamus. Nesfatin-1 colocalized also with oxytocin in the paraventricular nucleus and in the supraoptic nucleus of the hypothalamus

(Foo et al., 2008; Kohno et al., 2008; Noetzel et al., 2009). Refeeding of fasted rats led to the accumulation of c-Fos in neurons coexpressing nesfatin-1 and oxytocin (Kohno et al., 2008), indicating that the interaction between nesfatin-1 with oxytocin may be important for the effect of nesfatin-1 on food consumption. Indeed, it was shown that pretreatment with oxytocin receptor antagonists abolished the anorexigenic effect of nesfatin-1 in rodents (Maejima et al., 2009; Yosten & Samson, 2010b). In addition, treatment with nesfatin-1 stimulated the release of oxytocin from rodent neurons (Maejima et al., 2009) and passive immunoneutralization of nesaftin-1 led to an inhibition of oxytocin secretion (Maejima et al., 2009).

While it is clear that the actions of nesfatin-1 are dependent upon the central melanocortin system (Oh-I et al., 2006; Yosten & Samson, 2009), CRH-producing neurons (Stengel, Goebel, Wang, et al., 2009), and the central oxytocin system (Maejima et al., 2009; Yosten & Samson, 2010b), it is not known whether nesfatin-1-responsive circuits lie in series or in parallel. Nesfatin-1 colocalized with alpha-MSH, CRH, and oxytocin (Foo et al., 2008) and directly altered the membrane potential of CRH and oxytocin neurons (Price, Hoyda, Samson, & Ferguson, 2008), suggesting that nesfatin-1 may act locally to modulate the activity of all three neuronal cell types. However, the anorexigenic effect of exogenously applied nesfatin-1 is completely blocked by pretreatment with SHU9119 (Oh-I et al., 2006; Yosten & Samson, 2009), astressin2-B (Stengel, Goebel, Wang, et al., 2009), and the oxytocin receptor antagonists (Maejima et al., 2009; Yosten & Samson, 2010b), indicating that all three neuronal types are necessary for nesfatin-1's anorectic action. Identification of the nesfatin-1 receptor would yield important insight into the interaction of nesfatin-1 with the central melanocortin system, CRH-producing neurons, and the central oxytocin system.

3.2.2 Peripheral nesfatin-1 in the control of food intake and metabolism

Nesfatin-1 has been shown to circulate in the plasma of rodents (Mohan & Unniappan, 2012) and humans (Ari, Ozturk, Bez, Oktar, & Erduran, 2011; Deniz et al., 2012; Zhang et al., 2012), although the source of the circulating hormone remains unknown. Potential sources of plasma nesfatin-1 include the adipose tissue (Ramanjaneya et al., 2010; Tagaya, Miura, et al., 2012; Tagaya, Osaki, et al., 2012), the endocrine cells of the gastric mucosa and intestines (Mohan & Unniappan, 2012; Stengel, Goebel, Yakubov, et al., 2009; Zhang et al., 2010), and the endocrine pancreas, particularly the pancreatic beta cells (Foo et al., 2010; Gonzalez et al., 2009; Mohan &

Unniappan, 2012; Zhang et al., 2010). Although it is unclear whether circulating nesfatin-1 acts in the brain to influence food consumption, peripheral delivery of nesfatin-1 reduced food intake and body weight in rodents (Gonzalez et al., 2011). Two separate mechanisms for this effect have been proposed. First of all, it is known that nesfatin-1 is capable of crossing the blood–brain barrier via a nonsaturable mechanism (Pan, Hsuchou, & Kastin, 2007; Price, Samson, Niehoff, & Banks, 2007), and thus circulating nesfatin-1 could potentially act directly on feeding centers in the brain following diffusion out of the plasma into the parenchyma. However, it has also been demonstrated that nesfatin-1 can activate vagal afferent neurons, as measured by calcium mobilization (Iwasaki et al., 2009), suggesting an indirect modulation of central feeding circuits. Regardless of the mechanism, since nesfatin-1 is produced by adipocytes, it is reasonable to propose that nesfatin-1, like leptin, is an adipokine that relays metabolic information from the periphery to the brain.

Plasma levels of nesfatin-1 were shown to be elevated in several human conditions, including major depressive disorder (Ari et al., 2011), epilepsy (Aydin et al., 2009), and newly diagnosed type 2 diabetes (Zhang et al., 2012). Plasma levels of nesfatin-1 have been demonstrated to correlate with body mass index, insulin resistance, fasting blood glucose, and fasting insulin levels (Tan et al., 2011; Zhang et al., 2012), as well as with body weight and fat mass (Tan et al., 2011), suggesting that nesfatin-1, especially fat-derived nesfatin-1, may play an important role in human metabolism and food intake. Furthermore, plasma levels of nesfatin-1 were reduced in patients with restricting-type anorexia nervosa (Ogiso et al., 2011) and single nucleotide polymorphisms in the *NUCB2/NEFA* gene (rs1330A/G; rs214086G/C; rs214101C/T) have been associated with the susceptibility to obesity in adult human males (Zegers, Beckers, Mertens, Van Gaal, & Van Hul, 2011). However, further studies are necessary to determine the exact role of nesfatin-1 in the control of food intake in humans and whether the changes in plasma nesfatin-1 observed in obesity and anorexia are a cause or a consequence of these disorders.

3.2.3 Relationship between nesfatin-1-induced anorexia, autonomic activity, and fluid intake

In addition to modulation of food intake, nesfatin-1 increased mean arterial pressure (Tanida & Mori, 2011; Yosten & Samson, 2009) and stimulated renal sympathetic nerve activity (Tanida & Mori, 2011) in rodents. Like the effect of nesfatin-1 on appetite regulation, nesfatin-1-induced elevation in mean arterial pressure was dependent upon activation of central melanocortin receptors (Yosten & Samson, 2009) and central oxytocin receptors (Yosten & Samson, 2010b). Centrally administered nesfatin-1 also led to decreased gastroduodenal activity (Atsuchi et al., 2010) and gastric emptying (Goebel-Stengel et al., 2011; Stengel, Goebel, Wang, et al., 2009) via a CRH2 receptor-dependent mechanism (Stengel, Goebel, Wang, et al., 2009). Thus, the effect of nesfatin-1 on food intake may be due in part to sympathoactivation.

It has become increasingly clear that food intake and water consumption are intimately linked, despite the fact that these two processes are often studied in isolation out of necessity. It is not surprising then that the majority of peptides that influence food intake also modulate water drinking (e.g., neuronostatin (Samson et al., 2008), alpha-MSH (Yosten & Samson, 2010b), oxytocin (Yosten & Samson, 2010b)). Interestingly, the effect of nesfatin-1 on water intake (~70% reduction) appeared to be more pronounced than the effect on food consumption (~50% reduction) (Yosten & Samson, 2009). Additionally, nesfatin-1 abrogated water consumption in rats that were driven to drink by either a dipsogenic dose of angiotensin II or overnight fluid restriction, while morpholino-mediated knockdown of nesfatin-1 enhanced angiotensin II-induced water intake (Yosten, Redlinger, & Samson, 2012). Fluid restriction followed by rehydration also led to an increase in *NUCB2* gene expression (Yosten et al., 2012). Nesfatin-1 may regulate fluid homeostasis independently from the intake of energy and may represent an important regulatory mechanism in the integration of the two processes.

3.2.4 Physiological relevance of nesfatin-1 in the control of food intake and energy balance

Compromise of nesfatin-1 production or action using morpholino antisense molecules or an antibody directed against nesfatin-1, respectively, led to exaggerated food intake and body weight gain in male rats (Oh-I et al., 2006); thus, nesfatin-1 likely is a physiologically relevant regulator of appetite. However, the exact role of nesfatin-1 in this process remains to be elucidated. Identification of the as yet unknown nesfatin-1 receptor would be an important finding in determining the function of nesfatin-1 in normal and aberrant metabolic states. Nesfatin-1 increased calcium mobilization in several cell types, including neurons (Brailoiu et al., 2007; Iwasaki et al., 2009; Yoshida et al., 2010) and pancreatic beta cells (Nakata, Manaka, Yamamoto, Mori, & Yada, 2011), and nesfatin-1-induced calcium mobilization was blocked by exposure to pertussis toxin, suggesting that the nesfatin-1 receptor(s) was a GPCR coupled to Gi (Brailoiu et al., 2007). While many peptide hormones act as classical neurotransmitters, nesfatin-1 has not been observed in axon terminals (Foo et al., 2008). Nesfatin-1 has been observed, however, in secretory vesicles and in dendrites (Foo et al., 2008, Stengel, Goebel, Wang, et al., 2009; Stengel, Goebel, Yakubov, et al., 2009), leading many to speculate that nesfatin-1 is released dendritically to modulate the activity of local neurons in an autocrine or paracrine fashion (Foo et al., 2008; Yosten & Samson, 2009).

4. CONCLUSIONS

4.1. The proposed central POMC–CRH–OT feeding circuit

Neuronostatin and nesfatin-1 are two recently described neuropeptides that induce anorexia (Oh-I et al., 2006; Samson et al., 2008). While the effect of nesfatin-1 on food intake appears to be a primary, physiologically relevant action of the peptide (Oh-I et al., 2006), the anorexigenic activity of neuronostatin may be secondary to the activation of the sympathetic nervous system (Yosten et al., 2011). Interestingly, both peptides require the presence of functional central melanocortin receptors to exert their anorexigenic activities (Oh-I et al., 2006; Yosten & Samson, 2009, 2010a). Nesfatin-1 also interacts with CRH-producing neurons (Stengel, Goebel, Wang, et al., 2009, Stengel, Goebel, Yakubov, et al., 2009) and the central oxytocin system (Maejima et al., 2009; Yosten & Samson, 2010b), and these interactions reveal a potentially important central POMC–CRH–oxytocin feeding circuit, as well as provide insight into the structure of this circuit. For instance, while it is possible that the central melanocortin system and the central oxytocin system operate in parallel to simultaneously exert the effects of nesfatin-1, these two neuronal circuits may also act in series. Melanocortin agonists and oxytocin exert similar actions on a variety of physiological functions when injected into the brain, including the initiation of the yawning–stretching reflex and sexual behaviors (Sabatier, Caquineau, Douglas, et al., 2003). Central administrations of oxytocin (Michelini et al., 2003; Olson, Drutarosky, Chow, et al., 1991; Olson, Drutarosky, Stricker, et al., 1991; Wsol, Cudnoch-Jedrzejewska, Szczepanska-Sadowska, Kowalewski, & Puchalska, 2008) and melanocortin agonists (Cone, 2005) potently inhibit food intake and alter cardiovascular function. These similarities suggest a circuit in series.

Several lines of evidence support the hypothesis that oxytocin is a downstream mediator of the central melanocortin system. Intracerebroventricular administration of the melanocortin 3/4 receptor agonist, alpha-MSH led to c-Fos accumulation in oxytocin-producing neurons (Caquineau et al., 2006). Pretreatment with OVT reversed the anorexigenic effect of leptin (Blevins et al., 2004), a peptide that is dependent on the central melanocortin system to exert its activities (Dunbar & Lu, 1999). Additionally, alpha-MSH was shown to increase the dendritic release of oxytocin in the hypothalamus, but to inhibit the release of oxytocin from axon terminals in the posterior pituitary gland leading to a decrease in plasma OT levels (Sabatier, Caquineau, Dayanithi, et al., 2003). Nesfatin-1 may indeed increase dendritic release of oxytocin, as a recent report (Maejima et al., 2009) indicated that nesfatin-1 led to an increase in oxytocin secretion within the PVN and additional evidence indicates that nesfatin-1 does not affect basal plasma levels of oxytocin in conscious male rats (Yosten & Samson, 2010b).

CRF is another potential downstream mediator of the central melanocortin system, as the anorexigenic effect of the melanocortin agonist MTII was abolished by a CRF receptor antagonist (Lu, Barsh, Akil, & Watson, 2003). The anorexigenic effect of melanocortin agonists was reversed by pretreatment with the CRF receptor antagonist, astressin, in both mice (Kawashima et al., 2008) and chicks (Tachibana, Oikawa, Adachi, Boswell, & Furuse, 2007). While melanocortin agonists had no effect on CRF-deficient mice (Kawashima et al., 2008), centrally administered CRF significantly reduced food intake in mice lacking melanocortin 4 receptors (Marsh et al., 1999). Furthermore, treatment with leptin led to an increase in hypothalamic CRF content, and leptin-induced anorexia was attenuated by pretreatment with the CRF receptor antagonist, alpha-helical-CRF (Uehara, Shimizu, Ohtani, Sato, & Mori, 1998).

In addition to its role in mediating the anorexigenic effect of the central melanocortin system, the central oxytocin system may be also a downstream mediator of CRF. Pretreatment with the oxytocin receptor antagonist, OVT, abrogated CRF-induced anorexia (Olson, Drutarosky, Stricker, et al., 1991). Likewise, central administration of CRF led to an increase in oxytocin release, but did not affect the release of vasopressin (Bruhn, Sutton, Plotsky, & Vale, 1986). It is reasonable to postulate, then, that the central melanocortin system, CRF-producing neurons, and the central oxytocin system comprise a central circuit that is important for the control of food intake (Fig. 1.3).

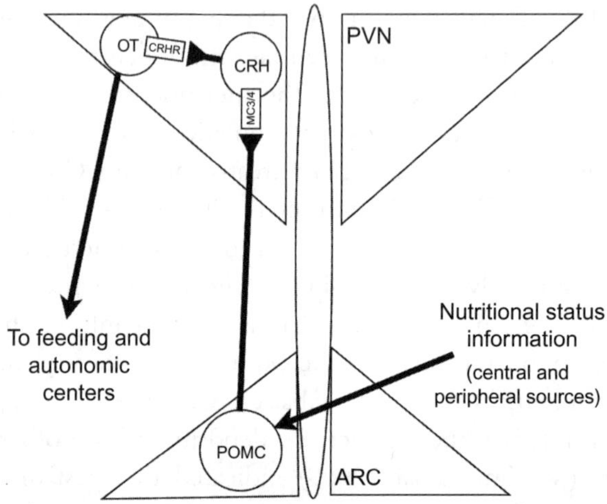

Figure 1.3 The POMC–CRH–OT feeding circuit. Nutritional status information, such as peripherally derived signals (e.g., leptin, nesfatin-1, and insulin) and centrally produced peptides (e.g., neuronostatin and nesfatin-1) interact with proopiomelanocortin (POMC) neurons in the arcuate nucleus of the hypothalamus (ARC), which produce alpha-MSH. POMC neurons project to the paraventricular nucleus of the hypothalamus (PVN), where alpha-MSH activates melanocortin 3/4 receptors (MC3/4) on corticotrophin-releasing hormone (CRH) neurons. CRH interacts with its receptor(s) (CRHR) on oxytocin (OT)-producing neurons, also situated in the PVN, which project to other feeding and autonomic centers, such as the brainstem and cortex.

4.2. Oxytocinergic and nonoxytocinergic-mediated anorexia

Unlike nesfatin-1, the anorexigenic effect of neuronostatin was not blocked by pretreatment with OVT (Yosten & Samson, 2010a). It is interesting that two peptides that exert similar activities and act via the central melanocortin system do not utilize the same downstream mediators. One explanation for this observation is that nesfatin-1 and neuronostatin interact with different subpopulations of POMC neurons, which project to different downstream neuronal circuits. Indeed, there is evidence that the cluster of POMC neurons originating in the arcuate nucleus of the hypothalamus is divided into neuronal subpopulations that express different sets of receptors and release different neurotransmitters. As noted previously, leptin is a peripherally produced anorexigen that is dependent on the central melanocortin system to exert its activity. However, only 67% of POMC neurons express the leptin receptor (Funahashi et al., 2003). Leptin stimulates transcription of POMC through activation of signal transducer and transcription 3 (STAT3) proteins, but the activated form of STAT3, phospho-STAT3 is detected only in 37% of POMC neurons treated with leptin (Munzberg, Huo, Nillni, Hollenberg, & Bjorbaek, 2003). There is also a subpopulation of POMC neurons that coexpress pituitary adenylate cyclase-activating polypeptide (PACAP) located in the ventrolateral arcuate nucleus that accounts for about 20% of POMC neurons (Durr et al., 2007). Perhaps POMC–PACAP coexpressing neurons are involved in mediating the increase in mean arterial pressure induced by neuronostatin, as PACAP has been shown to stimulate vasopressin secretion (Murase, Kondo, Otake, & Oiso, 1993). An additional subpopulation of POMC neurons, comprising about 37% of all POMC neurons, coexpress choline acetyltransferase, indicating that these neurons are cholinergic (Meister et al., 2006). These cholinergic POMC neurons are specifically located in the ventral aspect of the arcuate nucleus (Meister et al., 2006). These data suggest that not only do distinct groups of POMC neurons exist but also that they are organized regionally within the arcuate nucleus. It is possible that the projections of neuronostatin-responsive POMC neurons to nonoxytocinergic downstream circuits may reflect the observations that the primary effect of neuronostatin likely is not on food intake, but instead on the maintenance of cardiovascular function and sympathetic nervous system activity; however, further experimentation is required to confirm this hypothesis.

In conclusion, neuronostatin and nesfatin-1 are novel hormones that induce anorexia through related, but different neuronal pathways. While the central melanocortin system appears to play an important role in mediating the effects of both peptides, neuronostatin and nesfatin-1 utilize separate downstream circuits to exert their anorexigenic actions. The anorectic action of nesfatin-1 may be a primary, physiologically relevant effect of the peptide, but neuronostatin-induced anorexia may be secondary to autonomic activation. Further studies into the pharmacological and physiological actions of these peptides in both animals and humans could yield important information on the central control of appetite.

REFERENCES

Amico, J. A., Morris, M., & Vollmer, R. R. (2001). Mice deficient in oxytocin manifest increased saline consumption following overnight fluid deprivation. *The American Journal of Physiology*, *281*, R1368–R1373.

Ari, M., Ozturk, O. H., Bez, Y., Oktar, S., & Erduran, D. (2011). High plasma nesfatin-1 level in patients with major depressive disorder. *Progress in Neuropsychopharacology and Biological Psychiatry*, *35*, 497–500.

Arletti, R., Benelli, A., & Bertolini, A. (1989). Influence of oxytocin on feeding behavior in the rat. *Peptides*, *10*, 89–93.

Atsuchi, K., Asakawa, A., Ushikai, M., Ataka, K., Tsai, M., Koyama, K., et al. (2010). Centrally administered nesfatin-1 inhibits feeding behaviour and gastroduodenal motility in mice. *Neuroreport, 21,* 1008–1011.

Aydin, S., Dag, E., Ozkan, Y., Erman, F., Dagli, A. F., Kilic, N., et al. (2009). Nesfatin-1 and ghrelin levels in serum and saliva of epileptic patients: Hormonal changes can have a major effect on seizure disorders. *Molecular and Cellular Biochemistry, 328,* 49–56.

Bariohay, B., Roux, J., Tardivel, C., Trouslard, J., Jean, A., & Lebrun, B. (2009). Brain-derived neurotrophic factor/tropomyosin-related kinase receptor type B signaling is a downstream effector of the brainstem melanocortin system in food intake control. *Endocrinology, 150,* 2646–2653.

Berthoud, H. R. (2002). Multiple neural systems controlling food intake and body weight. *Neuroscience and Biobehavioral Reviews, 26,* 393–428.

Blevins, J. E., Schwartz, M. W., & Baskin, D. G. (2004). Evidence that paraventricular nucleus oxytocin neurons link hypothalamic leptin action to caudal brain stem nuclei controlling meal size. *The American Journal of Physiology, 287,* R87–R96.

Brailoiu, G. C., Dun, S. L., Brailoiu, E., Inan, S., Yang, J., Chang, J. K., et al. (2007). Nesfatin-1: Distribution and interaction with a G protein-coupled receptor in the rat brain. *Endocrinology, 148,* 5088–5094.

Bray, G. A., & York, D. A. (1997). Clinical review 90: Leptin and clinical medicine: A new piece in the puzzle of obesity. *The Journal of Clinical Endocrinology and Metabolism, 82,* 2771–2776.

Brown, M. R. (1988). Somatostatin-28 effects on central nervous system regulation of vasopressin secretion and blood pressure. *Neuroendocrinology, 47,* 556–562.

Bruhn, T. O., Sutton, S. W., Plotsky, P. M., & Vale, W. W. (1986). Central administration of corticotropin-releasing factor modulates oxytocin secretion in the rat. *Endocrinology, 119,* 1558–1563.

Brunner, L., Nick, H. P., Cumin, F., Chiesi, M., Baum, H. P., Whitebread, S., et al. (1997). Leptin is a physiologically important regulator of food intake. *International Journal of Obesity and Related Metabolic Disorders, 21,* 1152–1160.

Caquineau, C., Leng, G., Guan, X. M. M., Jiang, M., Van Der Ploeg, L., & Douglas, A. J. (2006). Effects of alpha-melanocyte-stimulating hormone on magnocellular oxytocin neurones and their activation at intromission in male rats. *Journal of Neuroendocrinology, 18,* 685–691.

Carlini, V. P., Ghersi, M., Gabach, L., Schioth, H. B., Perez, M. F., Ramirez, O. A., et al. (2011). Hippocampal effects of neuronostatin on memory, anxiety-like behavior and food intake in rats. *Neuroscience, 197,* 145–152.

Carretta, R., Fabris, B., Fischetti, F., Costantini, M., De Biasi, F., Muiesan, S., et al. (1989). Reduction of blood pressure in obese hyperinsulinaemic hypertensive patients during somatostatin infusion. *Journal of Hypertension,* 7, S196–S197.

Clegg, M., & Shafat, A. (2010). Energy and macronutrient composition of breakfast affect gastric emptying of lunch and subsequent food intake, satiety and satiation. *Appetite, 54,* 517–523.

Cone, R. D. (2005). Anatomy and regulation of the central melanocortin system. *Nature Neuroscience, 8,* 571–578.

Cone, R. D., Cowley, M. A., Butler, A. A., Fan, W., Marks, D. L., & Low, M. J. (2001). The arcuate nucleus as a conduit for diverse signals relevant to energy homeostasis. *International Journal of Obesity and Related Metabolic Disorders, 25,* S63–S67.

Culler, M. D., & Negro-Vilar, A. (1989). Passive immunoneutralization: A method for studying the regulation of basal and pulsatile hormone secretion. *Methods in Enzymology, 168,* 498–516.

Czimmer, J., Million, M., & Tache, Y. (2006). Urocortin 2 acts centrally to delay gastric emptying through sympathetic pathways while CRF and urocortin 1 inhibitory actions are vagal dependent in rats. *The American Journal of Physiology, 290,* G511–G518.

Daniel, P. M. (1976). Anatomy of the hypothalamus and pituitary gland. *Journal of Clinical Pathology Supplement*, 7, 1–7.

Deniz, R., Gurates, B., Aydin, S., Celik, H., Sahin, I., Baykus, Y., et al. (2012). Nesfatin-1 and other hormone alterations in polycystic ovary syndrome. *Endocrine*, *42*, 694–699 PMID: 22367584.

Dun, S. L., Brailoiu, G. C., Tica, A. A., Yang, J., Chang, J. K., Brailoiu, E., et al. (2010). Neuronostatin is co-expressed with somatostatin and mobilizes calcium in cultured rat hypothalamic neurons. *Neuroscience*, *166*, 455–463.

Dunbar, J. C., & Lu, H. (1999). Leptin-induced increase in sympathetic nervous and cardiovascular tone is mediated by proopiomelanocortin (POMC) products. *Brain Research Bulletin*, *50*, 215–221.

Durr, K., Norsted, E., Gomuc, B., Suarez, E., Hannibal, J., & Meister, B. (2007). Presence of pituitary adenylate cyclase-activating polypeptide (PACAP) defines a subpopulation of hypothalamic POMC neurons. *Brain Research*, *1186*, 203–211.

Fan, W., Boston, B. A., Kesterson, R. A., Hruby, V. J., & Cone, R. D. (1997). Role of melanocortinergic neurons in feeding and the agouti obesity syndrome. *Nature*, *385*, 165–168.

Ferguson, A. V., Latchford, K. J., & Samson, W. K. (2008). The paraventricular nucleus of the hypothalamus—A potential target for integrative treatment of autonomic dysfunction. *Expert Opinion on Therapeutic Targets*, *12*, 717–727.

Ferguson, A. V., & Samson, W. K. (2003). The orexin/hypocretin system: A critical regulator of neuroendocrine and autonomic function. *Frontiers in Neuroendocrinology*, *24*, 141–150.

Foo, K., Brauner, H., Ostenson, C.-G., & Broberger, C. (2010). Nucleobindin-2/nesfatin in the endocrine pancreas: Distribution and relationship to glycaemic state. *The Journal of Endocrinology*, *204*(3), 255–263.

Foo, K., Brismar, H., & Broberger, C. (2008). Distribution and neuropeptide coexistence of nucleobindin-2 mRNA/nesfatin-like immunoreactivity in the rat CNS. *Neuroscience*, *156*(3), 563–579.

Funahashi, H., Yamada, S., Kageyama, H., Takenoya, F., Guan, J. L., & Shioda, S. (2003). Co-existence of leptin- and orexin-receptors in feeding-regulating neurons in the hypothalamic arcuate nucleus-a triple labeling study. *Peptides*, *24*, 687–694.

Funckes, C. L., Minth, C. D., Deschenes, R., Magazin, M., Tavianini, M. A., Sheets, M., et al. (1983). Cloning and characterization of a mRNA-encoding rat preprosomatostatin. *The Journal of Biological Chemistry*, *258*, 8781–8787.

Goebel-Stengel, M., Wang, L., Stengel, A., & Tache, Y. (2011). Localization of nesfatin-1 neurons in the mouse brain and functional implication. *Brain Research*, *1396*, 20–34.

Gonzalez, R., Perry, R. L., Gao, X., Gaidhu, M. P., Tsushima, R. G., Ceddia, R. B., et al. (2011). Nutrient responsive nesfatin-1 regulates energy balance and induces glucose-stimulated insulin secretion in rats. *Endocrinology*, *152*, 3628–3637.

Gonzalez, R., Tiwari, A., & Unniappan, S. (2009). Pancreatic beta cells colocalize insulin and pronesfatin immunoreactivity in rodents. *Biochemistry and Biophysics Research Communications*, *381*, 643–648.

Grammatopoulos, D. K., & Chrousos, G. P. (2002). Functional characteristics of CRH receptors and potential clinical applications of CRH-receptor antagonists. *Trends in Endocrinology and Metabolism*, *13*, 436–444.

Heisler, L. K., Cowley, M. A., Kishi, T., Tecott, L. H., Fan, W., Low, M. J., et al. (2003). Central serotonin and melanocortin pathways regulating energy homeostasis. *Annals of the New York Academy of Science*, *994*, 169–174.

Huszar, D., Lynch, C. A., Fairchild-Huntress, V., Dunmore, J. H., Fang, Q., Berkemeier, L. R., et al. (1997). Targeted disruption of the melanocortin-4 receptor results in obesity in mice. *Cell*, *88*, 131–141.

Ingalls, A. M., Dickie, M. M., & Snell, G. D. (1950). Obese, a new mutation in the house mouse. *The Journal of Heredity*, *41*, 317–318.

Iwasaki, Y., Nakabayashi, H., Kakei, M., Shimizu, H., Mori, M., & Yada, T. (2009). Nesfatin-1 evokes Ca^{2+} signaling in isolated vagal afferent neurons via Ca^{2+} influx through N-type channels. *Biochemistry and Biophysics Research Communications*, *390*, 958–962.

Kawashima, S., Sakihara, S., Kageyama, K., Nigawara, T., & Suda, T. (2008). Corticotropin-releasing factor (CRF) is involved in the acute anorexic effect of alpha-melanocyte-stimulating hormone: A study using CRF-deficient mice. *Peptides*, *29*(12), 2169–2174.

Kerbel, B., & Unniappan, S. (2012). Nesfatin-1 suppresses energy intake, co-localises ghrelin in the brain and gut, and alters ghrelin, cholecystokinin and orexin mRNA expression in goldfish. *Journal of Neuroendocrinology*, *24*, 366–377.

Kishi, T., Aschkenasi, C. J., Lee, C. E., Mountjoy, K. G., Saper, C. B., & Elmquist, J. K. (2003). Expression of melanocortin 4 receptor mRNA in the central nervous system of the rat. *The Journal of Comparative Neurology*, *457*, 213–235.

Kohno, D., Nakata, M., Maejima, Y., Shimizu, H., Sedbazar, U., Yoshida, N., et al. (2008). Nesfatin-1 neurons in paraventricular and supraoptic nuclei of the rat hypothalamus coexpress oxytocin and vasopressin and are activated by refeeding. *Endocrinology*, *149*, 1295–1301.

Konczol, K., Bodnar, I., Zelena, D., Pinter, O., Papp, R. S., Palkovits, M., et al. (2010). Nesfatin-1/NUCB2 may participate in the activation of the hypothalamic-pituitary-adrenal axis in rats. *Neurochemistry International*, *57*, 189–197.

Loos, R. J. F., Lindgren, C. M., Li, S., Wheeler, E., Zhao, J. H., Prokopenko, I., et al. (2008). Common variants near MC4R are associated with fat mass, weight and risk of obesity. *Nature Genetics*, *40*, 768–775.

Lotter, E. C., Krinsky, R., McKay, J. M., Treneer, C. M., Porter, D., Jr., & Woods, S. C. (1981). Somatostatin decreases food intake of rats and baboons. *Journal of Comparative Physiology and Psychology*, *95*, 278–287.

Lu, X.-Y., Barsh, G. S., Akil, H., & Watson, S. J. (2003). Interaction between alpha-melanocyte-stimulating hormone and corticotropin-releasing hormone in the regulation of feeding and hypothalamo-pituitary-adrenal responses. *The Journal of Neuroscience*, *23*(21), 7863–7872.

Maejima, Y., Sedbazar, U., Suyama, S., Kohno, D., Onaka, T., Takano, E., et al. (2009). Nesfatin-1-regulated oxytocinergic signaling in the paraventricular nucleus causes anorexia through a leptin-independent melanocortin pathway. *Cell Metabolism*, *10*(5), 355–365.

Marsh, D. J., Hollopeter, G., Huszar, D., Laufer, R., Yagaloff, K. A., Fisher, S. L., et al. (1999). Response of melanocortin-4 receptor-deficient mice to anorectic and orexigenic peptides. *Nature Genetics*, *21*(1), 119–122.

Matsumura, K., Tsuchihashi, T., Abe, I., & Mitsuo, I. (2002). Central alpha-melanocyte-stimulating hormone acts at melanocortin-4 receptor to activate sympathetic nervous system in conscious rabbits. *Brain Research*, *948*, 145–148.

Meister, B., Gomuc, B., Suarez, E., Ishii, Y., Durr, K., & Gillberg, L. (2006). Hypothalamic proopiomelanocortin (POMC) neurons have a cholinergic phenotype. *The European Journal of Neuroscience*, *24*(10), 2731–2740.

Melmed, S. (1995). *The pituitary*. Cambridge, MA: Blackwell Science, Inc.

Michelini, L. C., Marcelo, M. C., Amico, J., & Morris, M. (2003). Oxytocinergic regulation of cardiovascular function: Studies in oxytoin-deficient mice. *The American Journal of Physiology*, *284*, H2269–H2276.

Miedlar, J. A., Rinaman, L., Vollmer, R. R., & Amico, J. A. (2007). Oxytocin gene deletion mice overconsume palatable sucrose solution but not palatable lipid emulsions. *The American Journal of Physiology*, *293*, R1063–R1068.

Mohan, H., & Unniappan, S. (2012). Ontogenic pattern of nucleobindin-2/nesfatin-1 expression in the gastroenteropancreatic tissues and serum of Sprague Dawley rats. *Regulatory Peptides, 175*, 61–69.

Munzberg, H., Huo, L., Nillni, E. A., Hollenberg, A. N., & Bjorbaek, C. (2003). Role of signal transducer and activator of transcription 3 in regulation of hypothalamic proopiomelanocortin gene expression by leptin. *Endocrinology, 144*, 2121–2131.

Murase, T., Kondo, K., Otake, K., & Oiso, Y. (1993). Pituitary adenylate cyclase-activating polypeptide stimulates arginine vasopressin release in conscious rats. *Neuroendocrinology, 57*, 1092–1096.

Nagase, H., Nakajima, A., Sekihara, H., York, D. A., & Bray, G. A. (2002). Regulation of feeding behavior, gastric emptying, and sympathetic nerve activity to interscapular brown adipose tissue by galanin and enterostatin: The involvement of vagal-central nervous system interactions. *Journal of Gastroenterology, 37*, 118–127.

Nakade, Y., Tsukamoto, K., Pappas, T. N., & Takahashi, T. (2006). Central glucagon like peptide-1 delays solid gastric emptying via central CRF and peripheral sympathetic pathway in rats. *Brain Research, 1111*, 117–121.

Nakata, M., Manaka, K., Yamamoto, S., Mori, M., & Yada, T. (2011). Nesfatin-1 enhances glucose-induced insulin secretion by promoting Ca(2+) influx through L-type channels in mouse islet beta cells. *Endocrine Journal, 58*, 305–313.

Neary, N. M., Small, C. J., Wren, A. M., Lee, J. L., Druce, M. R., Palmieri, C., et al. (2004). Ghrelin increases energy intake in cancer patients with impaired appetite: Acute, randomized, placebo-controlled trial. *The Journal of Clinical Endocrinology and Metabolism, 89*, 2832–2836.

Neumann, I. D. (2007). Stimuli and consequences of dendritic release of oxytocin within the brain. *Biochemical Society Transactions, 35*, 1252–1257.

Noetzel, S., Stengel, A., Inhoff, T., Goebel, M., Wisser, A. S., Bannert, N., et al. (2009). CCK-8S activates c-Fos in a dose-dependent manner in nesfatin-1 immunoreactive neurons in the paraventricular nucleus of the hypothalamus and in the nucleus of the solitary tract of the brainstem. *Regulatory Peptides, 157*, 84–91.

Ogiso, K., Asakawa, A., Amitani, H., Nakahara, T., Ushikai, M., Haruta, I., et al. (2011). Plasma nesfatin-1 concentrations in restricting-type anorexia nervosa. *Peptides, 32*, 150–153.

Oh-I, S., Shimizu, H., Satoh, T., Okada, S., Adachi, S., Inoue, K., et al. (2006). Identification of nesfatin-1 as a satiety molecule in the hypothalamus. *Nature, 443*, 709–712.

Olson, B. R., Drutarosky, M. D., Chow, M. S., Hruby, V. J., Stricker, E. M., & Verbalis, J. G. (1991). Oxytocin and an oxytocin agonist administered centrally decrease food intake in rats. *Peptides, 12*, 113–118.

Olson, B. R., Drutarosky, M. D., Stricker, E. M., & Verbalis, J. G. (1991). Brain oxytocin receptor antagonism blunts the effects of anorexigenic treatments in rats: Evidence for central oxytocin inhibition of food intake. *Endocrinology, 129*, 785–791.

Ozata, M., Ozdemir, I. C., & Licinio, J. (1999). Human leptin deficiency caused by a missense mutation: Multiple endocrine defects, decreased sympathetic tone, and immune system dysfunction indicate new targets for leptin action, greater central than peripheral resistance to the effects of leptin, and spontaneous correction of leptin-mediated defects. *The Journal of Clinical Endocrinology and Metabolism, 84*, 3686–3695.

Pan, W., Hsuchou, H., & Kastin, A. J. (2007). Nesfatin-1 crosses the blood-brain barrier without saturation. *Peptides, 28*(11), 2223–2228.

Price, C. J., Hoyda, T. D., Samson, W. K., & Ferguson, A. V. (2008). Nesfatin-1 influences the excitability of paraventricular nucleus neurones. *Journal of Neuroendocrinology, 20*(2), 245–250.

Price, T. O., Samson, W. K., Niehoff, M. L., & Banks, W. A. (2007). Permeability of the blood-brain barrier to a novel satiety molecule nesfatin-1. *Peptides, 28*(12), 2372–2381.

Puryear, R., Rigatto, K. V., Amico, J. A., & Morris, M. (2001). Enhanced salt intake in oxytocin deficient mice. *Experimental Neurology*, *171*, 323–328.

Ramanjaneya, M., Chen, J., Brown, J. E., Tripathi, G., Hallschmid, M., Patel, S., et al. (2010). Identification of nesfatin-1 in human and murine adipose tissue: A novel depot-specific adipokine with increased levels in obesity. *Endocrinology*, *151*, 3169–3180.

Reisine, T., & Bell, G. I. (1995). Molecular biology of somatostatin receptors. *Endocrinology Reviews*, *16*, 427–442.

Sabatier, N., Caquineau, C., Dayanithi, G., Bull, P., Douglas, A. J., Guan, X. M. M., et al. (2003). Alpha-melanocyte-stimulating hormone stimulates oxytocin release from the dendrites of hypothalamic neurons while inhibiting oxytocin release from their terminals in the neurohypophysis. *The Journal of Neuroscience*, *23*, 10351–10358.

Sabatier, N., Caquineau, C., Douglas, A. J., & Leng, G. (2003). Oxytocin released from magnocellular dendrites: A potential modulator of alpha-melanocyte-stimulating hormone behavioral actions? *Annals of the New York Academy of Sciences*, *994*, 218–224.

Samson, W. K., Zhang, J. V., Avsian-Kretchmer, O., Cui, K., Yosten, G. L. C., Klein, C., et al. (2008). Neuronostatin encoded by the somatostatin gene regulates neuronal, cardiovascular, and metabolic functions. *The Journal of Biological Chemistry*, *283*, 31949–31959.

Sinha, M. K., Opentanova, I., Ohannesian, J. P., Kolaczynski, J. W., Heiman, M. L., Hale, J., et al. (1996). Evidence of free and bound leptin in human circulation. Studies in lean and obese subjects an during short-term fasting. *The Journal of Clinical Investigation*, *98*, 1277–1282.

Stengel, A., Goebel, M., Wang, L., Rivier, J., Kobelt, P., Monnikes, H., et al. (2009). Central nesfatin-1 reduces dark-phase food intake and gastric emptying in rats: Differential role of corticotropin-releasing factor2 receptor. *Endocrinology*, *150*(11), 4911–4919.

Stengel, A., Goebel, M., Wang, L., Rivier, J., Kobelt, P., Monnikes, H., et al. (2010). Activation of brain somatostatin 2 receptors stimulates feeding in mice: Analysis of food intake microstructure. *Physiology and Behavior*, *101*, 614–622.

Stengel, A., Goebel, M., Yakubov, I., Wang, L., Witcher, D., Coskun, T., et al. (2009). Identification and characterization of nesfatin-1 immunoreactivity in endocrine cell types of the rat gastric oxyntic mucosa. *Endocrinology*, *150*(1), 232–238.

Su, S. F., Yang, A. M., Yang, S. B., Wang, N. B., Lu, S. S., Wang, H. H., et al. (2012). Intracerebroventricular administration of neuronostatin delays gastric emptying and gastrointestinal transit in mice. *Peptides*, *35*, 31–35.

Tachibana, T., Oikawa, D., Adachi, N., Boswell, T., & Furuse, M. (2007). Central administration of alpha-melanocyte-stimulating hormone changes lipid metabolism in chicks. *Comparative Biochemistry and Physiology*, *148*(2), 408–412.

Tagaya, Y., Miura, A., Okada, S., Ohshima, K., & Mori, M. (2012). Nucleobindin-2 is a positive modulator of EGF-dependent signals leading to enhancement of cell growth and suppression of adipocyte differentiation. *Endocrinology*, *153*, 3308–3319. PMID: 22514047.

Tagaya, Y., Osaki, A., Miura, A., Okada, S., Ohshima, K., Hashimoto, K., et al. (2012). Secreted nucleobindin-2 inhibits 3T3-L1 adipocyte differentiation. *Protein and Peptide Letters*, *19*, 997–1004. PMID: 22486620.

Takayanagi, Y., Kasahara, Y., Onaka, T., Takahashi, N., Kawada, T., & Nishimori, K. (2008). Oxytocin receptor-deficient mice developed late-onset obesity. *Neuroreport*, *19*, 951–955.

Tallam, L. S., da Silva, A. A., & Hall, J. E. (2006). Melanocortin-4 receptor mediates cardiovascular and metabolic actions of leptin. *Hypertension*, *48*, 58–64.

Tan, B. K., Hallschmid, M., Kern, W., Lehnert, H., & Randeva, H. S. (2011). Decreased cerebrospinal fluid/plasma ratio of the novel satiety molecule, nesfatin-1/NUCB-2, in obese humans: Evidence of nesfatin-1/NUCB-2 resistance and implications for obesity treatment. *The Journal of Clinical Endocrinology and Metabolism*, *96*, E669–E673.

Tanida, M., & Mori, M. (2011). Nesfatin-1 stimulates renal sympathetic nerve activity in rats. *Neuroreport*, *22*, 309–312.

Taylor, M. M., & Samson, W. K. (2001). Adrenomedullin and central cardiovascular regulation. *Peptides*, *22*(11), 1803–1807.

Toni, R., Malaguti, A., Benfenati, F., & Martini, L. (2004). The human hypothalamus: A morpho-functional perspective. *Journal of Endocrinological Investigation*, *27*(6 Suppl.), 73–94.

Uehara, Y., Shimizu, H., Ohtani, K., Sato, N., & Mori, M. (1998). Hypothalamic corticotropin-releasing hormone is a mediator of the anorexigenic effect of leptin. *Diabetes*, *47*, 890–893.

Vale, W., Brazeau, P., Grant, G., Nussey, A., Burgus, R., Rivier, J., et al. (1972). Preliminary observations on the mechanism of action of somatostatin, a hypothalamic factor inhibiting the secretion of growth hormone. *Comptes rendus hebdomadaires des seances de l'Academie des sciences*, *275*, 2913–2916.

Wsol, A., Cudnoch-Jedrzejewska, A., Szczepanska-Sadowska, E., Kowalewski, S., & Puchalska, L. (2008). Oxytocin in the cardiovascular responses to stress. *Journal of Physiology and Pharmacology*, *59*(Suppl. 8), 123–127.

Xu, B., Goulding, E. H., Zang, K., Cepoi, D., Cone, R. D., Jones, K. R., et al. (2003). Brain-derived neurotrophic factor regulates energy balance downstream of melanocortin-4 receptor. *Nature Neuroscience*, *6*, 736–742.

Yoshida, N., Maejima, Y., Sedbazar, U., Ando, A., Kurita, H., Damdindorj, B., et al. (2010). Stressor-responsive central nesfatin-1 activates corticotropin-releasing hormone, noradrenaline and serotonin neurons and evokes hypothalamic-pituitary-adrenal axis. *Aging*, *2*, 775–784.

Yosten, G. L. C., Pate, A. T., & Samson, W. K. (2011). Neuronostatin acts in brain to biphasically increase mean arterial pressure through sympathoactivation followed by vasopressin secretion: The role of melanocortin receptors. *The American Journal of Physiology*, *300*, R1194–R1199.

Yosten, G. L. C., Redlinger, L., & Samson, W. K. (2012). Evidence for a role of endogenous nesfatin-1 in the control of water drinking. *Journal of Neuroendocrinology*, *24*, 1078–1084. http://dx.doi.org/10.1111/j.1365-2826.2012.02304.x.

Yosten, G. L. C., & Samson, W. K. (2009). Nesfatin-1 exerts cardiovascular effects in brain: Possible interaction with the central melanocortin system. *The American Journal of Physiology*, *297*, R330–R336.

Yosten, G. L. C., & Samson, W. K. (2010a). The melanocortins, not oxytocin, mediate the anorexigenic and antidipsogenic effects of neuronostatin. *Peptides*, *31*, 1711–1714.

Yosten, G. L. C., & Samson, W. K. (2010b). The anorexigenic and hypertensive effects of nesfatin-1 are reversed by pretreatment with an oxytocin receptor antagonist. *The American Journal of Physiology*, *298*, R1642–R1647.

Yosten, G. L. C., & Samson, W. K. (2011). Evidence of a physiologic role for neuronostatin in baroreflex function. *The FASEB Journal*, *25*, 1075.17.

Zegers, D., Beckers, S., Mertens, I. L., Van Gaal, L. F., & Van Hul, W. (2011). Association between polymorphisms of the nesfatin gene, NUCB2, and obesity in men. *Molecular Genetics and Metabolism*, *103*, 282–286.

Zhang, A. Q., Li, X. L., Jiang, C. Y., Lin, L., Shi, R. H., Chen, J. D., et al. (2010). Expression of nesfatin-1/NUCB2 in rodent digestive system. *World Journal of Gastroenterology*, *16*, 1735–1741.

Zhang, Z., Li, L., Yang, M., Liu, H., Boden, G., & Yang, G. (2012). Increased plasma levels of nesfatin-1 in patients with newly diagnosed type 2 diabetes mellitus. *Experimental and Clinical Endocrinology and Diabetes*, *120*, 91–95.

CHAPTER TWO

Anorexia and Hypothalamic Degeneration

Ida A.K. Nilsson[*,†,‡,1], **Charlotte Lindfors**[*,†], **Martin Schalling**[*,†], **Tomas Hökfelt**[‡], **Jeanette E. Johansen**[*,†]

[*]Department of Molecular Medicine & Surgery, Karolinska Institutet, Stockholm, Sweden
[†]Center for Molecular Medicine, Karolinska University Hospital, Stockholm, Sweden
[‡]Department of Neuroscience, Karolinska Institutet, Stockholm, Sweden
[1]Corresponding author: e-mail address: ida.nilsson@ki.se

Contents

1. Introduction 28
   1.1 Anorexia 28
   1.2 Hypothalamic regulation of food intake 29
2. The *anx/anx* Mouse 30
   2.1 Phenotype: Original observations 30
   2.2 Neurochemical aberrances 32
   2.3 Activated microglia 35
   2.4 Microglial expression of MHC class I 36
   2.5 Neuronal expression of MHC class I 37
   2.6 Further signs of cell death/degeneration 38
   2.7 Mitochondrial complex I dysfunction 39
   2.8 On the *anx* mutation 40
3. General Aspects of Mechanisms Underlying Weight Disturbances 42
   3.1 Mitochondrial deficiencies and neurodegeneration 42
   3.2 Hypothalamic inflammation/neurodegeneration and food intake 45
   3.3 Hypothalamic neurogenesis and food intake 46
4. Neurodegeneration and Mitochondrial Dysfunction Related to Eating Disorders in Humans 48
5. Conclusions and Future Directions 49
Acknowledgments 49
References 50

Abstract

Anorexia, meaning poor appetite, occurs in many human conditions, for example, anorexia nervosa, cachexia, and failure to thrive in infants. A key player in the regulation of appetite/food intake in general, as well as conditions of anorexia, is the hypothalamus, in particular, the AGRP/NPY and POMC/CART neurons in the arcuate nucleus. In this chapter, we review the hypothalamic aberrances seen in the anorectic *anx/anx* mouse. This mouse displays deviations in neuropeptidergic/-transmitter systems,

Vitamins and Hormones, Volume 92
ISSN 0083-6729
http://dx.doi.org/10.1016/B978-0-12-410473-0.00002-7

including selective hypothalamic degeneration and inflammation that have been associated with mitochondrial dysfunction. In addition, we discuss data from other animal models, as well as clinical data relating hypothalamic inflammation/degeneration, neurogenesis, and mitochondrial dysfunction to conditions of disturbed regulation of food intake.

1. INTRODUCTION

1.1. Anorexia

Anorexia, literally meaning poor appetite, accompanies many conditions. In general, the term leads the thought to eating disorders and psychiatric diagnoses, primarily anorexia nervosa (AN; Bulik et al., 2006; Kaye, 2008). However, anorexia/wasting also occurs as a consequence of other diseases, for example, in different forms of cancer or infectious diseases. This type of wasting, called cachexia, is sometimes referred to as secondary anorexia. This has been described as a pathological state, in which lack of, or decreased, appetite is combined with increased energy expenditure leading to weight, muscle and adipose tissue loss, as well as weakness (Inui, 2002). HIV, cancer, inflammatory disorders, chronic kidney disease, and chronic heart failure are all examples of conditions commonly accompanied by cachexia (Tan & Fearon, 2008). During these conditions, when the patient is already struggling to cope with the primary disease, it can be deleterious, if he/she is further pushed into a catabolic state. In fact, 80% of patients with advanced stage cancer suffer from cachexia, which often is the actual cause of death (Ramos et al., 2004).

The causes for anorexia are not clear. However, genetics seem to play an important role. The heritability of AN is well established, for example, twin studies have reported a genetic contribution of 48–76% (Striegel-Moore & Bulik, 2007), indicating that genetic factors strongly contribute to its susceptibility. The genes involved are still unknown, even though some associations have been quite well established, for example, polymorphisms both in the opioid receptor gene (Bergen et al., 2003; Brown et al., 2007; Wang et al., 2011) and in the gene for the dopamine-metabolizing enzyme catechol-O-methyltransferase (Frisch et al., 2001; Rask-Andersen, Olszewski, Levine, & Schioth, 2010). Likewise, it is possible that some individuals are genetically predisposed to a higher risk of developing cachexia or more severe forms of cachexia. In order to understand why some people seem more susceptible to, or more severely affected by, anorexia and cachexia, we need to learn more about how food intake, that is, hunger and satiety, is regulated, as well as how environmental, genetic, and epigenetic factors interact and influence this regulation.

A particular anorectic condition, termed failure to thrive, occurs in children of young age. It describes an infant or a child whose growth is inadequate for its gender and age. Often, the infant has a decreased appetite, resulting in a decreased caloric intake. It appears as if the hypothalamus is not synchronized to the caloric requirements of the infant (Kasese-Hara, Wright, & Drewett, 2002; Shaoul et al., 2003). One to five percent of all pediatric hospital admissions have been estimated to be associated with failure to thrive (Kasese-Hara et al., 2002; Shaoul et al., 2003).

1.2. Hypothalamic regulation of food intake

In spite of major research efforts, we still lack decisive knowledge about the mechanisms controlling normal as well as abnormal food intake and energy metabolism, that is energy homeostasis. A key brain region in the energy homeostasis is the arcuate nucleus of the hypothalamus (Arc), and in particular, two neuronal populations located there (Baskin et al., 1999; Broberger, 2005; Broberger, & Hokfelt, 2001; Cone et al., 2001; Dietrich & Horvath, 2009; Druce & Bloom, 2003; Hillebrand, de Wied, & Adan, 2002; Kalra et al., 1999; Kalra & Kalra, 2003; Lawrence, Turnbull, & Rothwell, 1999; Meister, 2000; Morton & Schwartz, 2011; Saper, Chou, & Elmquist, 2002; Sawchenko, 1998; Schwartz, 2001; Schwartz, Woods, Porte, Seeley, & Baskin, 2000; van den Pol, 2003; Woods, Schwartz, Baskin, & Seeley, 2000).

One of these Arc populations is referred to as orexigenic due to the coexpression of food intake stimulating neuropeptides, neuropeptide Y (NPY; Tatemoto, 1982; Tatemoto, Carlquist, & Mutt, 1982) and agouti gene-related protein (AGRP; Shutter et al., 1997). NPY is expressed in multiple, widely distributed cell groups in the brain (Chronwall, 1985; Chronwall et al., 1985; de Quidt & Emson, 1986a,b) including the Arc, while AGRP is expressed exclusively in this nucleus (Broberger, Johansen, Johansson, Schalling & Hokfelt, 1998; Hahn, Breininger, Baskin, & Schwartz, 1998). AGRP is thus an ideal marker for studies on the distribution of Arc AGRP/NPY projections in the brain. The other population is referred to as anorexigenic because of the coexpression of the food intake-inhibiting cocaine- and amphetamine-regulated transcript (CART) peptide (Douglass, McKinzie, & Couceyro, 1995) and pro-opiomelanocortin (POMC), a precursor protein for, among others, α-melanocyte-stimulating hormone (α-MSH) and adrenocorticotropic hormone (ACTH; Mains, Eipper, & Ling, 1977; Roberts & Herbert, 1977).

Peripheral hormones circulating in relation to the energy status of the body, such as leptin and insulin, are able to enter Arc via a partly permeable blood–brain barrier in the Arc–median eminence complex (Broadwell & Brightman, 1976; Krisch & Leonhardt, 1978). Both AGRP/NPY and POMC/CART neurons express receptors for leptin as well as insulin, and binding of their ligands affects neuronal activity, inhibiting the former and activating the latter (Baskin, Blevins, & Schwartz, 2001; Kalra & Kalra, 2004; Meister, 2000; Schwartz et al., 2000).

The POMC/CART cells synthesize the excitatory neurotransmitter glutamate (Collin et al., 2003) and the AGRP/NPY neurons the inhibitory neurotransmitter gamma-aminobutyric acid (GABA; Horvath, Naftolin, & Leranth, 1992). Both populations send extensive projections to other hypothalamic areas, as well as to regions outside the hypothalamus (Bai et al., 1985; Baker & Herkenham, 1995; Broberger et al., 1998; Meister et al., 1989), where the signal is propagated further and contributes to an integrated response to the energy status (Broberger & Hokfelt, 2001; Elmquist, Coppari, Balthasar, Ichinose, & Lowell, 2005; Grill & Kaplan, 2002; Kalra et al., 2003; Wu & Palmiter, 2011). The AGRP/NPY neurons also innervate the POMC/CART neurons (Horvath et al., 1992; Fig. 2.1).

One way of studying these interactions and circuitries in general, and during disturbed eating behavior in particular, is to use animal models, where a mutation has created a phenotype with eating disturbance. While several models relating to overeating have been extensively studied (Coleman, 1978; Huszar et al., 1997; Kleyn et al., 1996; Lu et al., 1994; Naggert et al., 1995), most notably the $Lep^{ob/ob}$ mouse and the $Lep^{db/db}$ mouse with mutations affecting the leptin system (Chen et al., 1996; Chua et al., 1996; Coleman, 1973; Hummel, Dickie, & Coleman, 1966; Lee et al., 1996; Zhang et al., 1994), there are few models of anorexia. With the aim to understand appetite regulation we have, for more than 15 years, investigated the anorectic *anx/anx* mouse, which is a unique model for studying food intake and energy expenditure. Based on the results from our studies of the *anx/anx* mouse, we raise the possibility that hypothalamic inflammation and neurodegeneration, probably a consequence of a mitochondrial dysfunction, can lead to increased susceptibility to anorexia/cachexia.

2. THE *anx/anx* MOUSE

2.1. Phenotype: Original observations

The recessive *anorexia* mutation (*anx*) arose spontaneously at the Jackson Laboratory in 1976, and the anorectic *anx/anx* mouse was several years later

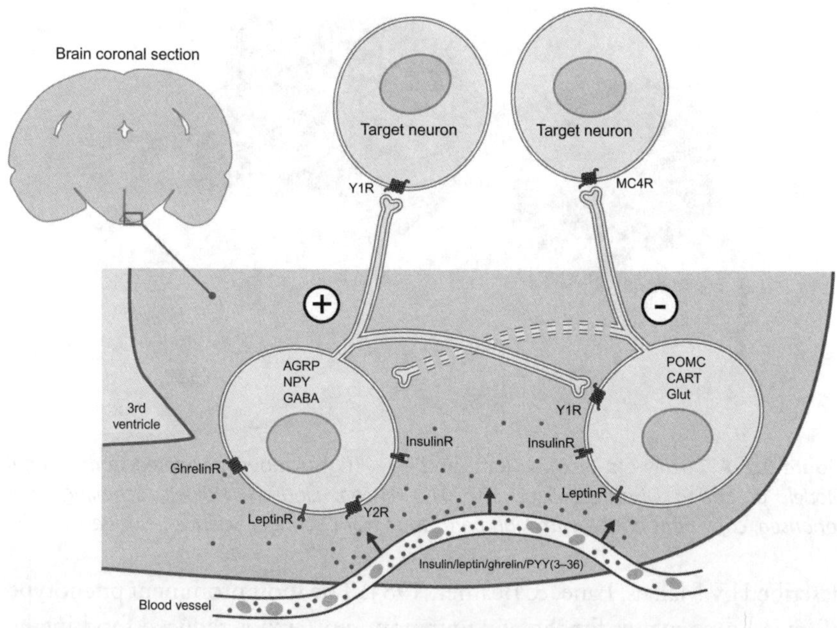

Figure 2.1 Schematic overview of the AGRP/NPY and POMC/CART neurons, their connectivity and regulation. The Arc is located in the most ventral, medial aspects of the hypothalamus bordering the third ventricle and the median eminence, and dorsally the ventromedial nucleus. It harbors a large number of neuron populations characterized by different neurochemical markers, in many cases coexisting (Everitt et al., 1986; Meister, 2007). There are two prominent cell groups that have received much attention due to their involvement in control of food intake: the NPY/AGRP neurons (ns), in part GABAergic (NAGns), and the POMC/CART neurons, in part glutamatergic (PCGns). In contrast to many other neurons in the Arc, they do not project into the median eminence, but their axons are directed into the brain targeting both more closely located nuclei such as the paraventricular nucleus, and the perifornical area, harboring neurons expressing orexin and the melanin-concentrating hormone (MCH), but also sending axons to the lower brain stem such as the solitary tract nucleus, an input station for the vagus nerve, and targets for blood born hormones like cholecystokinin, conveying both catabolic and anabolic information. The NAGns stimulate food intake, whereas the PCGns exert the opposite effect. They are reciprocally coupled, the former neurons releasing NPY acting on inhibitory postsynaptic Y1 receptors on the PCGns. These in turn innervate the NAGns activating melanocortin receptors (MCR3/4). Both neuron populations express leptin (cytokine receptor-type), insulin (tyrosine kinase-type), and ghrelin receptors. Since the arcuate nucleus is located partly outside the blood–brain barrier, leptin, insulin, ghrelin, and PYY(3–36) can access the arcuate neurons, even if they are large molecules. However, active transportation molecules may also be involved. For more detailed information and references, Dietrich and Horvath (2009), Porte, Baskin, & Schwartz, (2002), and Schwartz et al. (2000). *Adapted from Animal Models of Eating Disorders, Sept. 23 2012 Nilsson, Lindfors, Hökfelt, Schalling, and Johansen, copy right notice, with kind permission from Springer Science + Business Media.*

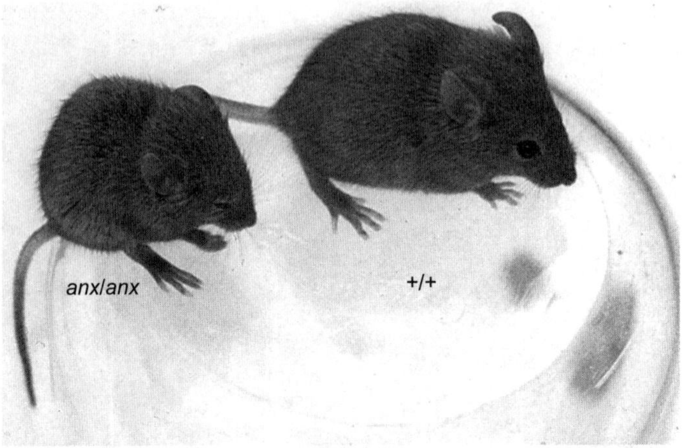

Figure 2.2 A 21-day-old *anx/anx* (left) and +/+ (right) mouse. *Adapted from Animal Models of Eating Disorders, Sept. 23 2012 Nilsson, Lindfors, Hökfelt, Schalling, and Johansen, copy right notice, with kind permission from Springer Science+Business Media.*

described by Maltais, Lane, & Beamer, 1984. The most prominent phenotype of mice homozygous for the *anx* mutation (*anx/anx*) is reduced food intake resulting in an emaciated appearance and death by 3–5 weeks of age. From at least postnatal day (P) 5, the *anx/anx* mouse eats less than normal littermates (+/+ and +/*anx*), despite free access to the mother as well as food and water (Maltais et al., 1984). Subsequently, the *anx/anx* mouse begins to deviate significantly from the normal growth curve from around P9 and weighs half as much as normal littermates by P21, approximately 4 versus 8 g (Fig. 2.2). The *anx/anx* mouse also displays other phenotypic traits, that is, hyperactivity and several neurological problems, such as head weaving, tremors, and uncoordinated gait. However, these traits are less prominent compared to the anorectic phenotype. No abnormalities in the gastrointestinal system or blood parameters, for example, hematocrit, hemoglobulin, or total red blood cell count, have been detected by histological/biochemical analyses. Neither have any abnormalities in other organs been detected using routine staining techniques (Maltais et al., 1984). The *anx* mutation thus seems to cause dysregulation of food intake and/or feeding behavioral systems.

2.2. Neurochemical aberrances

Immunohistochemistry (IHC) and *in situ* hybridization (ISH) studies of the anorectic *anx/anx* mouse brain have revealed several deviations in neuropeptidergic and -transmitter systems, in particular, related to hypothalamic circuitries important for the regulation of food intake and energy metabolism, that is, energy homeostasis, especially the AGRP/NPY and POMC/CART neurons (Broberger, Holmberg, Kuhar, & Hokfelt, 1999a; Broberger, Johansen, Schalling, & Hokfelt, 1997; Broberger et al., 1998, 1999b; Johansen et al., 2000; Nilsson, Lindfors, Fetissov, Hokfelt, & Johansen, 2008; Nilsson et al., 2011).

2.2.1 The NPY/AGRP system

Using IHC, we have revealed a reduced density of NPY- and AGRP-immunoreactive (ir) fibers in all projection areas studied, when comparing *anx/anx* and +/+ mice at P21 (Fig. 2.3). These areas include the paraventricular nucleus of hypothalamus (PVN), the lateral hypothalamic area (LHA), the dorsomedial hypothalamic nucleus (DMH), and Arc (Broberger et al., 1997, 1998). Normally, the AGRP system develops during the first 3 postnatal weeks in mice (Bouret, Draper, & Simerly, 2004a; Nilsson, Johansen, Schalling, Hokfelt, & Fetissov, 2005; Pinto et al., 2004), suggesting a critical period for the maturation of the neuronal mechanisms regulating food intake. We have shown that the AGRP system of the *anx/anx* mouse develops as in wild-type (WT) littermates (+/+) until around P12–15, when the normal increase in fiber density ceases, and even decreases during the following week (Nilsson et al., 2008). In addition, there is a dramatic increase in number and staining intensity of both AGRP- and NPY-ir cell bodies in *anx/anx* Arc at P21 (Fig. 2.3), a phenomenon seen in WT only after colchicine injection. Colchicine is a mitosis

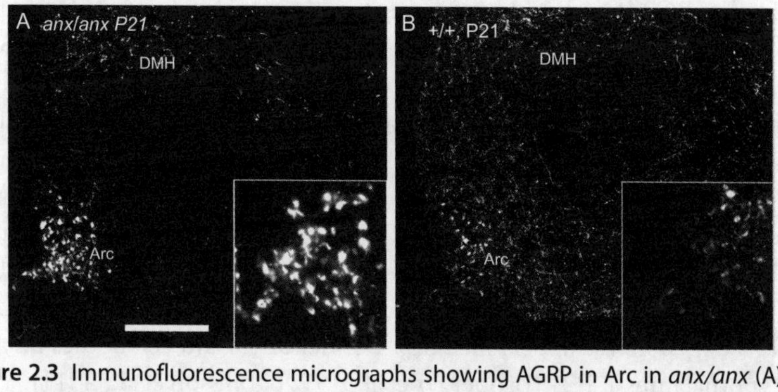

Figure 2.3 Immunofluorescence micrographs showing AGRP in Arc in *anx/anx* (A) and +/+ mouse (B) at P21. Note the reduced density of AGRP-ir fibers in Arc as well as DMH, and the increased intensity and number of AGRP-ir cell bodies in Arc (see insets) in the *anx/anx* mouse. Arc, arcuate nucleus; DMH, dorsomedial hypothalamus. Scale bar in A = 200 μm (applies to A and B). *Adapted from Nilsson et al. (2008).*

inhibitor and arrests centrifugal axonal transport, resulting in accumulation of newly synthesized molecules and organelles in the cell body (Dahlstrom, 1969; Karlsson & Sjostrand, 1970; Kreutzberg, 1969). These results would thus suggest a possible dysfunctional axonal transport in the *anx/anx* mouse, for example, due to derangement of microtubules.

ISH studies have revealed conflicting results regarding the mRNA levels of NPY and AGRP in the *anx/anx* Arc (Broberger et al., 1997; Fetissov et al., 2005; Jahng, Houpt, Kim, Joh, & Son, 1998). Broberger et al. (1997) concluded that there was no difference in mRNA levels of NPY in *anx/anx* when compared with +/+ mice at P21. This was confirmed by Jahng et al., 1998. However, a later study showed an increased expression of both AGRP and NPY mRNA in *anx/anx* mice at P21 (Fetissov et al., 2005). A reason for this discrepancy could be that the synthetic activity for NPY during early postnatal period is very high and that the autoradiographs in our early study were overexposed, resulting in saturation of the emulsion. With this in mind, several scenarios are possible: (i) dysfunctional axonal transport, as mentioned above; (ii) increased release, combined with a compensatory increase of synthesis/transcription, resulting in a decrease of AGRP (and NPY) in the nerve terminals and increased levels in the cell bodies; (iii) axonal degeneration leading to increased transcript levels (see below), followed by feedback-induced increase in neuropeptide synthesis.

2.2.2 The POMC/CART system

Deviations of the staining pattern have also been detected in the POMC/CART system in the *anx/anx* mouse at P21. ISH studies showed decreased numbers of POMC mRNA expressing neurons in *anx/anx* Arc (Broberger et al., 1999b). IHC using antibodies raised against α-MSH, one of the peptides synthesized from the precursor protein POMC, showed markedly attenuated ir fibers in *anx/anx* hypothalamus (Broberger et al., 1999b). This was accompanied by reduced numbers of ACTH-ir cell bodies (Broberger et al., 1999b), ACTH being another product generated from the POMC precursor. In addition, decreased CART mRNA levels, as well as reduced numbers of CART-ir cell bodies and fibers were seen (Johansen et al., 2000).

Of particular interest is the reduced density of NPY receptor (Y1)-LI as well as a degenerative appearance of Y1-ir dendrites and cell bodies in *anx/anx* hypothalamus at P21 (Broberger et al., 1999b; Nilsson et al., 2011). Y1 is mainly a postsynaptic receptor that normally decorates the soma and dendrites in many areas of the brain (Kopp et al., 2002; Zhang et al., 1994). Our results could thus indicate atrophy/degeneration of this neuronal population, similar to the situation for the AGRP/NPY neurons (Broberger et al., 1999b). However, in contrast to the reduction of the AGRP/NPY fiber staining, seen already at P15, the reduction in Y1-ir is apparent first at P21 (Nilsson et al., 2011). Thus, the reduction of the POMC system may, in fact, be a consequence of lost input from the AGRP/NPY system.

2.2.3 The serotonergic systems

Other studies have reported aberrances in serotonergic systems in the *anx/anx* mouse, including hyperinnervation of Arc, the olfactory bulb, frontal cortex, hippocampal formation, and cerebellum (Jahng et al., 1998; Son, Baker, Park, & Joh, 1994). An increased serotonergic innervation is in agreement with the anorectic phenotype of the *anx/anx* mouse, since there is evidence that serotonin decreases food intake (Meguid et al., 2000; Waldbillig, Bartness, & Stanley, 1981). Also, the motor disturbances occasionally detected in the *anx/anx* mouse, for example, head weaving, tremors, and uncoordinated gait, could be related to the serotonergic abnormalities. In fact, Maltais et al., 1984 reported that treating *anx/anx* mice with a serotonin antagonist attenuates their motor problems and that a serotonin precursor causes similar motor disturbances in 15-day-old normal mice. A possible explanation could be that not only serotonergic neurons in the forebrain are affected (Jahng et al., 1998; Son et al., 1994) but also the descending serotonergic neurons (Bowker, Westlund, & Coulter, 1981; Dahlstrom & Fuxe, 1964; Skagerberg & Bjorklund, 1985), which are involved in motoneuron control (Jacobs, van Praag, & Gage, 2000).

2.3. Activated microglia

A number of studies have suggested that hypothalamic inflammation is linked to the anorectic phenotype of the *anx/anx* mouse. Lachuer, Ouyang, Legras, Del Rio, & Barlow, 2005 performed a gene expression analysis of the hypothalamus and concluded that a hypothalamic inflammatory response is involved in the *anx* phenotype. In a following array study of the *anx/anx* hypothalamus, Mercader et al., 2008 reported that the most prominently affected pathways are related to cell death, cell morphology and cancer, centered around the proinflammatory cytokine tumor necrosis factor-α.

In the central nervous system (CNS), microglia cells are usually activated in response to, for example, neuroinflammation, neurodegeneration, and ischemia (Beyer, Gimsa, Eyupoglu, Hailer, & Nitsch, 2000; Streit, 2002; Streit, Graeber, & Kreutzberg, 1988). We have, in the *anx/anx* mouse, shown a strong activation of such cells in areas receiving projections from the food intake-regulating AGRP neurons, in particular, hypothalamic target regions (exemplified by MPO in Fig. 2.4). Here, activated microglia was detected

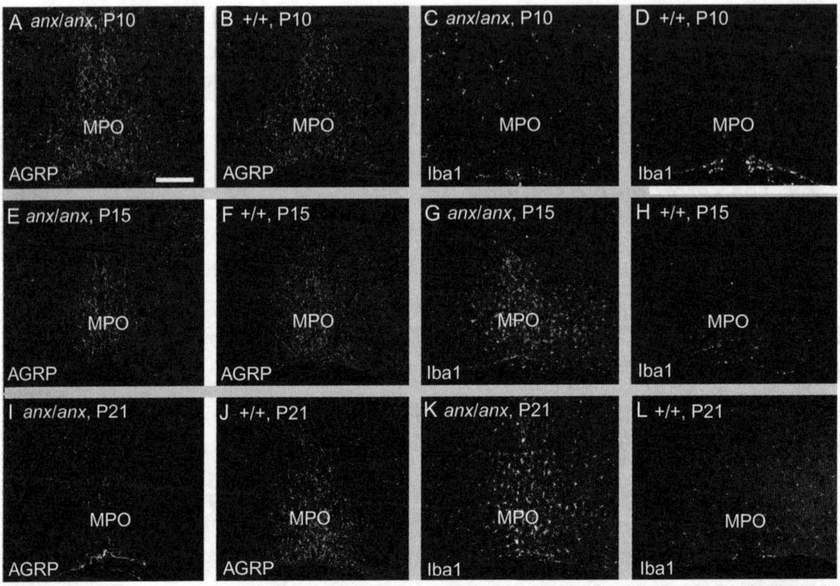

Figure 2.4 Immunofluorescence micrographs showing AGRP (A, B, E, F, I, and J) and Iba1, a marker of activated microglia (C, D, G, H, K, and L) in MPO of *anx/anx* (A, E, I, C, G, and K) and +/+ mice (B, F, J, D, H, and L) at P10 (A–D), P15 (E–H), and P21 (I–L). AGRP, agouti gene-related protein; Iba1, ionized calcium-binding adapter 1; MPO, medial preoptic area. Scale bar in A = 200 μm (applies to A–L).

already at P12, with a progressive increase reaching high levels at P21 (Fig. 2.4K and L; Nilsson et al., 2008). This correlates well with the reduction of AGRP fiber density, both temporally and spatially (Nilsson et al., 2008). Interestingly, in these regions, gliosis is induced by specific ablation of AGRP neurons (Wu, Howell, Cowley, & Palmiter, 2008). Thus, Wu et al., 2008 targeted expression of the diphtheria toxin receptor to AGRP-expressing neurons and subsequently administered the toxin, leading to a specific ablation of this neuron population (Wu et al., 2008). Taken together, these findings argue for inflammatory/degenerative processes in the *anx/anx* hypothalamus, possibly with a relation to the AGRP/NPY system.

2.4. Microglial expression of MHC class I

It has been shown that activated microglia become immunocompetent and gain ability to express high levels of major histocompatibility complex (MHC) class I protein (Neumann, 2001). Our studies show glial expression of MHC class I-related genes in several hypothalamic regions involved in food intake in the *anx/anx* mouse at P21, mostly in activated microglia (Fig. 2.5; Nilsson et al., 2011). Interestingly, microglial MHC class I expression

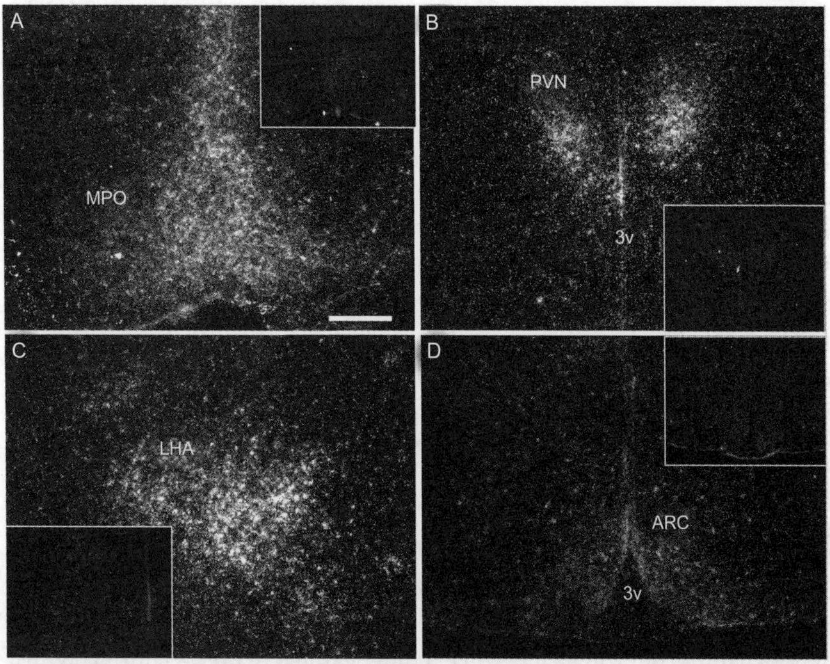

Figure 2.5 Autoradiographs showing MHC class I expression in MPO (A), PVN (B), LHA (C), and Arc (D) of *anx/anx* mice at P21. Note the total absence of labeling in +/+ mice (insets). 3v, third ventricle; Arc, arcuate nucleus; LHA, lateral hypothalamic area; MPO, medial preoptic area; PVN, paraventricular nucleus. Scale bar in A = 200 μm (applies to A–D).

is known to occur in regions with axonal degeneration (Akiyama, Itagaki, & McGeer, 1988; Moffett & Paden, 1994), and these results thus provide further support for such a process in the *anx/anx* hypothalamus.

2.5. Neuronal expression of MHC class I

MHC class I-related molecules were detected in arcuate neurons expressing AGRP/NPY and/or POMC/CART in the *anx/anx* mouse (Nilsson et al., 2011). Neuronal expression of MHC class I may facilitate removal of weak or dying neurons (Neumann, Cavalie, Jenne, & Wekerle, 1995; Neumann, Schmidt, Cavalie, Jenne, & Wekerle, 1997). Furthermore, these molecules seem essential for selective maintenance of synapses and regeneration after injury (Oliveira et al., 2004; Thams, Oliveira, & Cullheim, 2008). Accordingly, expression of MHC class I by neurons in the *anx/anx* Arc may aim at sparing these neurons from elimination of synaptic input, possibly facilitating regeneration.

Neuronal MHC class I expression can also occur as a result of abnormal neuronal activity (Corriveau, Huh, & Shatz, 1998; Neumann et al., 1997). Tetrodotoxin, a neurotoxin blocking action potentials and neuronal activity, causes a dramatic induction of MHC class I-related genes in all neurons (Neumann et al., 1997). Neuronal MHC class I expression has also been detected during extreme neuronal activity, for example, in hippocampal neurons in kainic acid-induced seizures (Corriveau et al., 1998). Thus, it is possible that the *anx/anx* AGRP/NPY and POMC/CART neurons, expressing MHC class I, may undergo degeneration as a result of abnormal neuronal activity. Furthermore, electrically active neurons are known to control the immune function of adjacent glia cells by suppressing glial expression of MHC class I (Neumann, 2001; Wekerle, 2005). MHC class I expression by microglia in the *anx/anx* hypothalamus may therefore reflect electrical inactivation of adjacent neurons.

2.6. Further signs of cell death/degeneration

The hypothesis on axonal degeneration in the *anx/anx* mouse is strengthened by the presence of activated caspase 6 in NPY fibers in the *anx/anx* hypothalamus (Nilsson et al., 2011). This enzyme is expressed during axonal degeneration, in contrast to caspase 3 which is involved in cell body apoptosis (Finn et al., 2000; Kuida et al., 1996; Nikolaev, McLaughlin, O'Leary, & Tessier-Lavigne, 2009), which we could not detect (Nilsson et al., 2011). Thus nerve endings, rather than cell bodies, appear to be more severely or earlier affected, at least in some types of degenerative processes in the *anx/anx* hypothalamus. In agreement, in Alzheimer's (Knobloch & Mansuy, 2008), Parkinson's (Orimo et al., 2008; Raff, Whitmore, & Finn, 2002), and Huntington's (Smith, Brundin, & Li, 2005) diseases, nerve endings have been documented to be affected prior to cell bodies.

Our immunohistochemical analyses indicate that the degeneration in *anx/anx* arcuate neurons may be of a hitherto little recognized type. We observed activated microglia that appeared to wrap around/embrace *anx/anx* Arc neurons similar to what has been termed *microglia-associated cell death* (Ribak, Shapiro, Perez, & Spigelman, 2009). This process differs from both necrosis and apoptosis and may not be detected by classical degenerative/apoptotic markers. Ribak et al. reported activated microglia in the granular layer of the dentate gyrus surrounding individual neuronal cell bodies in normal rats. Small openings in the neuronal plasma membrane and a watery cytoplasm and nucleoplasm as well as damaged organelles were observed. In the dentate gyrus, this process may balance the birth of relatively high number of neurons in this area, even in adulthood (Gould & McEwen, 1993; Jacobs, Martin-Cora, & Fornal, 2002).

Terminal dUTP nick end labeling (TUNEL) is a commonly used marker for programmed cell death (Gavrieli, Sherman, & Ben-Sasson, 1992). Significantly increased number of TUNEL-positive cells were detected in hypothalamus of the *anx/anx* mice compared with +/+ mice (Nilsson et al., 2011). Increased TUNEL-, as well as BrdU-labeling, indicative of proliferating cells, has been detected in dentate gyrus of the *anx/anx* mouse (Kim et al., 2001). Thus, since *microglia-associated cell death* escapes detection by classical apoptotic markers such as TUNEL, several apoptotic/cell death processes may simultaneously occur in the *anx/anx* hypothalamus.

Taken together, the data described above provide evidence for involvement of degenerative processes in the anorectic phenotype of the *anx/anx* mouse.

2.7. Mitochondrial complex I dysfunction

The oxidative phosphorylation system (OXPHOS), located in the mitochondrial inner membrane, is responsible for the generation of cellular energy, in the form of ATP. Dysfunction of OXPHOS, that is mitochondrial dysfunction, has been implicated in a variety of neurodegenerative disorders (Lin & Beal, 2006), for example, Parkinson's and Alzheimer's diseases (Ankarcrona, Mangialasche, & Winblad, 2010; Dawson & Dawson, 2002; Dumont & Beal, 2011; Ekstrand et al., 2007; Leonard & Schapira, 2000a; Morais & De Strooper, 2010). Critical in the degenerative process is reactive oxygen species (ROS), which can cause oxidative stress and cell death (Ott, Gogvadze, Orrenius, & Zhivotovsky, 2007; Sun & Chen, 1998). The majority of ROS is, even under normal conditions, produced by the OXPHOS in the mitochondrial inner membrane, but ROS production increases substantially during dysfunction of, in particular, complex I (CI; Ott et al., 2007).

We have reported that the anorexia and hypothalamic neurodegeneration of the *anx/anx* mouse are associated with mitochondrial dysfunction, especially CI deficiency, and increased production of ROS (Lindfors et al., 2011). A microarray and subsequent pathway analysis of hypothalamus from *anx/anx* and +/+ mice identified OXPHOS pathways, in particular, mitochondrial CI, as the most prominently affected one. Several genes related to mitochondria and oxidative stress were altered in expression levels in the *anx/anx* hypothalamus (Table 2.1). Furthermore, by histochemical methods, we detected increased hypothalamic levels of ROS and expression of antioxidants. By respirometry analyses, we saw a reduced mitochondrial respiration, in particular, via CI (Fig. 2.6), in hypothalamus of the *anx/anx* mouse suggesting CI deficiency (Lindfors et al., 2011).

Table 2.1 Selected mitochondria and oxidative stress related genes showing altered expression when comparing *anx/anx* with +/+ mice

Symbol	Entrez gene name	Fold change
Bcl2l11	BCL2-like 11 (apoptosis facilitator)	2.1
Atf4	Activating transcription factor 4 (tax-responsive enhancer element B67)	2.0
Gstm5	Glutathione *S*-transferase mu 5	1.8
Sod1	Superoxide dismutase 1, soluble	1.7
Ndufa5	NADH dehydrogenase (ubiquinone) 1 alpha subcomplex, 5 and 13 kDa	1.7
Cox6a1	Cytochrome *c* oxidase subunit VIa polypeptide 1	1.6
Ubb	Ubiquitin B	1.6
Cox4i1	Cytochrome c oxidase subunit IV isoform 1	1.6
Cox5b	Cytochrome c oxidase subunit Vb	1.5
Prdx1	Peroxiredoxin 1	1.5
Cox6c	Cytochrome *c* oxidase subunit VIc	1.5
Ndufc2	NADH dehydrogenase (ubiquinone) 1, subcomplex unknown, 2 and 14.5 kDa	1.5
Cox17	COX17 cytochrome c oxidase assembly homolog (*S. cerevisiae*)	1.4
Gpd2	Glycerol-3-phosphate dehydrogenase 2 (mitochondrial)	−1.4
Map2k4	Mitogen-activated protein kinase kinase 4	−1.6
Atp5f1	ATP synthase, H^+ transporting, mitochondrial F0 complex, subunit B1	−2.2
Ndufaf1	NADH dehydrogenase (ubiquinone) 1 alpha subcomplex, assembly factor 1	−2.2

Adapted from Lindfors et al. (2011).

2.8. On the *anx* mutation

We have mapped the *anx* mutation between markers *D2Mit133* and *Jojo5* corresponding to a 0.2 cM interval on chromosome 2 (Chr 2: bp 118, 889, 896–120, 175, 108; www.ensembl.org) (Lindfors et al., 2011). This interval includes approximately 40 identified genes, including the *Ndufaf1* gene (NADH dehydrogenase (ubiquinone) 1α-subcomplex, assembly factor 1).

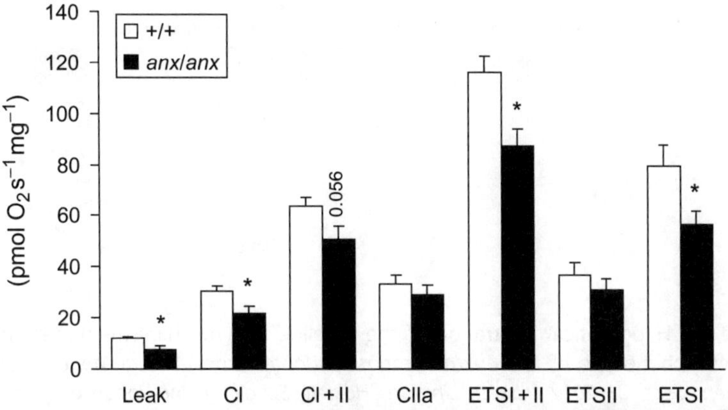

Figure 2.6 Hypothalamic complex I deficiency and mitochondrial dysfunction in the *anx/anx* mouse. Complex I respiratory capacity is impaired in *anx/anx* mice. Mitochondrial respiration was analyzed in hypothalamus samples ($n = 6$–9 per genotype). For basal O_2 flux from complex I of the respiratory chain, malate and pyruvate were added to the Oxygraph-2k chamber (Leak). To maximize oxidative phosphorylation from complex I, ADP and glutamate were added in sufficient amounts and in subsequent steps to couple electron transfer to ATP production, that is, coupled respiration from complex I (CI). To ascertain O_2 flux from complex I and II, succinate was added (CI + II). We calculated additional O_2 flux through complex II, subtracting CI from CI + II (CIIa). To reach maximal capacity of the electron transfer system by CI and II, the uncoupler FCCP was titrated to the chamber (ETSI + II). Complex I was inhibited by the addition of rotenone (ETSII). Electron transfer trough complex I was calculated by subtracting ETSII from ETSI + II. The remaining O_2 flux after inhibition of complex III with antimycin A (O_2 flux independent of the electron transfer system) was subtracted from each of the previous steps. Error bars represent standard error of mean. *Adapted from Lindfors et al. (2011).*

The *Ndufaf1* gene encodes one of several proteins important for the proper assembly of the 45/46 proteins that build up mitochondrial complex I (Smeitink, van den Heuvel, & DiMauro, 2001; Ugalde, Janssen, van den Heuvel, Smeitink, & Nijtmans, 2004; Ugalde et al., 2004; Vogel et al., 2005). Our microarray analysis revealed that *Ndufaf1* is approximately 50% downregulated in *anx/anx* hypothalamus, suggesting that *Ndufaf1* is equivalent to the *anx* gene. The downregulation of *Ndufaf1* was confirmed by real-time expression in five different tissues and by Western blot of hypothalamus. Still, the actual change in gene sequence linked to this down regulation has not been found (Lindfors et al., 2011). Interestingly, the *NDUFAF1* gene has also been implicated in human pathology. The genetic analysis of an 11-month-old baby with failure to thrive revealed mutations in this gene, resulting in markedly reduced levels of the NDUFAF1 protein, and reduced assembly as well as activity of CI (Dunning et al., 2007).

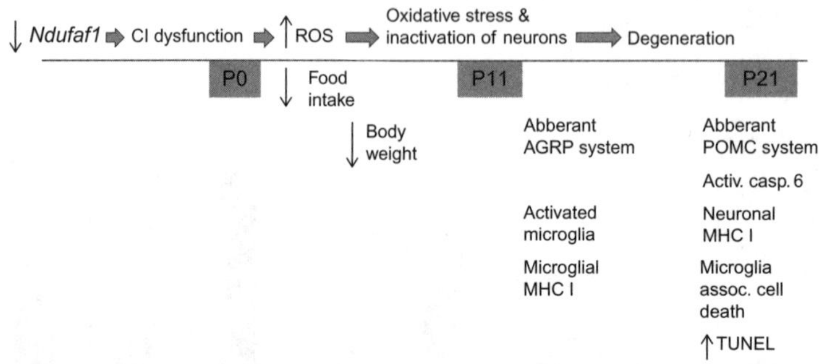

Figure 2.7 Hypothetical illustration of the timeline and mechanisms underlying the anorectic phenotype of the *anx/anx* mouse. *Adapted from Animal Models of Eating Disorders, Sept. 23 2012 Nilsson, Lindfors, Hökfelt, Schalling and Johansen, copy right notice, with kind permission from Springer Science + Business Media.*

Thus, the mutation underlying the *anx/anx* phenotype is not identified, even if a possible candidate gene now is under further scrutiny. In summary, we hypothesize that hypothalamic neurodegeneration, possibly caused/triggered by mitochondrial deficiency, could be one mechanism leading to anorexia/cachexia (Fig. 2.7).

3. GENERAL ASPECTS OF MECHANISMS UNDERLYING WEIGHT DISTURBANCES

3.1. Mitochondrial deficiencies and neurodegeneration

Disorders related to mitochondrial dysfunction present with a variety of clinical manifestations, for example, limb weakness, encephalomyopathies, myopathy, seizures, and lactic acidosis (Leonard & Schapira, 2000b). Deficiency of CI is the most common cause of OXPHOS dysfunctions and, interestingly, CI dysfunction has been shown to result in energy generation deficiencies, altered apoptotic signaling, and selective neurodegeneration, for example, in Parkinson's disease (Lazarou, Thorburn, Ryan, & McKenzie, 2009; Schapira, 2006). For example, chronic infusion of low doses of the CI inhibitor rotenone induces selective dopaminergic neurodegeneration and Parkinson-like symptoms in rats. The fact that the animals present with selective lesions and behavioral abnormalities may appear surprising, since the infusions cause a uniform CI inhibition throughout the brain (Betarbet et al., 2000). However, selective neuronal damage and gliosis, as observed in the *anx/anx* mouse (Nilsson et al., 2008), seem to occur in both human CI disorders (Distelmaier et al., 2009) as well as animal models with CI deficiencies, such as the *Ndufs4* knockout mouse (Quintana, Kruse, Kapur, Sanz, & Palmiter, 2010). This suggests that different brain areas are more or less sensitive to CI deficiency and/or oxidative stress, possibly resulting in the selective neuronal damage seen in both animal models and human patients with CI deficiencies. Moreover, both humans and animals with CI dysfunction share several phenotypes with the *anx/anx* mouse, including failure to thrive, dysphagia, weakness, and tremor (Chol et al., 2003; Finsterer, 2008; Kruse et al., 2008).

3.1.1 *Why is the NPY/AGRP system affected mainly in the* anx/anx *mouse?*

Mitochondrial deficiency, in particular CI deficiency, seems to be associated with selective neuronal damage/degeneration in a number of conditions (see above). The underlying mechanism(s) is still unclear, but some possible explanations for the selectivity will be discussed below.

In general, the electrical properties, as well as the structural and synaptic complexity of neurons, put an extraordinarily large demand on energy production by the OXPHOS. In particular, the axons and synaptic terminals require high amounts of ATP to rapidly restore ion gradients after depolarization and neurotransmitter release. This makes synapses highly susceptible to conditions such as increased stress, ischemia, and dramatic reduction in energy availability (Mattson & Liu, 2002), providing an explanation to the observation that degeneration of axons often precedes the death of the cell body (Knobloch et al., 2008; Orimo et al., 2008; Raff et al., 2002).

The Arc neurons are highly active during the early postnatal weaning period (van den Top & Spanswick, 2006) and are therefore probably particularly sensitive to CI deficiency and more prone to selective degeneration during this period. This could also be part of the reason why the Arc neurons are so severely and rather selectively affected in the *anx/anx* mouse.

3.1.2 *ATP sensitive K^+ channels: Kir 6.2/SUR1*

Another factor that could contribute to the neuronal vulnerability are the ATP- and sulfonylurea-sensitive $K^+{}_{-ATP}$ channels. Intracellular ATP closes the channel leading to membrane depolarization and links cell excitability with metabolic status (Ashcroft, 1988). Neuronal channels of this type have been suggested to have a strong neuroprotective effect (Blondeau, Plamondon, Richelme, Heurteaux, & Lazdunski, 2000). When intracellular ATP levels are low, due to for example metabolic stress, the $K^+{}_{-ATP}$ channels are and the membrane is hyperpolarized. This reduces neuronal activity and neurotransmitter release, an ATP-saving process, and could thus protect against excitotoxicity and calcium overload, a necessity in situations of metabolic stress (Ballanyi, 2004; Blondeau et al., 2000). However, *chronic* reduction in neuronal activity may lead to reduced expression of genes and proteins important for neuronal survival, such as neurotrophic factors (Chergui et al., 1997). Thus, transient activation of the $K^{+}{}_{-ATP}$ channels may be a short-term neuroprotective response to metabolic stress, whereas chronic $K^{+}{}_{-ATP}$ channel activation could have fatal consequences for the cell.

3.1.3 Expression of Kir 6.2/SUR1 by arcuate and substantia nigra neurons

The $K^{+}{}_{-ATP}$ channels consist of two types of subunits, the pore-forming, inwardly rectifying potassium channel (Kir 6-) family members and the regulatory sulfonylurea receptor (SUR) subunit. The complete channel consists of four subunits forming a tetramer (Ashcroft, 1988; Liss, Bruns, & Roeper, 1999). The most probable combination of $K^{+}{}_{-ATP}$ channels in Arc (both in NPY/AGRP and POMC/CART neurons) is Kir6.2/SUR1 (Dunn-Meynell, Rawson, & Levin, 1998; Ibrahim et al., 2003; Thomzig, Laube, Pruss, & Veh, 2005). Kir6.2/SUR1 expression is also found in a subpopulation of dopamine neurons in the substantia nigra, rendering these neurons a high sensitivity to rotenone by inhibition of mitochondrial CI (Liss et al., 1999). If hypothalamic neurodegeneration occurs also in rotenone-treated rodents remains to be explored. Interestingly, selective atrophy of the hypothalamus and the striatum was reported in a patient with a null mutation in the *NDUFA12L* gene, a gene encoding another CI assembly factor (Ogilvie, Kennaway, & Shoubridge, 2005), indicating that the hypothalamus could be sensitive to CI deficiency also in humans. It is thus possible that the reduced *Ndufaf1* expression and CI deficiency observed in the *anx/anx* mice could lead to hyperpolarization and inactivation of the Arc neurons.

As the nigral dopaminergic subpopulation of neurons projecting to striatum also expresses the Kir6.2/SUR1 combination, there might be degenerative signs also in this region of the *anx/anx* mouse. In fact, deviations in dopaminergic neurotransmission has been demonstrated in the *anx/anx* mouse striatum, that is, decreased levels of dopamine and its metabolites, homovanillic acid, and 3-methoxytyramine (Johansen et al., 2001). Furthermore, the striatal Na^{+}, K^{+}-ATPase activity, normally inhibited by dopamine, was shown to be upregulated in *anx/anx*, and isolated neostriatal neurons failed to respond to exogenous dopamine (Johansen et al., 2001). Interestingly, the levels of homovanillic acid in cerebrospinal fluid are reduced in both ill and recovered AN patients (Kaye, Frank, & McConaha, 1999). However, in our preliminary immunohistochemical analyses of *anx/anx* substantia nigra, using two markers (activated microglia and tyrosine hydroxylase), no obvious differences were seen. It is possible that changes in these markers would be detected, if the *anx/anx* mouse would survive longer and/or by using more sensitive approaches, for example, stereology.

3.2. Hypothalamic inflammation/neurodegeneration and food intake

Hypothalamic inflammation and neurodegeneration have been documented in other animal models with disturbed energy homeostasis. Inflammatory processes in the hypothalamus have been related to the impaired insulin signaling seen after feeding with high-fat diet (HFD; De Souza et al., 2005) and obese conditions (Milanski et al., 2009) as well as in cachexia (Durham, Dillon, & Sheffield-Moore, 2009). This process appears to be rapid, as hypothalamic inflammatory signaling is evident in both mice and rats already 1–3 days after introducing the HFD, even prior to substantial weight gain has occurred. Gliosis and markers suggestive of neuronal injury have subsequently been detected in Arc during the first week of HFD (Thaler et al., 2012). Furthermore, a study by Calegari et al., 2011 showed that hypothalamic inflammation impairs pancreatic islet function, thus providing the first evidence for a direct link between inflamed/dysfunctional hypothalamus and impaired insulin secretion. HFD also induces apoptosis of hypothalamic neurons (Moraes et al., 2009). These findings raise the possibility that diet-induced neurodegeneration may be involved in the etiology of obesity/metabolic disorders.

Mice that become obese due to the lack of the Ubb polyubiquitin gene develop selective hypothalamic degeneration, afflicting arcuate neurons controlling energy homeostasis. This has been attributed to the fact that Ubb-dependent protein degradation is required for axon remodeling to occur during development and after injury (Ryu, Garza, Lu, Barsh, & Kopito, 2008). Also, the mouse transgenic for E4B, a mammalian ubiquitin elongation factor, exhibits obesity and neurodegeneration, in particular in the hypothalamus, that is, PVN (Susaki & Nakayama, 2010).

Thus, paradoxically, conditions both of excess and lack of energy seem to be coupled to hypothalamic mechanisms involving inflammation/degeneration. A thorough evaluation of the mechanisms in the different conditions is needed to better understand the relationship between energy balance and hypothalamic inflammation and/or degeneration. It is possible that studies of the *anx/anx* mouse will contribute to further understanding of this paradox.

3.2.1 Experimental, selective ablation of hypothalamic neurons

Several studies with experimental ablation of hypothalamic neuronal populations have shown disturbances in energy homeostasis. Early studies by Olney and collaborators showed that monosodium glutamate destroys 80–90% of the neurons in Arc, including the ones regulating food intake, resulting in several endocrine dysfunctions and obesity (Cameron, Cutbush, & Opat, 1978; Coyle et al., 1981).

Specific ablation of the hypothalamic POMC neurons in mice causes obesity (Xu et al., 2005), although the phenotype is less dramatic than after knocking out the POMC gene (Challis et al., 2004). Interestingly, in contrast to monosodium glutamate treatment, simultaneous ablation of both the AGRP and POMC neurons leads to an even less obese phenotype (Xu et al., 2005), illustrating the complexity of these systems.

Adult ablation of AGRP neurons inhibits feeding and results in a lean/starvation phenotype (Bewick et al., 2005; Gropp et al., 2005; Luquet, Perez, Hnasko, & Palmiter, 2005). This starvation is independent of melanocortin signaling (Wu, Clark, & Palmiter, 2012), but has been attributed to a loss of GABAergic signaling, primarily in the parabrachial nucleus possibly resulting in unbalanced excitation of this nucleus (Wu, Boyle, & Palmiter, 2009; Wu, Howell, & Palmiter, 2008). Luquet et al., 2005 demonstrated that *neonatal* ablation of hypothalamic AGRP neurons has no effect on food intake or body weight. However, acute ablation of AGRP neurons, over a few days, gives rise to severe weight loss and starvation (Luquet et al., 2005), while a progressive ablation in adulthood, over months, results in a milder reduction in body weight (Xu et al., 2005). Thus, ablation of the Arc neurons influences food intake and body weight in a time- and neuronal type-dependent manner, and compensatory mechanisms are likely to occur during a temporally extended loss of neurons.

3.3. Hypothalamic neurogenesis and food intake

Neuronal death and neurodegeneration are closely linked to neurogenesis, a process now known to occur in several brain regions of the rodent brain (Alvarez-Buylla & Garcia-Verdugo, 2002; Gage, 2002), including the hypothalamus (Migaud et al., 2010). Moreover, there is an association between hypothalamic neurogenesis, combined with cell death and weight disturbances, in several rodent models. For example, the obese leptin-deficient $Lep^{ob/ob}$ mice display a pattern of reduced AGRP-expressing projections, resembling what is seen in the *anx/anx* mouse (Bouret et al., 2004a). By injecting $Lep^{ob/ob}$ mice postnatally with leptin, (Bouret, Draper, & Simerly, 2004b) normalized the development of these projections, indicating that leptin can act as neurotrophic factor on this hypothalamic circuit.

Kokoeva, Yin, & Flier, 2005 showed that ciliary neurotrophic factor (CNTF) induces weight loss in obese rodents, and that centrally administered CNTF stimulates cell proliferation/neurogenesis in the murine hypothalamus. The functional phenotype of these newborn neurons implies that they are relevant for energy homeostasis regulation. The authors suggest that hypothalamic neurogenesis could play a role in development of obesity by changing the energy-balance set point.

Furthermore, Pierce & Xu, 2010 showed that cell proliferation is increased in the hypothalamus of adult mice, in which AGRP neurons have been selectively ablated by deletion of mitochondrial transcription factor A (progressive ablation resulting in a small reduction in body weight; Xu et al., 2005). Some of these newly generated neurons differentiated into AGRP-neurons, as well as leptin-responsive neurons. Blocking this neurogenesis results in decreased food intake and adiposity, in the mutant, but not the WT mice (Pierce & Xu, 2010).

McNay, Briancon, Kokoeva, Maratos-Flier, & Flier, 2012 showed that Arc remodeling is inhibited in two animal models of obesity, diet-induced obesity (DIO) and the leptin-deficient Lep$^{ob/ob}$ mouse. This study also shows that Arc neurons involved in food intake regulation exhibit substantial turnover even in WT adult mice. Thus, more than half of the POMC and NPY neurons, which are present at 4 weeks of age, are replaced by ongoing neurogenesis during the subsequent 8 weeks in normal mice. However, in DIO mice, the number of newly generated Arc-cells, including neurons, was decreased. This was shown to be related to inhibited differentiation of stem-like cells into more proliferative progenitor-like cells and/or impaired survival of these cells.

The processes underlying remodeling of food intake regulating circuits described above are incompletely understood. Autophagy is a cellular degradation process that plays a role in cell elimination during neuronal development (Cecconi & Levine, 2008). Compromising autophagy in AGRP neurons leads to reduced AGRP levels, food intake, and adiposity. The same procedure in POMC neurons results in increased body weight and adiposity and alterations in maturation of POMC axonal processes (Coupe et al., 2012; Kaushik et al., 2012). Thus, autophagy may be critical for the proper development/remodeling of the Arc systems regulating food intake.

Finally, increased expression of neurotrophin tyrosine kinase receptor 3 (Ntrk3) has been detected in the *anx/anx* mouse hypothalamus, but not cortex (Mercader et al., 2008). Neurotrophins are factors that support the survival, development, and function of neurons (Bibel & Barde,

2000). This is interesting since both the *NTRK2* and *3* gene, as well as the ligand brain-derived neurotrophic factor, have also been associated with eating disorders/AN in humans (Mercader et al., 2008; Ribases et al., 2003; Ribases et al., 2004).

In summary, a number of factors/mechanism, among them leptin, CNTF, mitochondrial transcription factor A, neurotrophic factors, fasting, and autophagy seem to be critical in regulating remodeling, genesis, and survival of neurons in the hypothalamic energy balance-regulating circuitries.

4. NEURODEGENERATION AND MITOCHONDRIAL DYSFUNCTION RELATED TO EATING DISORDERS IN HUMANS

Indications for neurodegenerative processes have been detected also in humans with disturbed eating behavior. In patients with the restrictive type of AN, there is evidence of both a global reduction in white matter (WM), as well as focal reductions in gray matter, in hypothalamus and some other brain regions (Boghi et al., 2011). In addition, postmortem investigations and imaging studies have shown macroscopic anatomical changes in the brain of patients with AN (Artmann, Grau, Adelmann, & Schleiffer, 1985; Dolan, Mitchell, & Wakeling, 1988; Enzmann & Lane, 1977; Golden et al., 1996; Hoffman et al., 1989; Katzman et al., 1996; Miwa, Nakanishi, Kodama, & Kondo, 2004). Most commonly, these show cerebral and cerebellar gray and WM atrophy and ventricular/sulcal enlargement. Interestingly, Golden et al., 1996 detected enlargement of, in particular, the third ventricle, which is bordered by several hypothalamic regions, including the Arc, thus indicating hypothalamic degeneration as a possible process also in anorectic patients.

Huntington's disease is characterized by progressive neurodegeneration that primarily occurs in striatum and extends to other brain regions, including the hypothalamus (Hult, Schultz, Soylu, & Petersen, 2010; Ross & Tabrizi, 2011; Walker, 2007). Severe neuronal loss (>90%) occurs in the lateral hypothalamus, in particular involving orexin neurons (Aziz et al., 2008; Kremer et al., 1991; Kremer, Roos, Dingjan, Marani, & Bots, 1990) a also the POMC/CART system in Arc (van der Burg et al., 2008). These patients often show weight loss after disease onset, despite appropriate energy intake (Sanberg, Fibiger, & Mark, 1981). The neurodegeneration of hypothalamus in Huntington's disease has in fact been related to the metabolic disturbances seen in these patients (Gabery et al., 2010).

Hypothalamic pathologies have been detected in conditions of excess energy. In MRI studies of obese individuals, Thaler et al., 2012 detected gliosis in the mediobasal hypothalamus. Thus, gliosis in hypothalamic regions has been associated with obesity in both humans and rodents (De Souza et al., 2005; Milanski et al., 2009; Thaler, Choi, Schwartz, & Wisse, 2010; Thaler et al., 2012).

Leigh and Leigh-like syndromes comprise a group of disorders related to CI dysfunction with onset in early childhood and characterized by among other thing decreased food intake. Leigh syndrome is also referred to as subacute, necrotizing encephalopathy, a severe neurodegenerative disease affecting diencephalon, cerebellum, and/or the brainstem. Large variations in the clinical and genetic background of the syndrome exist, but all show a progressive decline of the CNS due to focal, necrotizing lesions of several brain regions.

5. CONCLUSIONS AND FUTURE DIRECTIONS

In this chapter, we have discussed neuropeptidergic/neurotransmitter disturbances, mitochondrial dysfunction and neurodegeneration/neuroinflammation that are related to the anorexia of the *anx/anx* mouse. We have also reviewed a possible role of such processes in other eating disorders, both in animal models and in humans, that is, anorexia, obesity, and failure to thrive. In addition, we have discussed hypothalamic neurogenesis and factors influencing such a process, all in relation to eating disorders.

We suggest that even subclinical CI dysfunction is a risk factor for the development of an anorectic condition. Our hypothesis is that the molecular mechanisms, in particular the neurodegeneration resulting from CI dysfunction, as documented in the *anx/anx* mouse, can be involved also in human conditions with disturbed food intake regulation, for example, AN, failure to thrive and cachexia. Studies on these patient groups are required to test this hypothesis.

ACKNOWLEDGMENTS

Part of the work presented in this chapter was supported by funding from Karolinska Institutet (KI), the Karolinska University Hospital, the AFA Insurance Company, National Institutes of Health Grant P40 RR001183, The Swedish Research Council, Hjärnfonden/Swedish Brain Foundation, Drottning Silvias Jubileums Fond, the Swedish Medical Association, and the following Foundations: Fredrik and Ingrid Thuring, Åhlén, Lennander, Marianne, and Marcus Wallenberg, Knut and Alice Wallenberg, Åke Wiberg, Magnus Bergvall, Torsten, and Ragnar Söderberg, and Erik and Edith Fernström, and unrestricted research grants from the Scandinavian Clinical Nutrition AB and Bringwell AB.

REFERENCES

Akiyama, H., Itagaki, S., & McGeer, P. L. (1988). Major histocompatibility complex antigen expression on rat microglia following epidural kainic acid lesions. *Journal of Neuroscience Research*, *20*, 147–157.

Alvarez-Buylla, A., & Garcia-Verdugo, J. M. (2002). Neurogenesis in adult subventricular zone. *The Journal of Neuroscience*, *22*, 629–634.

Ankarcrona, M., Mangialasche, F., & Winblad, B. (2010). Rethinking Alzheimer's disease therapy: Are mitochondria the key? *Journal of Alzheimer's Disease*, *20*(Suppl. 2), S579–S590.

Artmann, H., Grau, H., Adelmann, M., & Schleiffer, R. (1985). Reversible and non-reversible enlargement of cerebrospinal fluid spaces in anorexia nervosa. *Neuroradiology*, *27*, 304–312.

Ashcroft, F. M. (1988). Adenosine 5′-triphosphate-sensitive potassium channels. *Annual Review of Neuroscience*, *11*, 97–118.

Aziz, A., Fronczek, R., Maat-Schieman, M., Unmehopa, U., Roelandse, F., Overeem, S., et al. (2008). Hypocretin and melanin-concentrating hormone in patients with Huntington disease. *Brain Pathology*, *18*, 474–483.

Bai, F. L., Yamano, M., Shiotani, Y., Emson, P. C., Smith, A. D., Powell, J. F., et al. (1985). An arcuato-paraventricular and -dorsomedial hypothalamic neuropeptide Y-containing system which lacks noradrenaline in the rat. *Brain Research*, *331*, 172–175.

Baker, R. A., & Herkenham, M. (1995). Arcuate nucleus neurons that project to the hypothalamic paraventricular nucleus: Neuropeptidergic identity and consequences of adrenalectomy on mRNA levels in the rat. *The Journal of Comparative Neurology*, *358*, 518–530.

Ballanyi, K. (2004). Protective role of neuronal KATP channels in brain hypoxia. *The Journal of Experimental Biology*, *207*, 3201–3212.

Baskin, D. G., Blevins, J. E., & Schwartz, M. W. (2001). How the brain regulates food intake and body weight: The role of leptin. *Journal of Pediatric Endocrinology & Metabolism*, *14* (Suppl. 6), 1417–1429.

Baskin, D. G., Figlewicz Lattemann, D., Seeley, R. J., Woods, S. C., Porte, D., Jr., & Schwartz, M. W. (1999). Insulin and leptin: Dual adiposity signals to the brain for the regulation of food intake and body weight. *Brain Research*, *848*, 114–123.

Bergen, A. W., van den Bree, M. B., Yeager, M., Welch, R., Ganjei, J. K., Haque, K., et al. (2003). Candidate genes for anorexia nervosa in the 1p33-36 linkage region: Serotonin 1D and delta opioid receptor loci exhibit significant association to anorexia nervosa. *Molecular Psychiatry*, *8*, 397–406.

Betarbet, R., Sherer, T. B., MacKenzie, G., Garcia-Osuna, M., Panov, A. V., & Greenamyre, J. T. (2000). Chronic systemic pesticide exposure reproduces features of Parkinson's disease. *Nature Neuroscience*, *3*, 1301–1306.

Bewick, G. A., Gardiner, J. V., Dhillo, W. S., Kent, A. S., White, N. E., Webster, Z., et al. (2005). Post-embryonic ablation of AgRP neurons in mice leads to a lean, hypophagic phenotype. *The FASEB Journal*, *19*, 1680–1682.

Beyer, M., Gimsa, U., Eyupoglu, I. Y., Hailer, N. P., & Nitsch, R. (2000). Phagocytosis of neuronal or glial debris by microglial cells: Upregulation of MHC class II expression and multinuclear giant cell formation in vitro. *Glia*, *31*, 262–266.

Bibel, M., & Barde, Y. A. (2000). Neurotrophins: Key regulators of cell fate and cell shape in the vertebrate nervous system. *Genes & Development*, *14*, 2919–2937.

Blondeau, N., Plamondon, H., Richelme, C., Heurteaux, C., & Lazdunski, M. (2000). K(ATP) channel openers, adenosine agonists and epileptic preconditioning are stress signals inducing hippocampal neuroprotection. *Neuroscience*, *100*, 465–474.

Boghi, A., Sterpone, S., Sales, S., D'Agata, F., Bradac, G. B., Zullo, G., et al. (2011). In vivo evidence of global and focal brain alterations in anorexia nervosa. *Psychiatry Research*, *192*, 154–159.

Bouret, S. G., Draper, S. J., & Simerly, R. B. (2004a). Formation of projection pathways from the arcuate nucleus of the hypothalamus to hypothalamic regions implicated in the neural control of feeding behavior in mice. *The Journal of Neuroscience*, *24*, 2797–2805.

Bouret, S. G., Draper, S. J., & Simerly, R. B. (2004b). Trophic action of leptin on hypothalamic neurons that regulate feeding. *Science*, *304*, 108–110.

Bowker, R. M., Westlund, K. N., & Coulter, J. D. (1981). Origins of serotonergic projections to the spinal cord in rat: An immunocytochemical-retrograde transport study. *Brain Research*, *226*, 187–199.

Broadwell, R. D., & Brightman, M. W. (1976). Entry of peroxidase into neurons of the central and peripheral nervous systems from extracerebral and cerebral blood. *The Journal of Comparative Neurology*, *166*, 257–283.

Broberger, C. (2005). Brain regulation of food intake and appetite: Molecules and networks. *Journal of Internal Medicine*, *258*, 301–327.

Broberger, C., & Hokfelt, T. (2001). Hypothalamic and vagal neuropeptide circuitries regulating food intake. *Physiology & Behavior*, *74*, 669–682.

Broberger, C., Holmberg, K., Kuhar, M. J., & Hokfelt, T. (1999a). Cocaine- and amphetamine-regulated transcript in the rat vagus nerve: A putative mediator of cholecystokinin-induced satiety. *Proceedings of the National Academy of Sciences of the United States of America*, *96*, 13506–13511.

Broberger, C., Johansen, J., Brismar, H., Johansson, C., Schalling, M., & Hokfelt, T. (1999b). Changes in neuropeptide Y receptors and pro-opiomelanocortin in the anorexia (anx/anx) mouse hypothalamus. *The Journal of Neuroscience*, *19*, 7130–7139.

Broberger, C., Johansen, J., Johansson, C., Schalling, M., & Hokfelt, T. (1998). The neuropeptide Y/agouti gene-related protein (AGRP) brain circuitry in normal, anorectic, and monosodium glutamate-treated mice. *Proceedings of the National Academy of Sciences of the United States of America*, *95*, 15043–15048.

Broberger, C., Johansen, J., Schalling, M., & Hokfelt, T. (1997). Hypothalamic neurohistochemistry of the murine anorexia (anx/anx) mutation: Altered processing of neuropeptide Y in the arcuate nucleus. *The Journal of Comparative Neurology*, *387*, 124–135.

Brown, K. M., Bujac, S. R., Mann, E. T., Campbell, D. A., Stubbins, M. J., & Blundell, J. E. (2007). Further evidence of association of OPRD1 & HTR1D polymorphisms with susceptibility to anorexia nervosa. *Biological Psychiatry*, *61*, 367–373.

Bulik, C. M., Sullivan, P. F., Tozzi, F., Furberg, H., Lichtenstein, P., & Pedersen, N. L. (2006). Prevalence, heritability, and prospective risk factors for anorexia nervosa. *Archives of General Psychiatry*, *63*, 305–312.

Calegari, V. C., Torsoni, A. S., Vanzela, E. C., Araujo, E. P., Morari, J., Zoppi, C. C., et al. (2011). Inflammation of the hypothalamus leads to defective pancreatic islet function. *The Journal of Biological Chemistry*, *286*, 12870–12880.

Cameron, D. P., Cutbush, L., & Opat, F. (1978). Effects of monosodium glutamate-induced obesity in mice on carbohydrate metabolism in insulin secretion. *Clinical and Experimental Pharmacology & Physiology*, *5*, 41–51.

Cecconi, F., & Levine, B. (2008). The role of autophagy in mammalian development: Cell makeover rather than cell death. *Developmental Cell*, *15*, 344–357.

Challis, B. G., Coll, A. P., Yeo, G. S., Pinnock, S. B., Dickson, S. L., Thresher, R. R., et al. (2004). Mice lacking pro-opiomelanocortin are sensitive to high-fat feeding but respond normally to the acute anorectic effects of peptide-YY(3–36). *Proceedings of the National Academy of Sciences of the United States of America*, *101*, 4695–4700.

Chen, H., Charlat, O., Tartaglia, L. A., Woolf, E. A., Weng, X., Ellis, S. J., et al. (1996). Evidence that the diabetes gene encodes the leptin receptor: Identification of a mutation in the leptin receptor gene in db/db mice. *Cell*, *84*, 491–495.

Chergui, K., Svenningsson, P., Nomikos, G. G., Gonon, F., Fredholm, B. B., & Svennson, T. H. (1997). Increased expression of NGFI-A mRNA in the rat striatum

following burst stimulation of the medial forebrain bundle. *The European Journal of Neuroscience*, *9*, 2370–2382.
Chol, M., Lebon, S., Benit, P., Chretien, D., de Lonlay, P., Goldenberg, A., et al. (2003). The mitochondrial DNA G13513A MELAS mutation in the NADH dehydrogenase 5 gene is a frequent cause of Leigh-like syndrome with isolated complex I deficiency. *Journal of Medical Genetics*, *40*, 188–191.
Chronwall, B. M. (1985). Anatomy and physiology of the neuroendocrine arcuate nucleus. *Peptides*, *6*(Suppl. 2), 1–11.
Chronwall, B. M., DiMaggio, D. A., Massari, V. J., Pickel, V. M., Ruggiero, D. A., & O'Donohue, T. L. (1985). The anatomy of neuropeptide-Y-containing neurons in rat brain. *Neuroscience*, *15*, 1159–1181.
Chua, S. C., Jr., Chung, W. K., Wu-Peng, X. S., Zhang, Y., Liu, S. M., Tartaglia, L., et al. (1996). Phenotypes of mouse diabetes and rat fatty due to mutations in the OB (leptin) receptor. *Science*, *271*, 994–996.
Coleman, D. L. (1973). Effects of parabiosis of obese with diabetes and normal mice. *Diabetologia*, *9*, 294–298.
Coleman, D. L. (1978). Obese and diabetes: Two mutant genes causing diabetes-obesity syndromes in mice. *Diabetologia*, *14*, 141–148.
Collin, M., Backberg, M., Ovesjo, M. L., Fisone, G., Edwards, R. H., Fujiyama, F., et al. (2003). Plasma membrane and vesicular glutamate transporter mRNAs/proteins in hypothalamic neurons that regulate body weight. *The European Journal of Neuroscience*, *18*, 1265–1278.
Cone, R. D., Cowley, M. A., Butler, A. A., Fan, W., Marks, D. L., & Low, M. J. (2001). The arcuate nucleus as a conduit for diverse signals relevant to energy homeostasis. *International Journal of Obesity and Related Metabolic Disorders*, *25*(Suppl. 5), S63–S67.
Corriveau, R. A., Huh, G. S., & Shatz, C. J. (1998). Regulation of class I MHC gene expression in the developing and mature CNS by neural activity. *Neuron*, *21*, 505–520.
Coupe, B., Ishii, Y., Dietrich, M. O., Komatsu, M., Horvath, T. L., & Bouret, S. G. (2012). Loss of autophagy in pro-opiomelanocortin neurons perturbs axon growth and causes metabolic dysregulation. *Cell Metabolism*, *15*, 247–255.
Coyle, J. T., Bird, S. J., Evans, R. H., Gulley, R. L., Nadler, J. V., Nicklas, W. J., et al. (1981). Excitatory amino acid neurotoxins: Selectivity, specificity, and mechanisms of action. Based on an NRP one-day conference held June 30, 1980. *Neurosciences Research Program Bulletin*, *19*, 1–427.
Dahlstrom, A. (1969). Influence of colchicine axoplasmic transport of amine storage granules in rat sympathetic adrenergic nerves. *Acta Physiologica Scandinavica*, *76*, 33A–34A.
Dahlstrom, A., & Fuxe, K. (1964). Localization of monoamines in the lower brain stem. *Experientia*, *20*, 398–399.
Dawson, T. M., & Dawson, V. L. (2002). Neuroprotective and neurorestorative strategies for Parkinson's disease. *Nature Neuroscience*, *5*(Suppl.), 1058–1061.
de Quidt, M. E., & Emson, P. C. (1986a). Distribution of neuropeptide Y-like immunoreactivity in the rat central nervous system—I. Radioimmunoassay and chromatographic characterisation. *Neuroscience*, *18*, 527–543.
de Quidt, M. E., & Emson, P. C. (1986b). Distribution of neuropeptide Y-like immunoreactivity in the rat central nervous system—II. Immunohistochemical analysis. *Neuroscience*, *18*, 545–618.
De Souza, C. T., Araujo, E. P., Bordin, S., Ashimine, R., Zollner, R. L., Boschero, A. C., et al. (2005). Consumption of a fat-rich diet activates a proinflammatory response and induces insulin resistance in the hypothalamus. *Endocrinology*, *146*, 4192–4199.
Dietrich, M. O., & Horvath, T. L. (2009). Feeding signals and brain circuitry. *The European Journal of Neuroscience*, *30*, 1688–1696.

Distelmaier, F., Visch, H. J., Smeitink, J. A., Mayatepek, E., Koopman, W. J., & Willems, P. H. (2009). The antioxidant Trolox restores mitochondrial membrane potential and Ca2+-stimulated ATP production in human complex I deficiency. *Journal of molecular medicine (Berlin, Germany)*, *87*, 515–522.

Dolan, R. J., Mitchell, J., & Wakeling, A. (1988). Structural brain changes in patients with anorexia nervosa. *Psychological Medicine*, *18*, 349–353.

Douglass, J., McKinzie, A. A., & Couceyro, P. (1995). PCR differential display identifies a rat brain mRNA that is transcriptionally regulated by cocaine and amphetamine. *The Journal of Neuroscience*, *15*, 2471–2481.

Druce, M., & Bloom, S. R. (2003). Central regulators of food intake. *Current Opinion in Clinical Nutrition and Metabolic Care*, *6*, 361–367.

Dumont, M., & Beal, M. F. (2011). Neuroprotective strategies involving ROS in Alzheimer disease. *Free Radical Biology & Medicine*, *51*, 1014–1026.

Dunning, C. J., McKenzie, M., Sugiana, C., Lazarou, M., Silke, J., Connelly, A., et al. (2007). Human CIA30 is involved in the early assembly of mitochondrial complex I and mutations in its gene cause disease. *The EMBO Journal*, *26*, 3227–3237.

Dunn-Meynell, A. A., Rawson, N. E., & Levin, B. E. (1998). Distribution and phenotype of neurons containing the ATP-sensitive K+ channel in rat brain. *Brain Research*, *814*, 41–54.

Durham, W. J., Dillon, E. L., & Sheffield-Moore, M. (2009). Inflammatory burden and amino acid metabolism in cancer cachexia. *Current Opinion in Clinical Nutrition and Metabolic Care*, *12*, 72–77.

Ekstrand, M. I., Terzioglu, M., Galter, D., Zhu, S., Hofstetter, C., Lindqvist, E., et al. (2007). Progressive parkinsonism in mice with respiratory-chain-deficient dopamine neurons. *Proceedings of the National Academy of Sciences of the United States of America*, *104*, 1325–1330.

Elmquist, J. K., Coppari, R., Balthasar, N., Ichinose, M., & Lowell, B. B. (2005). Identifying hypothalamic pathways controlling food intake, body weight, and glucose homeostasis. *The Journal of Comparative Neurology*, *493*, 63–71.

Enzmann, D. R., & Lane, B. (1977). Cranial computed tomography findings in anorexia nervosa. *Journal of Computer Assisted Tomography*, *1*, 410–414.

Everitt, B. J., Meister, B., Hokfelt, T., Melander, T., Terenius, L., Rokaeus, A., et al. (1986). The hypothalamic arcuate nucleus-median eminence complex: Immunohistochemistry of transmitters, peptides and DARPP-32 with special reference to coexistence in dopamine neurons. *Brain Research*, *396*, 97–155.

Fetissov, S. O., Bergstrom, U., Johansen, J. E., Hokfelt, T., Schalling, M., & Ranscht, B. (2005). Alterations of arcuate nucleus neuropeptidergic development in contactin-deficient mice: Comparison with anorexia and food-deprived mice. *The European Journal of Neuroscience*, *22*, 3217–3228.

Finn, J. T., Weil, M., Archer, F., Siman, R., Srinivasan, A., & Raff, M. C. (2000). Evidence that Wallerian degeneration and localized axon degeneration induced by local neurotrophin deprivation do not involve caspases. *The Journal of Neuroscience*, *20*, 1333–1341.

Finsterer, J. (2008). Leigh and Leigh-like syndrome in children and adults. *Pediatric Neurology*, *39*, 223–235.

Frisch, A., Laufer, N., Danziger, Y., Michaelovsky, E., Leor, S., Carel, C., et al. (2001). Association of anorexia nervosa with the high activity allele of the COMT gene: A family-based study in Israeli patients. *Molecular Psychiatry*, *6*, 243–245.

Gabery, S., Murphy, K., Schultz, K., Loy, C. T., McCusker, E., Kirik, D., et al. (2010). Changes in key hypothalamic neuropeptide populations in Huntington disease revealed by neuropathological analyses. *Acta Neuropathologica*, *120*, 777–788.

Gage, F. H. (2002). Neurogenesis in the adult brain. *The Journal of Neuroscience*, *22*, 612–613.

Gavrieli, Y., Sherman, Y., & Ben-Sasson, S. A. (1992). Identification of programmed cell death in situ via specific labeling of nuclear DNA fragmentation. *The Journal of Cell Biology*, *119*, 493–501.

Golden, N. H., Ashtari, M., Kohn, M. R., Patel, M., Jacobson, M. S., Fletcher, A., et al. (1996). Reversibility of cerebral ventricular enlargement in anorexia nervosa, demonstrated by quantitative magnetic resonance imaging. *The Journal of Pediatrics*, *128*, 296–301.

Gould, E., & McEwen, B. S. (1993). Neuronal birth and death. *Current Opinion in Neurobiology*, *3*, 676–682.

Grill, H. J., & Kaplan, J. M. (2002). The neuroanatomical axis for control of energy balance. *Frontiers in Neuroendocrinology*, *23*, 2–40.

Gropp, E., Shanabrough, M., Borok, E., Xu, A. W., Janoschek, R., Buch, T., et al. (2005). Agouti-related peptide-expressing neurons are mandatory for feeding. *Nature Neuroscience*, *8*, 1289–1291.

Hahn, T. M., Breininger, J. F., Baskin, D. G., & Schwartz, M. W. (1998). Coexpression of Agrp and NPY in fasting-activated hypothalamic neurons. *Nature Neuroscience*, *1*, 271–272.

Hillebrand, J. J., de Wied, D., & Adan, R. A. (2002). Neuropeptides, food intake and body weight regulation: A hypothalamic focus. *Peptides*, *23*, 2283–2306.

Hoffman, G. W., Jr., Ellinwood, E. H., Jr., Rockwell, W. J., Herfkens, R. J., Nishita, J. K., & Guthrie, L. F. (1989). Cerebral atrophy in anorexia nervosa: A pilot study. *Biological Psychiatry*, *26*, 321–324.

Horvath, T. L., Naftolin, F., & Leranth, C. (1992). GABAergic and catecholaminergic innervation of mediobasal hypothalamic beta-endorphin cells projecting to the medial preoptic area. *Neuroscience*, *51*, 391–399.

Hult, S., Schultz, K., Soylu, R., & Petersen, A. (2010). Hypothalamic and neuroendocrine changes in Huntington's disease. *Current Drug Targets*, *11*, 1237–1249.

Hummel, K. P., Dickie, M. M., & Coleman, D. L. (1966). Diabetes, a new mutation in the mouse. *Science*, *153*, 1127–1128.

Huszar, D., Lynch, C. A., Fairchild-Huntress, V., Dunmore, J. H., Fang, Q., Berkemeier, L. R., et al. (1997). Targeted disruption of the melanocortin-4 receptor results in obesity in mice. *Cell*, *88*, 131–141.

Ibrahim, N., Bosch, M. A., Smart, J. L., Qiu, J., Rubinstein, M., Ronnekleiv, O. K., et al. (2003). Hypothalamic proopiomelanocortin neurons are glucose responsive and express K(ATP) channels. *Endocrinology*, *144*, 1331–1340.

Inui, A. (2002). Cancer anorexia-cachexia syndrome: Current issues in research and management. *CA: A Cancer Journal for Clinicians*, *52*, 72–91.

Jacobs, B. L., Martin-Cora, F. J., & Fornal, C. A. (2002). Activity of medullary serotonergic neurons in freely moving animals. *Brain Research. Brain Research Reviews*, *40*, 45–52.

Jacobs, B. L., van Praag, H., & Gage, F. H. (2000). Adult brain neurogenesis and psychiatry: A novel theory of depression. *Molecular Psychiatry*, *5*, 262–269.

Jahng, J. W., Houpt, T. A., Kim, S. J., Joh, T. H., & Son, J. H. (1998). Neuropeptide Y mRNA and serotonin innervation in the arcuate nucleus of anorexia mutant mice. *Brain Research*, *790*, 67–73.

Johansen, J. E., Broberger, C., Lavebratt, C., Johansson, C., Kuhar, M. J., Hokfelt, T., et al. (2000). Hypothalamic CART and serum leptin levels are reduced in the anorectic (anx/anx) mouse. *Brain Research. Molecular Brain Research*, *84*, 97–105.

Johansen, J. E., Teixeira, V. L., Johansson, C., Serrao, P., Berggren, P. O., Soares-Da-Silva, P., et al. (2001). Altered dopaminergic transmission in the anorexic anx/anx mouse striatum. *Neuroreport*, *12*, 2737–2741.

Kalra, S. P., Dube, M. G., Pu, S., Xu, B., Horvath, T. L., & Kalra, P. S. (1999). Interacting appetite-regulating pathways in the hypothalamic regulation of body weight. *Endocrine Reviews*, *20*, 68–100.

Kalra, S. P., & Kalra, P. S. (2003). Neuropeptide Y: A physiological orexigen modulated by the feedback action of ghrelin and leptin. *Endocrine*, *22*, 49–56.

Kalra, S. P., & Kalra, P. S. (2004). Overlapping and interactive pathways regulating appetite and craving. *Journal of Addictive Diseases*, *23*, 5–21.

Karlsson, J. O., & Sjostrand, J. (1970). Transport of neurotubular protein and the effect of colchicine on axonal transport. *Acta Physiologica Scandinavica. Supplementum*, *357*, 11–12.

Kasese-Hara, M., Wright, C., & Drewett, R. (2002). Energy compensation in young children who fail to thrive. *Journal of Child Psychology and Psychiatry*, *43*, 449–456.

Katzman, D. K., Lambe, E. K., Mikulis, D. J., Ridgley, J. N., Goldbloom, D. S., & Zipursky, R. B. (1996). Cerebral gray matter and white matter volume deficits in adolescent girls with anorexia nervosa. *The Journal of Pediatrics*, *129*, 794–803.

Kaushik, S., Rodriguez-Navarro, J. A., Arias, E., Kiffin, R., Sahu, S., Schwartz, G. J., et al. (2012). Autophagy in hypothalamic AgRP neurons regulates food intake and energy balance. *Cell Metabolism*, *14*, 173–183.

Kaye, W. (2008). Neurobiology of anorexia and bulimia nervosa. *Physiology & Behavior*, *94*, 121–135.

Kaye, W. H., Frank, G. K., & McConaha, C. (1999). Altered dopamine activity after recovery from restricting-type anorexia nervosa. *Neuropsychopharmacology*, *21*, 503–506.

Kim, M. J., Kim, Y., Kim, S. A., Lee, H. J., Choe, B. K., Nam, M., et al. (2001). Increases in cell proliferation and apoptosis in dentate gyrus of anorexia (anx/anx) mice. *Neuroscience Letters*, *302*, 109–112.

Kleyn, P. W., Fan, W., Kovats, S. G., Lee, J. J., Pulido, J. C., Wu, Y., et al. (1996). Identification and characterization of the mouse obesity gene tubby: A member of a novel gene family. *Cell*, *85*, 281–290.

Knobloch, M., & Mansuy, I. M. (2008). Dendritic spine loss and synaptic alterations in Alzheimer's disease. *Molecular Neurobiology*, *37*, 73–82.

Kokoeva, M. V., Yin, H., & Flier, J. S. (2005). Neurogenesis in the hypothalamus of adult mice: Potential role in energy balance. *Science*, *310*, 679–683.

Kopp, J., Xu, Z. Q., Zhang, X., Pedrazzini, T., Herzog, H., Kresse, A., et al. (2002). Expression of the neuropeptide Y Y1 receptor in the CNS of rat and of wild-type and Y1 receptor knock-out mice. Focus on immunohistochemical localization. *Neuroscience*, *111*, 443–532.

Kremer, H. P., Roos, R. A., Dingjan, G. M., Bots, G. T., Bruyn, G. W., & Hofman, M. A. (1991). The hypothalamic lateral tuberal nucleus and the characteristics of neuronal loss in Huntington's disease. *Neuroscience Letters*, *132*, 101–104.

Kremer, H. P., Roos, R. A., Dingjan, G., Marani, E., & Bots, G. T. (1990). Atrophy of the hypothalamic lateral tuberal nucleus in Huntington's disease. *Journal of Neuropathology and Experimental Neurology*, *49*, 371–382.

Kreutzberg, G. W. (1969). Neuronal dynamics and axonal flow. IV. Blockage of intra-axonal enzyme transport by colchicine. *Proceedings of the National Academy of Sciences of the United States of America*, *62*, 722–728.

Krisch, B., & Leonhardt, H. (1978). The functional and structural border of the neurohemal region of the median eminence. *Cell and Tissue Research*, *192*, 327–339.

Kruse, S. E., Watt, W. C., Marcinek, D. J., Kapur, R. P., Schenkman, K. A., & Palmiter, R. D. (2008). Mice with mitochondrial complex I deficiency develop a fatal encephalomyopathy. *Cell Metabolism*, 7, 312–320.

Kuida, K., Zheng, T. S., Na, S., Kuan, C., Yang, D., Karasuyama, H., et al. (1996). Decreased apoptosis in the brain and premature lethality in CPP32-deficient mice. *Nature*, *384*, 368–372.

Lachuer, J., Ouyang, L., Legras, C., Del Rio, J., & Barlow, C. (2005). Gene expression profiling reveals an inflammatory process in the anx/anx mutant mice. *Brain Research. Molecular Brain Research*, *139*, 372–376.

Lawrence, C. B., Turnbull, A. V., & Rothwell, N. J. (1999). Hypothalamic control of feeding. *Current Opinion in Neurobiology, 9*, 778–783.

Lazarou, M., Thorburn, D. R., Ryan, M. T., & McKenzie, M. (2009). Assembly of mitochondrial complex I and defects in disease. *Biochimica et Biophysica Acta, 1793*, 78–88.

Lee, G. H., Proenca, R., Montez, J. M., Carroll, K. M., Darvishzadeh, J. G., Lee, J. I., et al. (1996). Abnormal splicing of the leptin receptor in diabetic mice. *Nature, 379*, 632–635.

Leonard, J. V., & Schapira, A. H. (2000a). Mitochondrial respiratory chain disorders I: Mitochondrial DNA defects. *Lancet, 355*, 299–304.

Leonard, J. V., & Schapira, A. H. (2000b). Mitochondrial respiratory chain disorders II: Neurodegenerative disorders and nuclear gene defects. *Lancet, 355*, 389–394.

Lin, M. T., & Beal, M. F. (2006). Mitochondrial dysfunction and oxidative stress in neurodegenerative diseases. *Nature, 443*, 787–795.

Lindfors, C., Nilsson, I. A., Garcia-Roves, P. M., Zuberi, A. R., Karimi, M., Donahue, L. R., et al. (2011). Hypothalamic mitochondrial dysfunction associated with anorexia in the anx/anx mouse. *Proceedings of the National Academy of Sciences of the United States of America, 108*, 18108–18113.

Liss, B., Bruns, R., & Roeper, J. (1999). Alternative sulfonylurea receptor expression defines metabolic sensitivity of K-ATP channels in dopaminergic midbrain neurons. *The EMBO Journal, 18*, 833–846.

Lu, D., Willard, D., Patel, I. R., Kadwell, S., Overton, L., Kost, T., et al. (1994). Agouti protein is an antagonist of the melanocyte-stimulating-hormone receptor. *Nature, 371*, 799–802.

Luquet, S., Perez, F. A., Hnasko, T. S., & Palmiter, R. D. (2005). NPY/AgRP neurons are essential for feeding in adult mice but can be ablated in neonates. *Science, 310*, 683–685.

Mains, R. E., Eipper, B. A., & Ling, N. (1977). Common precursor to corticotropins and endorphins. *Proceedings of the National Academy of Sciences of the United States of America, 74*, 3014–3018.

Maltais, L. J., Lane, P. W., & Beamer, W. G. (1984). Anorexia, a recessive mutation causing starvation in preweanling mice. *The Journal of Heredity, 75*, 468–472.

Mattson, M. P., & Liu, D. (2002). Energetics and oxidative stress in synaptic plasticity and neurodegenerative disorders. *Neuromolecular Medicine, 2*, 215–231.

McNay, D. E., Briancon, N., Kokoeva, M. V., Maratos-Flier, E., & Flier, J. S. (2012). Remodeling of the arcuate nucleus energy-balance circuit is inhibited in obese mice. *The Journal of Clinical Investigation, 122*, 142–152.

Meguid, M. M., Fetissov, S. O., Varma, M., Sato, T., Zhang, L., Laviano, A., et al. (2000). Hypothalamic dopamine and serotonin in the regulation of food intake. *Nutrition, 16*, 843–857.

Meister, B. (2000). Control of food intake via leptin receptors in the hypothalamus. *Vitamins and Hormones, 59*, 265–304.

Meister, B. (2007). Neurotransmitters in key neurons of the hypothalamus that regulate feeding behavior and body weight. *Physiology & Behavior, 92*, 263–271.

Meister, B., Ceccatelli, S., Hokfelt, T., Anden, N. E., Anden, M., & Theodorsson, E. (1989). Neurotransmitters, neuropeptides and binding sites in the rat mediobasal hypothalamus: Effects of monosodium glutamate (MSG) lesions. *Experimental Brain Research, 76*, 343–368.

Mercader, J. M., Lozano, J. J., Sumoy, L., Dierssen, M., Visa, J., Gratacos, M., et al. (2008). Hypothalamus transcriptome profile suggests an anorexia-cachexia syndrome in the anx/anx mouse model. *Physiological Genomics, 35*, 341–350.

Mercader, J. M., Saus, E., Aguera, Z., Bayes, M., Boni, C., Carreras, A., et al. (2008). Association of NTRK3 and its interaction with NGF suggest an altered cross-regulation of the neurotrophin signaling pathway in eating disorders. *Human Molecular Genetics, 17*, 1234–1244.

Migaud, M., Batailler, M., Segura, S., Duittoz, A., Franceschini, I., & Pillon, D. (2010). Emerging new sites for adult neurogenesis in the mammalian brain: A comparative study between the hypothalamus and the classical neurogenic zones. *The European Journal of Neuroscience, 32*, 2042–2052.

Milanski, M., Degasperi, G., Coope, A., Morari, J., Denis, R., Cintra, D. E., et al. (2009). Saturated fatty acids produce an inflammatory response predominantly through the activation of TLR4 signaling in hypothalamus: Implications for the pathogenesis of obesity. *The Journal of Neuroscience, 29*, 359–370.

Miwa, H., Nakanishi, I., Kodama, R., & Kondo, T. (2004). Cerebellar atrophy in a patient with anorexia nervosa. *The International Journal of Eating Disorders, 36*, 238–241.

Moffett, C. W., & Paden, C. M. (1994). Microglia in the rat neurohypophysis increase expression of class I major histocompatibility antigens following central nervous system injury. *Journal of Neuroimmunology, 50*, 139–151.

Moraes, J. C., Coope, A., Morari, J., Cintra, D. E., Roman, E. A., Pauli, J. R., et al. (2009). High-fat diet induces apoptosis of hypothalamic neurons. *PloS One, 4*, e5045.

Morais, V. A., & De Strooper, B. (2010). Mitochondria dysfunction and neurodegenerative disorders: Cause or consequence. *Journal of Alzheimer's Disease, 20*(Suppl. 2), S255–S263.

Morton, G. J., & Schwartz, M. W. (2011). Leptin and the central nervous system control of glucose metabolism. *Physiological Reviews, 91*, 389–411.

Naggert, J. K., Fricker, L. D., Varlamov, O., Nishina, P. M., Rouille, Y., Steiner, D. F., et al. (1995). Hyperproinsulinaemia in obese fat/fat mice associated with a carboxypeptidase E mutation which reduces enzyme activity. *Nature Genetics, 10*, 135–142.

Neumann, H. (2001). Control of glial immune function by neurons. *Glia, 36*, 191–199.

Neumann, H., Cavalie, A., Jenne, D. E., & Wekerle, H. (1995). Induction of MHC class I genes in neurons. *Science, 269*, 549–552.

Neumann, H., Schmidt, H., Cavalie, A., Jenne, D., & Wekerle, H. (1997). Major histocompatibility complex (MHC) class I gene expression in single neurons of the central nervous system: Differential regulation by interferon (IFN)-gamma and tumor necrosis factor (TNF)-alpha. *The Journal of Experimental Medicine, 185*, 305–316.

Nikolaev, A., McLaughlin, T., O'Leary, D. D., & Tessier-Lavigne, M. (2009). APP binds DR6 to trigger axon pruning and neuron death via distinct caspases. *Nature, 457*, 981–989.

Nilsson, I., Johansen, J. E., Schalling, M., Hokfelt, T., & Fetissov, S. O. (2005). Maturation of the hypothalamic arcuate agouti-related protein system during postnatal development in the mouse. *Brain Research. Developmental Brain Research, 155*, 147–154.

Nilsson, I., Lindfors, C., Fetissov, S. O., Hokfelt, T., & Johansen, J. E. (2008). Aberrant agouti-related protein system in the hypothalamus of the anx/anx mouse is associated with activation of microglia. *The Journal of Comparative Neurology, 507*, 1128–1140.

Nilsson, I. A., Thams, S., Lindfors, C., Bergstrand, A., Cullheim, S., Hokfelt, T., et al. (2011). Evidence of hypothalamic degeneration in the anorectic anx/anx mouse. *Glia, 59*, 45–57.

Ogilvie, I., Kennaway, N. G., & Shoubridge, E. A. (2005). A molecular chaperone for mitochondrial complex I assembly is mutated in a progressive encephalopathy. *The Journal of Clinical Investigation, 115*, 2784–2792.

Oliveira, A. L., Thams, S., Lidman, O., Piehl, F., Hokfelt, T., Karre, K., et al. (2004). A role for MHC class I molecules in synaptic plasticity and regeneration of neurons after axotomy. *Proceedings of the National Academy of Sciences of the United States of America, 101*, 17843–17848.

Orimo, S., Uchihara, T., Nakamura, A., Mori, F., Ikeuchi, T., Onodera, O., et al. (2008). Cardiac sympathetic denervation in Parkinson's disease linked to SNCA duplication. *Acta Neuropathologica, 116*, 575–577.

Ott, M., Gogvadze, V., Orrenius, S., & Zhivotovsky, B. (2007). Mitochondria, oxidative stress and cell death. *Apoptosis, 12*, 913–922.

Pierce, A. A., & Xu, A. W. (2010). De novo neurogenesis in adult hypothalamus as a compensatory mechanism to regulate energy balance. *The Journal of Neuroscience*, *30*, 723–730.

Pinto, S., Roseberry, A. G., Liu, H., Diano, S., Shanabrough, M., Cai, X., et al. (2004). Rapid rewiring of arcuate nucleus feeding circuits by leptin. *Science*, *304*, 110–115.

Porte, D., Jr., Baskin, D. G., & Schwartz, M. W. (2002). Leptin and insulin action in the central nervous system. *Nutrition Reviews*, *60*, S20–S29 discussion S68–S84, S85–S87.

Quintana, A., Kruse, S. E., Kapur, R. P., Sanz, E., & Palmiter, R. D. (2010). Complex I deficiency due to loss of Ndufs4 in the brain results in progressive encephalopathy resembling Leigh syndrome. *Proceedings of the National Academy of Sciences of the United States of America*, *107*, 10996–11001.

Raff, M. C., Whitmore, A. V., & Finn, J. T. (2002). Axonal self-destruction and neurodegeneration. *Science*, *296*, 868–871.

Ramos, E. J., Suzuki, S., Marks, D., Inui, A., Asakawa, A., & Meguid, M. M. (2004). Cancer anorexia-cachexia syndrome: Cytokines and neuropeptides. *Current Opinion in Clinical Nutrition and Metabolic Care*, *7*, 427–434.

Rask-Andersen, M., Olszewski, P. K., Levine, A. S., & Schioth, H. B. (2010). Molecular mechanisms underlying anorexia nervosa: Focus on human gene association studies and systems controlling food intake. *Brain Research Reviews*, *62*, 147–164.

Ribak, C. E., Shapiro, L. A., Perez, Z. D., & Spigelman, I. (2009). Microglia-associated granule cell death in the normal adult dentate gyrus. *Brain Structure & Function*, *214*, 25–35.

Ribases, M., Gratacos, M., Armengol, L., de Cid, R., Badia, A., Jimenez, L., et al. (2003). Met66 in the brain-derived neurotrophic factor (BDNF) precursor is associated with anorexia nervosa restrictive type. *Molecular Psychiatry*, *8*, 745–751.

Ribases, M., Gratacos, M., Fernandez-Aranda, F., Bellodi, L., Boni, C., Anderluh, M., et al. (2004). Association of BDNF with anorexia, bulimia and age of onset of weight loss in six European populations. *Human Molecular Genetics*, *13*, 1205–1212.

Roberts, J. L., & Herbert, E. (1977). Characterization of a common precursor to corticotropin and beta-lipotropin: Identification of beta-lipotropin peptides and their arrangement relative to corticotropin in the precursor synthesized in a cell-free system. *Proceedings of the National Academy of Sciences of the United States of America*, *74*, 5300–5304.

Ross, C. A., & Tabrizi, S. J. (2011). Huntington's disease: From molecular pathogenesis to clinical treatment. *Lancet Neurology*, *10*, 83–98.

Ryu, K. Y., Garza, J. C., Lu, X. Y., Barsh, G. S., & Kopito, R. R. (2008). Hypothalamic neurodegeneration and adult-onset obesity in mice lacking the Ubb polyubiquitin gene. *Proceedings of the National Academy of Sciences of the United States of America*, *105*, 4016–4021.

Sanberg, P. R., Fibiger, H. C., & Mark, R. F. (1981). Body weight and dietary factors in Huntington's disease patients compared with matched controls. *The Medical Journal of Australia*, *1*, 407–409.

Saper, C. B., Chou, T. C., & Elmquist, J. K. (2002). The need to feed: Homeostatic and hedonic control of eating. *Neuron*, *36*, 199–211.

Sawchenko, P. E. (1998). Toward a new neurobiology of energy balance, appetite, and obesity: The anatomists weigh in. *The Journal of Comparative Neurology*, *402*, 435–441.

Schapira, A. H. (2006). Etiology of Parkinson's disease. *Neurology*, *66*, S10–S23.

Schwartz, M. W. (2001). Brain pathways controlling food intake and body weight. *Experimental Biology and Medicine (Maywood, N.J.)*, *226*, 978–981.

Schwartz, M. W., Woods, S. C., Porte, D., Jr., Seeley, R. J., & Baskin, D. G. (2000). Central nervous system control of food intake. *Nature*, *404*, 661–671.

Shaoul, R., Kessel, A., Toubi, E., Lanir, A., Glazer, O., & Jaffe, M. (2003). Leptin and cytokines levels in children with failure to thrive. *Journal of Pediatric Gastroenterology and Nutrition*, *37*, 487–491.

Shutter, J. R., Graham, M., Kinsey, A. C., Scully, S., Luthy, R., & Stark, K. L. (1997). Hypothalamic expression of ART, a novel gene related to agouti, is up-regulated in obese and diabetic mutant mice. *Genes & Development, 11*, 593–602.

Skagerberg, G., & Bjorklund, A. (1985). Topographic principles in the spinal projections of serotonergic and non-serotonergic brainstem neurons in the rat. *Neuroscience, 15*, 445–480.

Smeitink, J., van den Heuvel, L., & DiMauro, S. (2001). The genetics and pathology of oxidative phosphorylation. *Nature Reviews. Genetics, 2*, 342–352.

Smith, R., Brundin, P., & Li, J. Y. (2005). Synaptic dysfunction in Huntington's disease: A new perspective. *Cellular and Molecular Life Sciences, 62*, 1901–1912.

Son, J. H., Baker, H., Park, D. H., & Joh, T. H. (1994). Drastic and selective hyperinnervation of central serotonergic neurons in a lethal neurodevelopmental mouse mutant, Anorexia (anx). *Brain Research. Molecular Brain Research, 25*, 129–134.

Streit, W. J. (2002). Microglia as neuroprotective, immunocompetent cells of the CNS. *Glia, 40*, 133–139.

Streit, W. J., Graeber, M. B., & Kreutzberg, G. W. (1988). Functional plasticity of microglia: A review. *Glia, 1*, 301–307.

Striegel-Moore, R. H., & Bulik, C. M. (2007). Risk factors for eating disorders. *The American Psychologist, 62*, 181–198.

Sun, A. Y., & Chen, Y. M. (1998). Oxidative stress and neurodegenerative disorders. *Journal of Biomedical Science, 5*, 401–414.

Susaki, E., & Nakayama, K. I. (2010). An animal model manifesting neurodegeneration and obesity. *Aging (Albany NY), 2*, 453–456.

Tan, B. H., & Fearon, K. C. (2008). Cachexia: Prevalence and impact in medicine. *Current Opinion in Clinical Nutrition and Metabolic Care, 11*, 400–407.

Tatemoto, K. (1982). Neuropeptide Y: Complete amino acid sequence of the brain peptide. *Proceedings of the National Academy of Sciences of the United States of America, 79*, 5485–5489.

Tatemoto, K., Carlquist, M., & Mutt, V. (1982). Neuropeptide Y—A novel brain peptide with structural similarities to peptide YY and pancreatic polypeptide. *Nature, 296*, 659–660.

Thaler, J. P., Choi, S. J., Schwartz, M. W., & Wisse, B. E. (2010). Hypothalamic inflammation and energy homeostasis: Resolving the paradox. *Frontiers in Neuroendocrinology, 31*, 79–84.

Thaler, J. P., Yi, C. X., Schur, E. A., Guyenet, S. J., Hwang, B. H., Dietrich, M. O., et al. (2012). Obesity is associated with hypothalamic injury in rodents and humans. *The Journal of Clinical Investigation, 122*, 153–162.

Thams, S., Oliveira, A., & Cullheim, S. (2008). MHC class I expression and synaptic plasticity after nerve lesion. *Brain Research Reviews, 57*, 265–269.

Thomzig, A., Laube, G., Pruss, H., & Veh, R. W. (2005). Pore-forming subunits of K-ATP channels, Kir6.1 and Kir6.2, display prominent differences in regional and cellular distribution in the rat brain. *The Journal of Comparative Neurology, 484*, 313–330.

Ugalde, C., Janssen, R. J., van den Heuvel, L. P., Smeitink, J. A., & Nijtmans, L. G. (2004). Differences in assembly or stability of complex I and other mitochondrial OXPHOS complexes in inherited complex I deficiency. *Human Molecular Genetics, 13*, 659–667.

Ugalde, C., Vogel, R., Huijbens, R., Van Den Heuvel, B., Smeitink, J., & Nijtmans, L. (2004). Human mitochondrial complex I assembles through the combination of evolutionary conserved modules: A framework to interpret complex I deficiencies. *Human Molecular Genetics, 13*, 2461–2472.

van den Pol, A. N. (2003). Weighing the role of hypothalamic feeding neurotransmitters. *Neuron, 40*, 1059–1061.

van den Top, M., & Spanswick, D. (2006). Integration of metabolic stimuli in the hypothalamic arcuate nucleus. *Progress in Brain Research, 153*, 141–154.

van der Burg, J. M., Bacos, K., Wood, N. I., Lindqvist, A., Wierup, N., Woodman, B., et al. (2008). Increased metabolism in the R6/2 mouse model of Huntington's disease. *Neurobiology of Disease, 29*, 41–51.

Vogel, R. O., Janssen, R. J., Ugalde, C., Grovenstein, M., Huijbens, R. J., Visch, H. J., et al. (2005). Human mitochondrial complex I assembly is mediated by NDUFAF1. *The FEBS Journal, 272*, 5317–5326.

Waldbillig, R. J., Bartness, T. J., & Stanley, B. G. (1981). Increased food intake, body weight, and adiposity in rats after regional neurochemical depletion of serotonin. *Journal of Comparative and Physiological Psychology, 95*, 391–405.

Walker, F. O. (2007). Huntington's disease. *Lancet, 369*, 218–228.

Wang, K., Zhang, H., Bloss, C. S., Duvvuri, V., Kaye, W., Schork, N. J., et al. (2011). A genome-wide association study on common SNPs and rare CNVs in anorexia nervosa. *Molecular Psychiatry, 16*, 949–959.

Wekerle, H. (2005). Planting and pruning in the brain: MHC antigens involved in synaptic plasticity? *Proceedings of the National Academy of Sciences of the United States of America, 102*, 3–4.

Woods, S. C., Schwartz, M. W., Baskin, D. G., & Seeley, R. J. (2000). Food intake and the regulation of body weight. *Annual Review of Psychology, 51*, 255–277.

Wu, Q., Boyle, M. P., & Palmiter, R. D. (2009). Loss of GABAergic signaling by AgRP neurons to the parabrachial nucleus leads to starvation. *Cell, 137*, 1225–1234.

Wu, Q., Clark, M. S., & Palmiter, R. D. (2012). Deciphering a neuronal circuit that mediates appetite. *Nature, 483*, 594–597.

Wu, Q., Howell, M. P., Cowley, M. A., & Palmiter, R. D. (2008). Starvation after AgRP neuron ablation is independent of melanocortin signaling. *Proceedings of the National Academy of Sciences of the United States of America, 105*, 2687–2692.

Wu, Q., Howell, M. P., & Palmiter, R. D. (2008). Ablation of neurons expressing agouti-related protein activates fos and gliosis in postsynaptic target regions. *The Journal of Neuroscience, 28*, 9218–9226.

Wu, Q., & Palmiter, R. D. (2011). GABAergic signaling by AgRP neurons prevents anorexia via a melanocortin-independent mechanism. *European Journal of Pharmacology, 660*, 21–27.

Xu, A. W., Kaelin, C. B., Morton, G. J., Ogimoto, K., Stanhope, K., Graham, J., et al. (2005). Effects of hypothalamic neurodegeneration on energy balance. *PLoS Biology, 3*, e415.

Zhang, X., Bao, L., Xu, Z. Q., Kopp, J., Arvidsson, U., Elde, R., et al. (1994). Localization of neuropeptide Y Y1 receptors in the rat nervous system with special reference to somatic receptors on small dorsal root ganglion neurons. *Proceedings of the National Academy of Sciences of the United States of America, 91*, 11738–11742.

Zhang, Y., Proenca, R., Maffei, M., Barone, M., Leopold, L., & Friedman, J. M. (1994). Positional cloning of the mouse obese gene and its human homologue. *Nature, 372*, 425–432.

CHAPTER THREE

The Role of Ghrelin in Anorexia–Cachexia Syndromes

Bobby Guillory[*,1], **Andres Splenser**[*,1], **Jose Garcia**[*,†,2]
[*]Division of Diabetes, Endocrinology and Metabolism, Michael E DeBakey Veterans Affairs Medical Center, Baylor College of Medicine, Houston, Texas, USA
[†]Department of Molecular and Cell Biology, Huffington Center on Aging, Baylor College of Medicine, Houston, Texas, USA
[1]These authors contributed equally to this chapter
[2]Corresponding author: e-mail address: jgarcia1@bcm.edu

Contents

1. Introduction 62
2. Discovery of Ghrelin 63
3. Ghrelin, GHS-R1a, and GOAT 64
4. Mechanisms of Action of Ghrelin 66
   4.1 Ghrelin, muscle, and the GH-IGF-1 axis 66
   4.2 Ghrelin and appetite regulation 69
   4.3 Ghrelin and lipid metabolism 69
   4.4 Ghrelin and inflammation 71
5. Ghrelin and Sarcopenia of Aging 72
6. Ghrelin and Cancer Cachexia 73
   6.1 Safety of ghrelin and GHS in the setting of cancer 82
7. Ghrelin and COPD-Induced Cachexia 83
8. Ghrelin and Anorexia Nervosa 85
9. Ghrelin and CHF-Induced Cachexia 87
10. Ghrelin and ESRD 89
11. AIDS-Associated Cachexia 90
12. RA-Associated Cachexia 91
13. Conclusions 93
Acknowledgments 93
References 93

Abstract

Anorexia, sarcopenia, and cachexia are common complications of many chronic conditions including cancer, rheumatoid arthritis, HIV infection, aging, and chronic lung, heart, or kidney disease. Currently, there is no effective treatment for muscle atrophy or wasting conditions although they typically take a significant toll on the quality of life of patients and are associated with poor prognosis and decreased survival. Ghrelin affects multiple key pathways in the regulation of body weight, body composition, and appetite in the

Vitamins and Hormones, Volume 92 2013 Published by Elsevier Inc.
ISSN 0083-6729
http://dx.doi.org/10.1016/B978-0-12-410473-0.00003-9

setting of cachexia that may lead to an increase in appetite and growth hormone secretion and a reduction in energy expenditure and inflammation. The net effect is increased lean body mass and fat mass preservation. In this chapter, we review the mechanisms of action of ghrelin and present the available data in animal models and human trials using ghrelin or ghrelin mimetics in different settings of cachexia.

1. INTRODUCTION

Cachexia has been defined as weight loss >5% over a 6-month period in the absence of simple starvation, a BMI <20 and weight loss >2%, or as severe body weight, fat and muscle loss, and increased protein catabolism due to underlying diseases (Muscaritoli et al., 2010). Anorexia, defined as a decrease in appetite and food intake, and cachexia are frequently seen in the setting of cancer, acquired immune deficiency syndrome (AIDS), chronic obstructive pulmonary disease (COPD), congestive heart failure (CHF), rheumatoid arthritis (RA), and end-stage renal disease (ESRD), and are associated with decreased quality of life and increased morbidity and mortality (Ashby, Choi, & Bloom, 2008; Ashitani, Matsumoto, & Nakazato, 2009; Tisdale, 2002; von Haehling, Lainscak, Springer, & Anker, 2009). Sarcopenia, the functional impairment of muscle loss associated with aging (Ruegg & Glass, 2011), is also associated with poor prognosis and decreased functional performance. Despite the significant burden that these symptoms represent to patients, no effective therapies are currently available and these symptoms often remain underdiagnosed and untreated. Moreover, off-label treatments used such as appetite stimulants are largely ineffective and are associated with potentially serious side effects (i.e., adrenal insufficiency, hypogonadism, deep venous thrombosis, etc.).

Since its discovery in 1999, ghrelin has been postulated as a treatment of many catabolic conditions. Ghrelin is the endogenous ligand for the growth hormone secretagogue receptor (AKA ghrelin receptor, GHS-R1a; Kojima et al., 1999; Smith et al., 1997). Others and we have shown that activation of the GHS-R1a or ghrelin receptor by ghrelin or ghrelin mimetics (growth hormone secretagogues, GHS) induces GH secretion (Takaya et al., 2000) and increases food intake and body weight in humans (Garcia & Polvino, 2007; Wren et al., 2001a). In animal models of cachexia, ghrelin also reduces fat oxidation and increases adiposity (Tschop, Smiley, & Heiman, 2000). Ghrelin administration decreases energy expenditure in noncancer human and animal models (Vestergaard et al., 2008). Moreover, ghrelin mimetics increase body weight and reverse the negative nitrogen balance induced by starvation independently of their orexigenic effects. These findings suggest that ghrelin's effects are not entirely mediated through an increase in appetite and that other mechanisms, such as a decrease in energy expenditure, are involved (Murphy et al., 1998). The purpose of this chapter is to review the mechanisms of action, potential therapeutic role of ghrelin in the setting of anorexia, cachexia, and sarcopenia, and present the murine and human studies where ghrelin has been used in these conditions.

2. DISCOVERY OF GHRELIN

Preceding the discovery of ghrelin, Cyril Bowers et al. discovered small synthetic molecules which exhibited potent GH-releasing activity in cultured pituitary cells and that could be administered orally, later referred to as GHS (Bowers, Momany, Reynolds, & Hong, 1984; Bowers et al., 1981; Smith et al., 1997). GHS acts at the hypothalamic and pituitary level causing GH secretion (Korbonits & Grossman, 1995). GHS is derived from the met-enkephalin molecule which is an opioid-like peptide that lacks opioid activity and is believed to play a major role in locomotor behavior (Babbini & Davis, 1972; Camanni, Ghigo, & Arvat, 1998). Early *in vitro* data demonstrated that molecules such as the GHS GH-releasing peptide (GHRP)-6 modulate the release of GH by binding to a specific GTP-linked receptor. This receptor, located in the plasma membrane of cells that release GH in the anterior pituitary gland, was first identified by Smith et al. and it was named GHS-R1a (Smith, Feighner, Prendergast, Guan, & Howard, 1999). GHS-R1a, an orphan receptor at the time of its discovery, is the receptor for ghrelin and it is widely expressed in various tissues: hypothalamic–pituitary, cardiovascular, immune, gastrointestinal, and reproductive systems (Cruz & Smith, 2008; Kojima et al., 1999). Eventually, Kojima et al. identified the acylated peptide ghrelin as the endogenous ligand for the GHS-R1a (Bowers, 2001; Horvath, Diano, Sotonyi, Heiman, & Tschop, 2001; Kojima et al., 1999). "Ghre" means to "grow" in Proto-Indo-European languages and with the addition of "lin" the word "ghrelin" was derived. Currently, there are two major bioactivities attributed to the actions of ghrelin: stimulation of growth hormone secretion and regulation of energy balance (Bowen, Noakes, & Clifton, 2007). Ghrelin also stimulates gut motility, regulates insulin levels, and promotes carbohydrate utilization, adiposity, and food intake (Cummings & Overduin, 2007; Inui, 2001; Kojima & Kangawa, 2005; Kojima et al., 1999). Ghrelin has also been implicated in regulating heart and gonadal function

(Lee, Wang, Englander, Kojima, & Greeley, 2002; Tena-Sempere et al., 2002; Wang, Lee, Englander, & Greeley, 2002). Higher expression of total ghrelin is observed in patients with Prader–Willi syndrome, a genetic disorder characterized by mental retardation and hyperphagia leading to severe obesity (Cummings et al., 2002). Circulating levels of total ghrelin are also higher in cases of anorexia and cachexia and are decreased in obese individuals (Muccioli et al., 2002; Tschop, Weyer et al., 2001). Furthermore, plasma ghrelin levels are negatively correlated with body mass index (BMI); body fat mass; and plasma leptin, insulin, and glucose levels (Muccioli et al., 2002; Ukkola, 2003).

3. GHRELIN, GHS-R1a, AND GOAT

Ghrelin is the only identified systemic hormone that promotes feeding. It is primarily secreted by the stomach and duodenum but has also been detected at lower levels in the pituitary, hypothalamus, colon, lung, heart, pancreas, kidney, and testis (Kojima et al., 1999). Ghrelin is a highly conserved molecule in vertebrates (Kojima & Kangawa, 2005) and it is synthesized as a preprohormone, 117-amino acid peptide that is proteolytically cleaved to yield an acyl peptide containing 28 amino acids that bind GSH-R1a. The human and mouse ghrelin gene is located in chromosome 3, and the human form is made up of four exons and three introns. The genetic structure of the human and rat ghrelin gene is very similar to the mouse gene (Kishimoto et al., 2003). Ghrelin is synthesized in the gastric fundus in the oxyntic gland by A-like cells, which exhibit granules resembling those in pancreatic A cells (Pearse, Coulling, Weavers, & Friesen, 1970; Solcia, Capella, Vassallo, & Buffa, 1975). These cells are positioned in the proximity of capillaries and have no contact with the lumen of the oxyntic gland, indicating that secretion occurs in the plasma and not in the intestinal tract. Circulating ghrelin exists in several forms. The most abundant form is the nonacylated form (des-octanoyl ghrelin, unacylated ghrelin, UAG). Ghrelin is acylated by a membrane-bound *O*-acyl transferase, named ghrelin *O*-acyl transferase (GOAT). This step is required for serine-209 acylation and transport of the Wnt3a, a protein modifier of proliferation and differentiation (Gutierrez et al., 2008; Logan & Nusse, 2004; Takada et al., 2006; Yang, Brown, Liang, Grishin, & Goldstein, 2008). GOAT is a conserved structure in vertebrates and is synthesized in the stomach and pancreas, but minimally expressed in the brain (Gutierrez et al., 2008; Yang et al., 2008). Other studies with small interfering RNA molecules demonstrated that GOAT is the transferase responsible for acylation and bioactivity of ghrelin on serine-3 (Gutierrez et al., 2008). Studies with GOAT knockout mice ($GOAT^{-/-}$) showed that in the absence of GOAT there was no detectable AG synthesized, indicating the requirement for GOAT for acylation and activation of ghrelin (Gutierrez et al., 2008; Kang et al., 2012). Further processing of ghrelin is accomplished by an endoprotease belonging to the subtilisin-like prohormone family, prohormone convertase 1/3, which converts proghrelin to ghrelin (Zhu, Cao, Voogd, & Steiner, 2006). This posttranslational acylation of ghrelin is essential not only for GHS-R1a binding (Granata, Isgaard, Alloatti, & Ghigo, 2011) but also for the hormone to exert its many endocrine functions such as increasing GH secretion from the pituitary, increasing food intake, and regulation of energy homeostasis (Hosoda, Kojima, Matsuo, & Kangawa, 2000; Van der Lely, Tschop, Heiman, & Ghigo, 2004). Both forms of ghrelin, acylated and des-acyl ghrelins, rise gradually in the plasma in the absence of food intake (Tschop et al., 2000). However, only AG binds GHS-R1a causing GH secretion. UAG has not been shown to bind GHS-R1a but may be biologically active. Data suggest that UAG is involved in ghrelin's antiproliferative effects on some human cancer lines (Cassoni et al., 2004; Volante et al., 2003). For example, UAG and AG both inhibited, in a dose-dependent manner, the proliferation of human metastatic prostate cell lines DU-145 and PC-3 (Cassoni et al., 2004, 2001). Interestingly, a recent manuscript suggests that a novel ghrelin isoform (In1-ghrelin) is eight times overexpressed in the human breast cancer cell line MDA-MB-231, when compared to control noncancerous mammary tissue, and may have a significant pathophysiological role in breast cancer (Gahete et al., 2011). Acylated ghrelin has been shown to stimulate ACTH, lactotroph, corticotroph, prolactin, and glucocorticoid production, and to influence sleep and behavior (Horvath et al., 2001; Muccioli et al., 2002). Physiologically, the half-life of AG is approximately 15 min, and it appears not necessary for embryologic development since ghrelin *null* mice ($Ghrl^{-/-}$) are born phenotypically normal, similar in size, body composition, food intake, and reproduction compared with wild-type mice (Sun, Ahmed, & Smith, 2003; Sun, Wang, Zheng, & Smith, 2004). However, it has been reported that ghrelin receptor null mice ($Ghsr^{-/-}$) have impaired abilities to integrate sleep and thermoregulatory responses to metabolic challenges such as cold temperature and fasting, suggesting that there may be independent, noncanonical functions between $Ghrl^{-/-}$ and $Ghsr^{-/-}$ (Szentirmai, Kapas, Sun, Smith, & Krueger, 2009).

The only identified receptor for ghrelin to date is the GHS-R1a which only binds AG. Animal studies with GHS-R1a knockout mice demonstrated that ghrelin injections did not increase food intake or GH in the absence of this receptor (Sun et al., 2004; Zigman et al., 2005). The GHS-R1a receptor is a seven-domain transmembrane G-protein-coupled receptor, which contains 366 amino acids and contains disulfide bonds (Howard et al., 1996). There is 92–96% sequence homology in GHS-R1a between human, rat, pig, and sheep (Palyha et al., 2000). The highest concentrations of GHS-R1a are detected in the pituitary, hypothalamus, pancreas, testis, thyroid, spleen, myocardium, adrenal glands, and stomach (Albarran-Zeckler, Sun, & Smith, 2011; Gnanapavan et al., 2002). A few groups have reportedly found GHS-R1a in skeletal muscle and white adipose tissue (Davies et al., 2009; Soares, Garcia-Souza, Lacerda-Miranda, & Moura, 2012), but these results have not been confirmed by other groups including ours. However, the widespread expression of ghrelin peripherally and limited locations of the GHS-R1a raise the question that ghrelin may be acting on a different receptor peripherally (Gnanapavan et al., 2002). A recent study suggests that acylated ghrelin and UAG induce differentiation of C2C12 mouse skeletal muscle myoblast into myotubes although they do not express GHS-R1a which raises the possibility of an alternate receptor (Filigheddu et al., 2007).

4. MECHANISMS OF ACTION OF GHRELIN

4.1. Ghrelin, muscle, and the GH-IGF-1 axis

Ghrelin is a powerful stimulant for the release of growth hormone (GH; Kojima et al., 1999; Takaya et al., 2000), and this leads to an increase in the production of insulin-like growth factor-1 (IGF-1). The potency of ghrelin, as measured by its GH-releasing capability, is higher than and partially additive to that of growth hormone-releasing hormone (GHRH), suggesting ghrelin's potential therapeutic use as a GH secretagogue (Takaya et al., 2000). The GH/IGF-1 axis is involved in many metabolic events occurring during development (Ding, List, Bower, & Kopchick, 2011), and it also plays an important role in normal well-being during aging and life span (Fontana, Partridge, & Longo, 2010). More importantly, this axis is one of the primary anabolic pathways in skeletal muscle.

GH is a 191-amino acid single peptide primarily secreted from the anterior pituitary, and its release can be stimulated not only by GHRH and ghrelin but also by changes in the metabolic milieu including hypoglycemia, high insulin levels, stress, exercise, and deep sleep (Elijah, Branski, Finnerty, & Herndon, 2011). GH modulates cellular metabolism and mediates its effect on somatic growth through binding to its transmembrane G-protein-coupled receptor, the growth hormone receptor, inducing multiple signaling pathways, primarily IGF-1 in target organs (Cannata, Vijayakumar, Fierz, & LeRoith, 2010; Kopchick & Andry, 2000). The IGF family consists of the mitogenic and anabolic ligands, IGF-1, IGF-2, and insulin (Rinderknecht & Humbel, 1978). IGF-1 is a 70-kDa unstable molecule with a half-life of approximately 10 min. The majority of IGF-1 is bound to one of the six accessory proteins, IGF binding proteins 1–6 (IGFBPs 1–6; Humbel, 1990). The rodent IGF-1 structure is composed of six exons and five introns, and shares approximately 50% homology with the insulin structure (Rinderknecht & Humbel, 1978; Shavlakadze, White, Davies, Hoh, & Grounds, 2005; Shavlakadze, Winn, Rosenthal, & Grounds, 2005). Studies have shown that IGF-1 transcripts are not tissue restricted. For example, transcripts that initiate at Exon 2 are expressed primarily in the liver and are GH sensitive. In contrast, Exon 1-initiating transcripts are expressed in multiple tissues and have been shown to be less affected by circulating GH levels (LeRoith & Roberts, 1991). Both IGFs are synthesized and secreted by hepatocytes and various muscle types, including cardiac and skeletal muscles.

There is animal and human data suggesting that GH and IGF-1 work synergistically in the balance between catabolism and anabolism in respect to skeletal muscle. Studies have shown that both GH and IGF-1 treatments increased body weight (lean body mass and fluid mass; Moller & Jorgensen, 2009; Velloso, 2008). Furthermore, when GH levels are reduced or elevated, IGF-1 is similarly reduced or elevated, confirming both hormones' overlapping yet independent effect on growth. Transgenic animals driven by a myosin light chain promoter of the IGF-1 gene (mIGF-1) in myotubes showed significant skeletal muscle hypertrophy compared to wild-type age-matched young and old littermates (Musaro et al., 2001). Animal studies with induced CHF showed that GH activates nuclear factor kappa-B (NF-κB), promoting increased levels of antiapoptotic factor Bcl-2. Simultaneously, caspases and bax were reduced enhancing cell survival (Jeay, Sonenshein, Postel-Vinay, & Baixeras, 2000).

It remains unclear whether GH acts directly on skeletal muscle to stimulate growth or if these effects are mediated exclusively through IGF-1. GH increases the expression of IGF-1 in muscles of rats leading to growth, and exogenous IGF-1 increases skeletal muscle protein synthesis in mice and humans (Bark, McNurlan, Lang, & Garlick, 1998; Fryburg, 1994; Isgaard,

Carlsson, Isaksson, & Jansson, 1988). However, recent data suggest that there may be IGF-1-independent effects of GH on growth and metabolism. For example, GH alone stimulates mouse myoblast differentiation and muscle growth in the absence of IGF-1 expression probably by increasing satellite cell activation (Imanaka et al., 2008). Furthermore, differentiating between the two hormones in terms of their growth-promoting properties is challenging due to common or overlapping signaling pathways involving both hormones (Ding et al., 2011). To date, there are limited data that differentiate the actions of GH and IGF-1 in various disease processes (Dominici et al., 2005). Regardless of the mechanism of action, the GH/IGF-1 axis is critical to growth, development, and adaptation to different metabolic states.

Recent studies have focused on downstream mediators of an IGF-1 pathway: protein kinase B (PKB/AKT), Forkhead box (FOXO), and the E3 ubiquitin ligases that mediate proteolysis atrogin-1 and muscle ring finger-1 (MuRF1; Bodine et al., 2001; Stitt et al., 2004; Yoshida, Semprun-Prieto, Sukhanov, & Delafontaine, 2010). When IGF-1 binds to its IGF-1 receptor on the plasma membrane, this activates tyrosine kinase phosphorylation which includes insulin receptor substrate (IRS). IRS serves as an accessory docking protein to recruit and activate PI3K which phosphorylates and activates AKT (White, 2002; Withers et al., 1999). Phosphorylation of FOXO by AKT/PKB on multiple sites leads to the inactivation of FOXO preventing its translocation into the nucleus and binding to atrogin-1 and MuRF1 DNA sequence (Reed, Sandesara, Senf, & Judge, 2012). Dephosphorylated FOXO (active form) is shuttled through the nuclear pore (reversible step) where it is able to bind DNA initiating transcription of atrogin-1 and MuRF1 (Barthel, Schmoll, & Unterman, 2005; Glauser & Schlegel, 2007). FOXO is regulated predominantly through the ubiquitin proteasome pathway and to a lesser degree by phosphorylation and acetylation (Vogt, Jiang, & Aoki, 2005). During anorexia, sarcopenia, and cachexia, there is an increase in protein degradation mediated through this pathway. The FOXO family of genes has also been implicated in gene metabolism, apoptosis, atrophy, and cell-cycle progression (Carlsson & Mahlapuu, 2002). Animal studies have demonstrated that DNA binding FOXO was blocked in the muscles of mice by dominant-negative plasmids which decreased the expression of atrogin-1 and MuRF1 decreasing muscle fiber atrophy (Reed et al., 2012). This investigation suggested the requirement for FOXO in muscle protein degradation. Another study showed that mice lacking Atrogin-1 (*MAFbx*$^{-/-}$) and MuRF-1 (*MuRF1*) show reduced atrophy (Stitt et al., 2004). Interestingly, recent data demonstrated that the ghrelin mimetic BIM-28131 decreased atrogin-1 and

MuRF1 in a CHF-induced cachectic rat model supporting the therapeutic role of ghrelin in treating anorexia and cachexia syndrome (Palus et al., 2011). It remains to be determined whether these effects are mediated centrally—via GH—or peripherally and whether they are GHS-R1a dependent or independent.

4.2. Ghrelin and appetite regulation

Ghrelin is known to stimulate food intake and to increase body weight in rodents (Wren et al., 2000), and it also increases food intake in both lean and obese humans (Druce et al., 2005). Ghrelin administration stimulates food intake within 1 h and continuous administration results in sustained feeding (Smith, Jiang, & Sun, 2005). In fact, ghrelin administered centrally or peripherally stimulates food intake more effectively than any peptide besides neuropeptide Y (NPY; Asakawa et al., 2001; Wren et al., 2001b).

Food intake is controlled by the hypothalamic arcuate nucleus containing orexigenic neurons expressing NPY and agouti-related protein (AGRP) and anorexigenic neurons that release proopiomelanocortin (Huda, Wilding, & Pinkney, 2006). NPY and AGRP are coexpressed in subsets of neurons in the arcuate nucleus of the hypothalamus (Hahn, Breininger, Baskin, & Schwartz, 1998), and ghrelin-containing neurons in the arcuate nucleus extend projections to these NPY and AGRP neurons (Cowley et al., 2003). In these neurons, GHS-R1a is coexpressed with AGRP and NPY and their activation promotes a positive energy balance through stimulation of food intake and decreased energy expenditure (Barsh, He, & Gunn, 2002; Willesen, Kristensen, & Romer, 1999). Central administration of ghrelin in fed and fasted rodents causes significant increases in mRNA of neuropeptides AgRP and NPY (Kamegai et al., 2001), and inhibition of endogenous NPY and AGRP by anti-NPY and anti-AGRP intracerebroventricular injections of antibodies abolished ghrelin-induced feeding (Chen et al., 2004; Nakazato et al., 2001). Leptin, which is an anorexigenic hormone secreted by adipocytes in proportion to fat mass, is also inhibited with the rise in ghrelin expression. All these studies support that NPY and AGRP are required for the orexigenic effects of ghrelin and that these effects are mediated in the arcuate nucleus of the hypothalamus.

4.3. Ghrelin and lipid metabolism

Ghrelin favors adiposity through activation of lipogenic pathways in the central nervous system (Cowley et al., 2003). Ghrelin has been identified in the hypothalamic, pituitary, dorsal vagal complex, nucleus of the solitary, and dorsal motor nucleus of the vagus; Korbonits & Grossman, 1995; Zigman, Jones, Lee, Saper, & Elmquist, 2006). Central administration of ghrelin—acting through agouti-related peptide (AgRP)/NPY neurons—blocked melanocortin receptors 3–4 leading to increased lipid storage and adiposity (Theander-Carrillo et al., 2006). Ghrelin also appears to activate AMPK increasing its phosphorylation (Nogueiras, Lopez, & Dieguez, 2010). This pathway is critical for the central regulation of lipid metabolism (Varela et al., 2011). Moreover, these effects of ghrelin administration centrally on lipid metabolism have been shown to be GH dependent (Maccario et al., 2000). Studies with dwarf rats show that chronic ghrelin administration regulates lipid metabolism by increasing the expression of the lipogenic enzymes acetyl-CoA carboxylase, fatty acid synthase, and succinyl co-A dehydrogenase-1 (Sangiao-Alvarellos et al., 2009). Central ghrelin administration on rats regulates adipocyte metabolism by shifting nutrients toward fat storage favoring glucose and triglyceride uptake. This was accomplished by increasing lipogenesis as well as inhibiting lipid oxidation in white adipocyte. Interestingly, animals administered ghrelin peripherally (at doses equal to those of studies using centrally administered ghrelin) have none of the observed effects on adipocyte metabolism seen with central administration. This suggests that the effects of ghrelin on adipocytes are centrally mediated (Theander-Carrillo et al., 2006). However, Barazzoni et al. showed that chronic peripheral ghrelin infusion in rats influenced expression of lipogenic enzymes, gluconeogenesis, and lipid oxidation in liver and muscle tissues (Barazzoni et al., 2005). The authors suggest that these differences could be explained by the concentration and type of ghrelin administered.

Ghrelin also reduces uncoupling protein-1 and -3 in brown adipose tissue (BAT), thereby decreasing thermogenesis and energy expenditure. The mechanism of action for these effects is not clear, but ghrelin may mediate these indirectly by suppressing sympathetic activity (Yasuda, Masaki, Kakuma, & Yoshimatsu, 2003). This investigation also showed that BAT temperature is temporarily decreased in ghrelin-treated animals compared to control animals although rectal temperature was not affected (Yasuda et al., 2003). A recent study suggested that both ghrelin and des-acyl ghrelin possess a direct leptin-releasing activity in retroperitoneal (RP) adipocytes. Des-acyl ghrelin also enhances RP adipocyte differentiation suggesting a role in adipogenesis. This specific effect was not observed with acyl ghrelin (Giovambattista, Gaillard, & Spinedi, 2008) suggesting that the mechanism mediating these effects is GHS-R1a independent. Although the role of ghrelin on lipid metabolism in humans has not been well established, when exogenous ghrelin was intravenously infused to humans, lipolysis was stimulated and free fatty acids (FFA) were increased (Vestergaard et al., 2007, 2008). In summary, ghrelin has been shown to increase adiposity in a number of animal models. The mechanisms involved include centrally mediated increases in food intake and decreases in energy expenditure as well as direct effects on lipolytic and lipid synthesis pathways. *In vitro* studies also suggest a role of ghrelin directly on adipocytes although the exact mechanism has not been completely characterized.

4.4. Ghrelin and inflammation

Inflammation has been postulated as a key mediator in the setting of cachexia. Markers of inflammation including tumor necrosis factor-α (TNF-α), interleukin (IL)-1, IL-6, and interferon-γ (IFN-γ) may play a central pathogenic role in the decreased food intake and increased energy expenditure seen in most chronic conditions associated with the anorexia and cachexia syndrome (Plata-Salaman, 2001). Increased cytokines in the hypothalamus result in the activation of anorexigenic pathways and subsequent decrease in food intake (Laviano, Meguid, & Rossi-Fanelli, 2003). Inflammation may also play a role in the development of muscle atrophy. One major pathway involved in proteolysis is NF-κB which leads to an increase in inflammatory cytokines including TNF-α and skeletal muscle atrophy (Li & Reid, 2000; Wyke, Russell, & Tisdale, 2004). This is relevant because ghrelin administration in rodents and humans has been shown to decrease inflammatory markers (Balasubramaniam et al., 2009; Garcia, Cata, Dougherty, & Smith, 2008; Hillman, Tong, & Tschop, 2011; Itoh et al., 2004). Nevertheless, the role of ghrelin and GHS on the immune system remains unclear. Ghrelin has been shown to activate lymphocyte development and prevent age-associated thymic involution. Ghrelin and GHS-R1a are expressed by resident and resting activated human T-cell and have been shown to mediate anti-inflammatory signals in various cells (Dixit et al., 2004, 2007; Li et al., 2004). Ghrelin treatment in 14-month-old mice enhanced thymic size and cellularity, thus improving immunity. No significant T-cell increase was exhibited in younger mice (Dixit et al., 2007). Ghrelin has also been shown to attenuate excessive inflammation and reduce organ injury in the gut after ischemia/reperfusion through activation of the cholinergic anti-inflammatory pathway (Wu et al., 2009). Furthermore, ghrelin inhibits the production of anorectic proinflammatory cytokines, IL-1β, IL-6, and TNF-α therefore limiting and possibly inhibiting the inflammatory process induced by administration of lipopolysaccharides (Dixit et al., 2004). In other studies, exogenously administered ghrelin was reported to suppress the expression and/or production of cytokines regardless of the pathology (Hattori, 2009; Smith et al., 2005).

In summary, ghrelin affects multiple pathways that are known to be key in the regulation of body weight, body composition, and appetite in the setting of cachexia. These include orexigenic and anorexigenic pathways in the arcuate nucleus of the hypothalamus, the GH/IGF-1 pathway, adipocyte and skeletal muscle metabolism and inflammation. We will now review the data on the potential therapeutic role of ghrelin in the setting of cachexia.

5. GHRELIN AND SARCOPENIA OF AGING

Age-related sarcopenia refers to the loss of muscle mass and muscle strength that is associated with aging. Although not the norm, a number of elderly individuals even without chronic illness suffer from sarcopenia of aging. A number of processes have been reported in the mechanism of sarcopenia in aging including decreased appetite, reduced levels of anabolic hormones such as GH and IGF-1, increased muscle cell apoptosis, and increased proinflammatory cytokines such as TNF-α and IL-1 and IL-6 (Hall, Ma, Marco, & Gallouzi, 2011).

Although to date there are no published studies evaluating the role of ghrelin during aging in animals, Nass et al. looked at the effects of placebo versus the GHS MK-677 in 65 healthy, nonsarcopenic elderly (60–81) men and women over a 2-year period on a randomized, placebo-controlled, double-blinded, and modified crossover study. Among the key findings of this study were a 1.8- and 1.5-fold increase in pulsatile 24 h GH and IGF-1 secretion, respectively, compared to placebo. Fat-free mass, appendicular skeletal muscle mass (lean limb), abdominal subcutaneous (SC) fat, and body weight also increased with MK-677 treatment. Moreover, skeletal muscle mass increased and evaluation of muscle strength showed an increase in shoulder flexion total work. No difference in strength of knee extension or flexion among groups was noted, and there was no change in functional capacity (measured with 30-m walk, 6-min walk, ability to sit/stand from a chair, or stair climbing) or quality of life between groups (Nass et al., 2008). These results, however, need to be interpreted carefully as they reflect a healthy nonsarcopenic population and they may not be applicable to the general elderly population which often has other chronic medical conditions or to the sarcopenic elderly population. Also, the study was likely underpowered to detect changes in functional capacity. The absence of functional improvement with GH therapy has also been noted in other studies, indicating that increasing growth hormone levels in elderly subjects is not sufficient to treat sarcopenia (Nass, Johannsson, Christiansen, Kopchick, & Thorner, 2009). Future larger studies focusing on sarcopenic elderly individuals are warranted to determine if strength and functional capacity will respond to ghrelin treatment or if combination therapy (i.e., with nutritional supplements) will be effective. An interesting target population may be those individuals at risk for fractures. Falls in the elderly are as frequent as 0.3–1.6 per person annually among community living, generally healthy elderly people of age <65 (Rubenstein, 2006). In addition, about 5% of these falls induce a fracture or require hospitalization, and in the case of hip fractures, are associated with a five- to eightfold higher risk for all-cause mortality during the first 3 months after fracture (Haentjens et al., 2010). Therefore, attempts at decreasing or reversing muscle loss could improve strength, balance, and directly decrease risk for falls. Also, improving energy balance and protein intake with ghrelin may not only prevent sarcopenia but also improve healing and recovery in an elderly patient with underlying sarcopenia undergoing surgery. Future studies are also needed to differentiate the effects of ghrelin therapy compared to growth hormone therapy in strength and muscle mass. Studies evaluating the effects of ghrelin on healing return to functional status, and mortality in sarcopenic patients with hip or other fractures are also warranted.

6. GHRELIN AND CANCER CACHEXIA

The most promising intervention of ghrelin in cachexia is that in the setting of cancer. Anorexia/cachexia in cancer have been partly explained by elevated proinflammatory cytokines such as IFN-γ, TNF-α, IL-1β, and IL-6 (Guney, Ozel Turkcu, Hicsonmez, Nalca Andrieu, & Kurtman, 2007). Different mouse models have been utilized for cancer-induced cachexia: CD2F1 mice inoculated with colon-26 adenocarcinoma cells, C57BL/6 mice injected with Lewis lung carcinoma tumor cells, $Apc^{Min/+}$ mouse (heterozygotes for a mutation in the *adenomatous polyposis coli* (*Apc*) gene leading to spontaneous development of intestinal and colon adenomas), and G361—a human melanoma cell line—inoculated into nude mice. Early studies looking at the G361 human melanoma cell line mouse models in nude mice with cachexia demonstrated an increase in ghrelin biosynthesis and secretion measured by ghrelin peptide and mRNA in the stomach and plasma concentration, respectively, with the progression of cachexia in mice (Hanada et al., 2004). Similarly, using the SEKI (human melanoma cell line mouse) model of cancer cachexia and vehicle mice were treated with ghrelin intraperitoneal twice a day for 6 days. In both SEKI and sham-inoculated mice, ghrelin administration increased body weight, white adipose tissue, and daily food intake. No significant difference in tumor size was observed between the saline- and ghrelin-administered groups (Hanada et al., 2003). The latter study only looked at leukemia inhibitory factor, which was similar between SEKI and vehicle mice, but no other inflammatory markers or assessments of LBM or muscle mass were assessed. DeBoer et al. used F344/NTacfBR rats implanted with methylcholanthrene sarcoma as an animal model of cancer cachexia and continuously administered either ghrelin or BIM-28131 (a synthetic GHS) via SC osmotic mini-pumps versus saline. Results showed that both ghrelin and BIM-28131 at high doses increased food intake, weight gain, and retention of lean body mass (DeBoer et al., 2007). In addition, there was no change in tumor mass among any of the treatment groups. De Boer et al. also showed that treatment with ghrelin and GHS in a rat model increased gene expression of AgRP and NPY, two orexigenic neuropeptides produced in the arcuate nucleus of the hypothalamus. As mentioned before, this central hypothalamic effect has been postulated as ghrelin's main orexigenic effect. In C57BL/6 mice also injected with methylcholanthrene-induced sarcoma (MCG-101), ghrelin administration improved weight gain and lean body mass preservation. These effects were attributed to the orexigenic neuropeptides (NPY in the hypothalamus) and anti-inflammatory effects of ghrelin, respectively (Wang et al., 2006). Again, tumor growth was not altered by exogenous ghrelin treatment. Finally, in nude mice bearing human melanoma cells, ghrelin administration led to an increase in total body weight, increased average single-day food intake in both tumor-implanted and sham animals (Hanada et al., 2003). No significant difference in tumor size was noted with or without ghrelin treatment. In murine models of cancer, therefore, it appears that ghrelin administration successfully diminishes cachexia, increases appetite, and preserves lean muscle mass without affecting tumor growth (Table 3.1).

In humans, many have reported increased plasma ghrelin levels in individuals with low BMI compared to those with normal or higher BMIs (Soriano-Guillen, Barrios, Campos-Barros, & Argente, 2004; Tanaka, Naruo, Nagai, et al., 2003). A large Japanese study of 638 subjects evaluated ghrelin levels and their relation to other factors. Study results revealed, in a nonobese population with mean BMI of 23.8 kg/m^2, an inverse relationship between ghrelin and age, BMI, waist circumference, fasting plasma glucose, and insulin

Table 3.1 Summary of studies using ghrelin or GHS in animal models of cachexia

Animal model	Regimen	Results	References
Cancer cachexia			
Five-week-old female BALB/c-mice human melanoma cells	IP ghrelin 10.1 μg twice a day for 6 days	– Increased body weight – Increased food intake – No effect on tumor size	Hanada et al. (2003)
C57BL/6 mice SC with methylcholanthrene-induced sarcoma (MCG-101)	IP ghrelin low dose = 10 μg and high dose = 20 μg versus 100 μl saline daily for 4 days	– Weight gain – LBM preservation – No effect on tumor size	Wang et al. (2006)
F344/NTacfBR male rats implanted with methylcholanthrene sarcoma	SC osmotic pumps ghrelin low dose = 168 μg/kg/d or high dose = 1680 μg/kg/d or BIM-28131 daily for 5 days	– Increased food intake – Weight gain – Retention of LBM – No effect on tumor size	DeBoer et al. (2007)
Sprague–Dawley rats treated with cisplatin	IP ghrelin 0.8 mg/kg daily	– Ghrelin prevented the decrease in food intake, weight, and IGF-1	Garcia, Graham, Kumor, and Polvino (2007)
CHF-associated cachexia			
Wistar rats with MI induced by LAD ligation	SC ghrelin (100 μg/kg) or saline twice daily for 3 weeks	– Increased body weight – Higher cardiac output – Increased diastolic thickness of the noninfarcted posterior wall – Inhibited LV enlargement – Increased LV fractional shortening in CHF rats	Nagaya et al. (2001)

Continued

Table 3.1 Summary of studies using ghrelin or GHS in animal models of cachexia—cont'd

Animal model	Regimen	Results	References
Sprague–Dawley rats pressure-overload CHF was created by abdominal aortic banding in rats	SC hexarelin (GHSR agonist, dose 100 μg/kg) twice daily for 3 weeks	– Increased body weight – Improved LVEF and remodeling in CHF – Decreased LV end-diastolic pressure and dimension	Xu et al. (2005)
Sprague–Dawley rats infarcted via LAD ligation	SC ghrelin (low dose = 168 μg/kg/d vs. high dose 336 μg/kg/d SC) three times daily for 2 weeks	– Increased body weight – Increased LBM and FM – No effect on LVEF or change of LV diameters	Akashi et al. (2009)
Sprague–Dawley rats with MI	SC ghrelin (100 μg/kg) twice daily for 2 weeks	– Attenuated LV enlargement induced by MI – Decreased LV end-diastolic pressure – Suppressed the MI-induced increase in heart rate and plasma N.E. concentration to the similar levels as in controls	Soeki et al. (2008)
Cachexia and renal disease			
Nephrectomized rats (surgical model of CKD)	SC ghrelin continuous mini-osmotic pumps ghrelin vs. BIM-28125 and BIM-28131 (GHS-R1a agonist) versus saline at a rate of 0.5 μl/h for 14 days[a]	– Increased weight and food intake – Increased LBM and decreased muscle protein degradation – Decrease in proinflammatory cytokines – Increase in IL-10 (anti-inflammatory cytokine) – Decrease in muscle catabolism (via decrease in 14-kDa actin fragment)	Deboer et al. (2008)
Rheumatoid arthritis, COPD, Anorexia nervosa, CHF Aging, or AIDS-associated cachexia			
No studies			

BW, body weight; CHF, congestive heart failure; CKD, chronic kidney disease; E, epinephrine; IGF-1, insulin-like growth factor-1; IP, intraperitoneal; FM, fat mass; GH, growth hormone; LAD, left anterior descending artery; LBM, lean body mass; LV, left ventricle; LVEF, left ventricular ejection fraction; LOS, length of stay; MI, myocardial infarction; NE, noreipnephrine; SC, subcutaneous; TNF-α, tumor necrosis factor alpha.

[a]Ghrelin dose not reported.

levels among other variables (Nanjo et al., 2011). These observations led to the hypothesis that ghrelin levels would also be elevated in other settings of negative energy balance such as cancer cachexia. Subsequent studies have proven this in different types of cancer with cachexia including both small cell and nonsmall cell lung cancer (Karapanagiotou et al., 2009), breast and colorectal cancer (Wolf et al., 2006), and multiple cancer types combined (Fouladiun et al., 2005; Garcia et al., 2005). Although the majority of the studies evaluating ghrelin levels in cancer cachexia do show an increase in ghrelin levels, not all studies have proved the above hypothesis particularly in patients with gastrointestinal malignancies (Kemik et al., 2010). For example, Huang et al. looked at ghrelin levels in gastric cancer or colorectal cancer patients compared to controls and did not find a difference in ghrelin concentrations when matching for BMI (Huang, Fan, Ge, Zhu, & Tu, 2007). However, it is worth noting that the latter study included 58 patients with gastric cancer and 20 with colorectal cancer, 83% had a history of radical surgery, and only 31 of the 78 patients had cachexia. Similarly, a small study of 30 patients in Greece with mainly pancreatic and gastric cancer compared to 27 healthy, age- and gender-matched control subjects found a similarly low level of ghrelin in cancer patients compared to controls (Legakis, Stathopoulos, Matzouridis, & Stathopoulos, 2009). Therefore, it is possible that in patients with GI malignancies and particularly those involving the stomach, ghrelin levels may be diminished as a direct result of cancer affecting ghrelin-secreting areas of the GI tract. In addition, patients with history of radical surgery may have had part of their gastric mucosa resected leading to decreased ghrelin production. The majority of evidence, however, indicates that total ghrelin levels are elevated—approximately 25% above normal in a variety of cancers causing cachexia: lung, breast, colon, and prostate cancers (Garcia et al., 2005; Shimizu et al., 2003; Wolf et al., 2006). Our group has also demonstrated high levels of acyl ghrelin in patients with cancer cachexia. Interestingly, ghrelin elevation in many of these cancer cachexia patients is still associated with poor appetite and weight loss. This has led some to postulate a possible state of ghrelin resistance or a net anorectic effect of other processes in cancer cachexia that cannot be overcome even by reactive increases in endogenous ghrelin production (Garcia et al., 2005). Nevertheless, others and we have postulated that administration of supraphysiologic doses of exogenous ghrelin or ghrelin mimetics may still have a beneficial effect in this setting in spite of the already elevated circulating ghrelin levels. This would be analogous to the effects of administering insulin in individuals with type 2 diabetes where its effects are still present even in the presence of insulin resistance.

There are a few published studies testing the effects of ghrelin in cancer patients (Table 3.2). Neary et al. looked at seven cancer patients with anorexia and found that energy intake was increased by 31% and the perceived pleasantness of the meal (measured via a visual analog score) by 23% with ghrelin administration compared to controls (Neary et al., 2004). In another randomized, double-crossover study, 21 patients with advanced incurable cancer and anorexia were randomized to receive low dose or high dose of intravenous ghrelin × 50 min versus placebo. A marked increase in energy intake was observed with ghrelin infusion compared with placebo, and every patient ate more (Strasser et al., 2008). Ghrelin was well tolerated even in the high dose treatment arm, and no increases in the rate of tumor progression were noted although follow-up was only 2 weeks after ghrelin therapy. Researchers also found an increase in these patient's meal appreciation score with ghrelin treatment. This latter finding holds clinical promise as patients with cancer cachexia and particularly those on chemotherapy often complain of food losing its appeal or taste. The mechanism responsible for this improvement in meal appreciation may be related to ghrelin's positive effects on reward as it has previously been described in animals (Dickson et al., 2011). Lundholm et al. also tested the effects of ghrelin in a group of 31 patients with solid gastrointestinal tumors and weight loss. Patients were randomized to receive low dose (0.5 μg/kg) or high dose (10 μg/kg) daily subcutaneously for 8 weeks. Results showed increased appetite scores and decreased whole body fat loss with a trend for high-dose ghrelin to improve energy balance, and there were no adverse effects or change in tumor markers between groups (Lundholm et al., 2011). Given that ghrelin is a peptide with a very short half-life (<30 min) that needs to be administered parenterally, several groups including ours are investigating the potential role of ghrelin mimetics (GHS) in this setting. These molecules are nonpeptidic agonists of the ghrelin receptor GHS-R1a that have a long half-life that allows for once-a-day administration. In a randomized, double-blind, placebo-controlled, multiple-dose, dose-escalation study conducted in three sequential panels of healthy volunteers, subjects who received the orally active ghrelin mimetic and GHS anamorelin (formerly known as RC-1291) had a mean increase in weight from baseline after 6 days of treatment of about 1.2 kg compared to placebo (Garcia & Polvino, 2007). Based on this, a randomized, placebo-controlled, double-blind phase II study of anamorelin versus placebo was performed in individuals with incurable cancer and cachexia. Preliminary results show that anamorelin increased appetite, handgrip strength, and body weight compared to placebo with

Table 3.2 Summary of human studies using ghrelin or GHS in cachexia

Population	Regimen	Results	References
Aging/sarcopenia			
Healthy elderly 60–81-years-old	MK-677 25 mg oral (ghrelin mimetic) versus placebo once daily for 1–2 years	– 1.8- and 1.5-fold increase in pulsatile 24-h growth hormone and IGF-1 secretion – Increased fat mass – Increased appendicular muscle mass – Improved shoulder flexion – No change in knee flexion/extension	Nass et al. (2008)
Cancer cachexia			
Breast cancer ($n=5$) Melanoma ($n=1$) Colon CA ($n=1$) versus 7 healthy controls	IV ghrelin infusion 16.8 μg/kg/min for 3 h once	– Energy intake was increased by 31% – Increase of 23% in the perceived pleasantness of the meal	Neary et al. (2004)
Twenty-one subjects with advanced incurable cancer Ten subjects low dose Eleven subjects high dose	IV ghrelin low dose = 2 μg/kg or high dose = 8 μg/kg over 1 h versus placebo for 2 days (7 days apart)	– Increased energy intake – Increased meal appreciation score – No effect on tumor size	Strasser et al. (2008)
31 patients with weight loss and solid GI tumors Fourteen subjects low dose Seventeen subjects high dose	SC ghrelin low dose = 0.5 μg/kg or high dose = 10 μg/kg daily or daily for 8 weeks	– Increased appetite scores – Decreased whole body fat loss – Trend for improved energy balance – No effect on tumor size	Lundholm et al. (2011)
Twenty-nine patients with solid organ tumors	GHSR agonist anamorelin 50 mg once daily	– Increased body mass – Increased hand grip strength – No effect on disease progression	Garcia et al. preliminary results

Continued

Table 3.2 Summary of human studies using ghrelin or GHS in cachexia—cont'd

Population	Regimen	Results	References
Forty-two patients with stage II–III esophageal cancer on cisplatin neo-adjuvant chemotherapy	IV ghrelin infusion 3 μg/kg twice daily vs. placebo(saline) for 1 week	– Increased food intake – Better quality-of-life score – Less nausea and vomiting from chemo – Less toxicity from chemotherapy – Reduced LOS – No difference in tumor response to chemotherapy	Hiura et al. (2012)
COPD cachexia			
Seven patients with COPD and cachexia	IV ghrelin infusion 2 μg/kg twice daily versus placebo (saline) for 3 weeks	– Increased GH and IGF-1 – Stimulated feeding – Increased BW and LBM – Decreased SNS activity with decreased N.E. levels – Increased peripheral and respiratory muscle strength – Increased Karnofsky performance status	Nagaya et al. (2005)
Anorexia nervosa			
Five patients with ANRT	IV ghrelin infusion 3 μg/kg twice a day for 14 days	– Increased daily energy intake by 20% – Improved epigastric discomfort – 40% weight gain	Hotta et al. (2009)
Four patients with purging and five with restrictive AN, six partially recovered AN patients	IV ghrelin infusion 16.8 μg/kg/min for 300 min once	– No effect on appetite	Miljic et al. (2006)

CHF cachexia			
NYHA stage III–IV CHF patients: 10 were randomized to human ghrelin (8 had cardiac cachexia) and 8 to placebo (6 with cardiac cachexia)	IV ghrelin 2 μg/kg twice a day for 3 weeks	– Increased food intake, LBM, and grip strength – Trend favoring body weight increase – Decreased plasma N.E. and Epinephrine – Increased LVEF ejection and LV mass – Decreased LV end-systolic volume – Improved exercise capacity (increase in peak workload and peak VO_2) – Improved (NYHA) functional class in 4/10 pts	Nagaya et al. (2004)
Ghrelin and ESRD			
Twelve malnourished HD patients	SC ghrelin once daily for 1 week	– Increased food intake – No change in IL-6 or TNF-α	Ashby et al. (2009)
Nine malnourished PD patients	SC ghrelin 12.2 μg/kg SC ghrelin vs. placebo once daily for 1 week	– Increased energy intake within 30 min of injection – No change in appetite (VAS) – Trend for enhanced meal enjoyment	Wynne et al. (2005)
AIDS, rheumatoid arthritis–cachexia			
No studies			

BW, body weight; CHF, congestive heart failure; CKD, chronic kidney disease; E, epinephrine; ESRD, end-stage renal disease; IGF-1, insulin-like growth factor-1; IP, intraperitoneal; IV, intravenous; FM, fat mass; GH, growth hormone; LAD, left anterior descending artery; LBM, lean body mass; LV, left ventricle; LVEF, left ventricular ejection fraction; LOS, length of stay; MI, myocardial infarction; NE, noreipnephrine; SC, subcutaneous; TNF-α, tumor necrosis factor alpha; VAS, visual analog scale.

good tolerability (Garcia, Kumor, & PolvinoGarcia, 2007). As expected, this intervention also increased circulating IGF-1 and IGFBP-3 which are known to be decreased in this setting (Garcia et al., 2005). A recent randomized, placebo-controlled phase II study enrolled 42 patients with advanced esophageal cancer, and the aim of this study was to elucidate the effect of exogenous ghrelin on patients with esophageal cancer receiving cisplatin-based neo-adjuvant chemotherapy (Hiura et al., 2012). Patients were randomized 1:1 to receive IV infusion of ghrelin or placebo twice daily for 7 consecutive days. Ghrelin therapy led to improved food intake, significantly better global health status scores (quality-of-life evaluation scale), less nausea/vomiting reports compared to placebo, and decreased loss of appetite. Also, ghrelin treatment led to less toxicity from chemotherapy (as assessed by need to have dose modification) and reduced length of hospital stay from 23.5 days in control to 18.4 days in treatment group. There was no difference in objective tumor response rate to chemotherapy.

6.1. Safety of ghrelin and GHS in the setting of cancer

Although ghrelin or ghrelin mimetic therapy in the setting of cancer cachexia has many potential benefits, there are also some concerns about the safety of these agents in this setting. The GHS-R1a is expressed in many normal and tumoral tissues including breast, thyroid, and prostate. However, activation of this receptor in tumor cell lines *ex vivo* has yielded conflicting results. Ghrelin mimetics have induced proliferation of certain tumor cell lines but growth inhibition in others (Cassoni et al., 2000, 2001). Administration of a growth factor such as ghrelin or GH to tumor-bearing individuals raises potential concerns of stimulation of tumor growth, particularly through elevation of IGF-1. However, when whole animal tumor growth studies have been conducted to evaluate the effect of increasing GH tone, the results have generally indicated a beneficial effect (Bartlett, Charland, & Torosian, 1994; Bartlett, Stein, & Torosian, 1995; Wolf, Ng, Weksler, Burt, & Brennan, 1994). There have been publications implicating IGF-1 in oncogenic potential; in addition, there have been reports indicating the therapeutic potential of the major binding protein, IGFBP-3, in attenuating oncogenic behavior either via its ability to bind IGF-1 or via direct, IGF-independent actions. Consequently, it may be that the balanced effect of a growth hormone-based intervention to increase both IGF-1 and IGFBP-3 may be responsible, in part, for some of the apparent discrepancies. Hanada et al. (Hanada et al., 2003) tested the effects of ghrelin in a mouse model of cancer cachexia injected with human melanoma cells. In this experiment, cachexia was reversed by the administration of ghrelin and tumor size remained unchanged, decreasing the tumor/carcass ratio. In summary, the composite preclinical literature indicates beneficial effects of ghrelin-based intervention in cancer-related weight loss models and that ghrelin increases lean body mass without affecting disease progression relative to the untreated state. Preliminary clinical data to date show that ghrelin maintains its GH secretagogue and orexigenic effect in the setting of cancer. However, more studies to evaluate the effects of ghrelin administration to different cancer types are needed to asses fully concerns for tumor growth and other possible deleterious effects of therapy.

7. GHRELIN AND COPD-INDUCED CACHEXIA

Unwanted muscle wasting and weight loss leading to cachexia that may or may not be accompanied by caloric deficiency (i.e., starvation) are frequently seen in COPD and particularly emphysema. Ghrelin is a very promising agent for treating cachexia due to its known anti-inflammatory effects, preservation of lean body mass, and ability to decrease sympathetic activity, all of which play a role in causing cachexia in COPD. Although there are animal models for COPD/emphysema, not many of them have been able to successfully mimic the systemic effects or the cachexia and muscular effects seen with this condition. However, a recent study by Rinaldi et al. used nose-only exposure to cigarette smoke in C57BL6 mice for 3–6 months and was able to cause lung injury similar to what is seen in COPD/emphysema. Most importantly, after 6 months of cigarette smoke exposure, a shift from muscle fiber type IIa (oxidative) to IIX/b (glycolytic) was observed and 20% reduction of force at high stimulation frequencies were noted in the soleus muscle (Rinaldi et al., 2012). Another study using C57Bl6 mice exposed to cigarette smoke also found significantly higher TNF-α levels after chronic smoke exposure, and a tendency for higher proinflammatory cytokines such as IL-1β, IL-3, and IL-17. Chronic smoke exposure also decreased body weight gain, lowered soleus muscle weight with a lower proportion of oxidative type-IIA and higher proportion of glycolytic type-IIB muscle fibers compared to controls (Gosker et al., 2009). Another group induced emphysema in adult male mice strain A/J by local injection of elastase into the lungs (classic model for pulmonary emphysema; Fermoselle, Sanchez, & Barreiro, 2011). The mice that developed emphysema were noted to have lower total body weight and lower weight of the diaphragm and gastrocnemius. In the diaphragm, myosin content was lower and myostatin, FoxO1, and extracellular signal-regulated kinase (ERK) 1/2 signaling pathways were increased compared to controls. The gastrocnemius of emphysematous mice showed lower levels of myostatin, but c-Jun-amino-terminal kinase-interacting protein and NF-κB signaling pathways were increased. Therefore, these mouse models of COPD/emphysema support that cachexia associated with this respiratory condition is accompanied by weight loss, skeletal muscle loss, and increased inflammation. Nevertheless, ghrelin or GHS administration has not been used in any animal model of COPD-induced cachexia.

Human studies have shown elevated ghrelin levels in patients with COPD who were underweight (Ying et al., 2008). Although hypoxia does not seem to have an effect on ghrelin regulation (Chaiban, Bitar, & Azar, 2008), circulating TNF-α and IL-6 concentrations were significantly higher in underweight COPD patients compared to normal weight (NW) controls. Another trial of 73 patients with COPD compared to healthy smokers as controls found that 17 of the 73 patients had significantly lower BMI and tended to have less muscle mass. These cachectic subjects also exhibited elevated muscle TNF-α mRNA levels and TNF-α-impaired muscle oxyphen (a marker of skeletal muscle dysfunction and muscle loss) mediated via NF-κB (Remels et al., 2010). Nagaya et al. showed that ghrelin administration increased GH and IGF-1 in 7 patients with COPD and cachexia (Nagaya et al., 2005). Administration of ghrelin also stimulated feeding in six of the seven patients, increased body weight and lean body mass, and attenuated sympathetic nerve activity by causing a marked decrease in plasma norepinephrine levels. Most importantly, ghrelin significantly increased peripheral and respiratory muscle strength, Karnofsky performance status score, and the distance walked in 6 min after 3 weeks twice daily IV infusion of ghrelin (370 ± 30 to 432 ± 35 m; $p < 0.05$; Nagaya et al., 2005). Some of these effects could be GH dependent, particularly due to the elevation seen in GH/IGF-1. However, non-GH-dependent mechanisms for ghrelin's anticachexia effects in COPD also appear to be at play including the hormone's known orexigenic action and inhibitory effect on sympathetic drive (Nagaya et al., 2005; Schols, 2002). Finally, there is also evidence that ghrelin may have immune modulatory function. For instance, intravenous ghrelin treatment for 3 weeks in patients with COPD reduced both neutrophil counts in sputum samples and also the volume of sputum (Kodama, Ashitani, Matsumoto, Kangawa, & Nakazato, 2008). This may suggest that in COPD ghrelin may also have a direct effect on sputum production which is key in the pathophysiology of COPD and COPD exacerbations. More randomized control studies are needed to determine if ghrelin therapy decreases disease progression, improves functional capacity, and even may lead to decreased COPD exacerbations and hospitalization in this patient population.

8. GHRELIN AND ANOREXIA NERVOSA

In anorexia nervosa restrictive type (ANRT), patients experience excess loss of weight as a result of severe and selective caloric restriction (Fairburn & Harrison, 2003). It has also been shown that with the undernutrition seen in AN total ghrelin levels (in addition to increased ratio of des-acyl ghrelin to acyl ghrelin) are higher than controls (Misra et al., 2005; Otto et al., 2001; Tanaka et al., 2003; Uehara et al., 2011). A meta-analysis that included 24 out of 28 studies assessing GI hormones in the setting of eating disorders found 8 studies looking at anorexia nervosa (AN) and ghrelin levels. Four of these studies looked at ghrelin levels in ANRT and all four demonstrated an increase in baseline ghrelin concentrations compared to healthy subjects (Prince, Brooks, Stahl, & Treasure, 2009). It therefore appears that total ghrelin, mostly in the form of des-acyl ghrelin, is elevated in ANRT. As expected, hospitalization and refeeding in ANRT patients lead to a decrease in ghrelin levels (particularly des-acyl ghrelin), and 8 weeks after refeeding, des-acyl levels were even lower than in control subjects. Finally, the ratio of acyl ghrelin to total ghrelin increased 8 weeks after refeeding (Koyama et al., 2010). It is therefore possible that the elevation in total and des-acyl ghrelin seen in AN is in the form of inactive ghrelin which is not able to bind to the GHS-R1a receptor in the pituitary to affect appetite and energy metabolism. A recent study looked at genetic variation of GOAT and the association with AN. Research looked at the association of six tagging single nucleotide polymorphisms (tag SNPs), which were predicted to cover 96% of the common genetic variability of GOAT plus 50 kb of the 5′ and 3′ flanking region, in 543 German patients with AN compared to 612 German normal and underweight healthy controls. This study showed an association of the G/G genotype at SNP rs10096097 with AN based on a recessive mode of inheritance indicating that there may be genetic variation in GOAT responsible for AN (Muller et al., 2011). Again, this genetic variation in GOAT activity may lead to less formation of acylated ghrelin and therefore impaired appetite and energy homeostasis.

Laboratory examinations of the stomach in patients with AN reveal atrophy of the mucosa, alteration of peristalsis, and delayed emptying time (Hillman et al., 2011). Interestingly, Hotta et al. showed that patients with AN have a mean increase in daily energy intake of almost 20% compared to pretreatment period during ghrelin infusion in a study of five patients with AN. Ghrelin infusion improved epigastric discomfort or constipation in four out of five patients and hunger scores evaluated by visual analogue scale questionnaires also increased significantly after ghrelin infusion. At the end of this study, 80% of patients had significant increase in energy intake and 40% (2 out of 5) actually gained weight (Hotta et al., 2009). The authors also point out that although ghrelin levels were not measured at follow-up, one out of the five patients treated with ghrelin had return of normal menses 6 months after treatment indicating return to normal function of some of the hypothalamic–pituitary axis and possibly indicating more prolonged effects of ghrelin therapy. However, another study using a onetime ghrelin infusion of 5 pmol/kg/min for 5 h found no difference in hunger score between ANRT or partially recovered AN patients and controls using a visual analog scale (VAS) to asses hunger (Miljic et al., 2006). Food intake was not measured in this study, and also it is unclear if measuring hunger via VAS in AN patients is reliable in a disease where hunger is often downplayed. It is also possible that a onetime infusion may not be sufficient to counteract the many factors that play a role in ANRT (such as anxiety, depression, and obsessive–compulsive disorder), and that a longer duration of ghrelin therapy is needed to see changes in appetite. Finally, AN subjects voluntarily restrict caloric intake and minimized their hunger both of which make subjective hunger assessment and response to intervention very difficult. The lack of response to ghrelin therapy in both appetite and body composition in AN has led some to postulate blunted GH response to ghrelin in AN. Similar to other states of malnutrition, AN may lead to peripheral GH resistance and decreased IGF-1 (Gianotti et al., 2002; Terashi et al., 2011). GH increases not only due to the effects of ghrelin but also due to the absence of negative inhibition by IGF-1 on GH release. It has been previously shown that elevated ghrelin levels can desensitize the growth hormone stimulatory effect of ghrelin (Camina et al., 2004), but whether this occurs in AN patients who also have elevated GH levels and low IGF-1 has not been demonstrated. The term ghrelin resistance has also been used to explain this apparent absence or blunted response of AN patients to ghrelin in regard with appetite and GH release. For instance, Broglio et al. showed higher basal morning ghrelin and GH levels and lower IGF-1 levels in AN compared to normal women. The GH response to GHRH in AN was significantly higher than that in NW, but in AN subjects, the GH response to ghrelin was significantly lower than in NW (Broglio et al., 2004). This indicates less ghrelin responsiveness or ghrelin resistance. Similarly, a study of 15 young women (9 with AN, 6 with history of AN who remained amenorrheic but had regained some body weight) compared to 10 thin women without AN or amenorrhea was given an IV ghrelin infusion over 5 h. After ghrelin infusion, researchers found AN patients to be less sensitive to ghrelin in terms of GH response and appetite than healthy controls (Miljic et al., 2006). Mixed results have also been shown in relation to ghrelin secretion response to meal ingestions. For instance, some studies have shown a blunted response in the secretion of ghrelin following meal ingestion or oral glucose administration in underweight AN patients compared to controls (Nedvidkova et al., 2003; Tanaka, Naruo, Yasuhara, et al., 2003), while others have shown more pronounced decreases in ghrelin secretion after a meal (Nakahara et al., 2007; Stock et al., 2005). Finally, it has been demonstrated in women that hyperinsulinemia causes ghrelin to decrease much more significantly in AN patients compared to thin and obese control women. This might lead to earlier or increased feeling of satiety in AN patients after even a small carbohydrate-rich meal (Karczewska-Kupczewska et al., 2010).

There are no long-term studies on the treatment of restrictive AN with either ghrelin or ghrelin mimetics. Aside from its orexigenic effects, however, it is unclear if treatment with agents that activate the GHS-R1a would have any effect on AN by increasing GH level further and possibly raising IGF-1. Also, the anti-inflammatory and antisympathetic nervous system effects of GHS may help in this chronic condition or prove to be useless in a condition often associated with many psychological factors resulting in severe caloric restriction and weight loss. On the other hand, AN patients also suffer from loss of LBM, and long-term studies in patients with restrictive AN on ghrelin may show preservation of LBM and muscle mass, even without changes in food intake, and help prevent some of the more serious complications seen in AN such as cardiac cachexia or arrhythmias, amenorrhea, and accelerated bone loss. Although ANRT is a complicated and multifactorial disorder, the potential benefits of ghrelin therapy in these patients may go beyond just improvement in appetite. As Murphy et al. showed, GHS therapy can prevent weight loss in the setting of caloric restriction even in the absence of increased food intake (Murphy et al., 1998). More studies are needed to evaluate short- and long-term effects of ghrelin or GHS on these outcomes.

9. GHRELIN AND CHF-INDUCED CACHEXIA

CHF is another chronic medical condition associated with unintentional weight loss and muscle wasting. Epidemiologic studies have shown that in patients with end-stage CHF, cachexia and weight loss are strong independent risk factors associated with increased mortality (Anker et al., 1997). Interestingly, after cardiac transplantation in CHF patients, it appears that there is no effect of body weight change on survival (Clark et al., 2007). Elevations in circulating ghrelin have been documented in CHF patients and believed to be a compensatory mechanism in response to anabolic/catabolic imbalance (Nagaya, Uematsu, Kojima, Date, et al., 2001). It is important to also keep in mind that ghrelin appears to have direct cardiovascular (CV) effects in addition to antiwasting properties in CHF.

In rat models of heart failure, ghrelin administration increases left ventricular (LV) ejection fraction and LV mass. Also, CHF rats treated with ghrelin showed a greater increase in body weight than those given placebo (Nagaya, Uematsu, Kojima, Ikeda, et al., 2001). Similarly, in another rat model of CHF induced via abdominal aortic banding for 9 weeks, rats were treated with GHRP-1, -2, and -6 and hexarelin (100 μg/kg), subcutaneously twice daily for 3 weeks compared to saline. GHRP treatment significantly improved LV ejection fraction, LV end-systolic pressure, and cardiac remodeling. Mean body weight in animals was significantly higher in the four CHF-GHRP groups than in the CHF-saline group. Finally, norepinephrine, renin, angiotensin II, aldosterone, atrial natriuretic peptide, and endothelin-1 decreased significantly in CHF-GHRP groups compared with the CHF-saline group reflecting a diminished neurohormonal stress response (Xu et al., 2005). In a different rat model of CHF, heart failure was established by ligation of the left anterior descending coronary artery inducing myocardial infarction (MI) and eventually heart failure. Twenty-eight days after surgery, infarcted rats were randomized to several treatment arms ranging from continuous infusion of human ghrelin via SC pump infusion to placebo versus SC injections three times daily of low-dose human ghrelin (50 nmol/kg/d) or high-dose ghrelin (100 nmol/kg/d; Akashi et al., 2009). This study showed increase in body weight, fat mass (noted after 55 days of treatment) and increased lean body mass in rats with CHF treated with continuous and three times daily ghrelin infusion. However, this study did not show any changes in LVEF or cardiac function. In another murine model of CHF and MI, ghrelin treatment significantly attenuated LV enlargement. In addition, there was a significant decrease in LV end-diastolic pressure and less MI-induced increase in heart rate and plasma norepinephrine concentration in ghrelin-treated mice compared to controls. This highlights not only the effects of ghrelin on sympathetic tone but also the possible cardio-protective effects of ghrelin (Soeki et al., 2008).

In humans, ghrelin induces vasodilation *in vitro* (Wiley & Davenport, 2002), decreases system vascular resistance in patients with CHF, increases cardiac output, inhibits sympathetic nerve activity, and stimulates feeding (Nagaya, Miyatake, et al., 2001). Ghrelin and des-acyl ghrelin also inhibit apoptosis of primary adult and H9c2 cardiac myocytes and endothelial cells *in vitro* through activation of ERK 1/2 and Akt serine kinases (Baldanzi et al., 2002). In a clinical study of NYHA stage III–IV CHF patients, 10 subjects (8 had cardiac cachexia) were randomized to receive ghrelin (2 μg/kg twice a day) intravenously and 8 were in the control group (6 of which had cardiac cachexia). Ghrelin treatment for 3 weeks increased food intake; there was a trend favoring body weight increase, and increased lean body mass and hand grip strength were noted. From a CV standpoint, there was a significant decrease in plasma norepinephrine and epinephrine, increased LV ejection fraction, increased LV mass, and decreased LV end-systolic volume. Furthermore, ghrelin improved exercise capacity in patients with CHF, as indicated by an increase in peak workload and peak VO_2, and even improved New York Heart Association (NYHA) functional class in 4 out of 10 patients (Nagaya et al., 2004).

In conclusion, it appears that in the setting of CHF ghrelin has many mechanisms to counteract cachexia including increased appetite and energy intake, anti-inflammatory effects, and increasing GH levels. Ghrelin also decreases sympathetic nerve outflow, a key pathologic abnormality in CHF, and inhibits apoptosis of cardiac myocytes and endothelial cells (Akamizu & Kangawa, 2011; Nagaya & Kangawa, 2006). Future studies involving larger groups of patients are needed to determine the potential role of ghrelin as a treatment for CHF cachexia.

10. GHRELIN AND ESRD

In chronic kidney disease (CKD) and ESRD rat models and human studies, anorexia, weight loss with significant LBM loss, increased muscle catabolism, increased energy expenditure, and increased inflammation have all been reported (Bailey et al., 1996; Benigni & Remuzzi, 2001; Chertow, Ackert, Lew, Lazarus, & Lowrie, 2000; Du et al., 2004; Kaysen et al., 2004; Mitch, 2002; Pickering et al., 2002). In addition, just like other chronic diseases associated with cachexia, the presence of cachexia in CKD is associated with worse quality of life and increased morbidity and mortality (Bologa et al., 1998; Chertow, Johansen, Lew, Lazarus, & Lowrie, 2000; Dwyer et al., 2002). In patients with ESRD, conflicting results for circulating ghrelin concentrations have been reported. Aygen et al. recently reported elevations in both serum and salivary total and acyl ghrelin in prehemodialysis (HD) ESRD patients in comparison to post-HD and age-matched healthy controls

(Aygen et al., 2009). However, Iglesias et al. indicated that patients undergoing HD had similar total ghrelin concentrations to the control group, and that only peritoneal dialysis (PD) patients had a significantly lower total ghrelin concentrations at baseline compared to others (Iglesias et al., 2006). These mixed results are likely due to different factors in ESRD/CKD patients including use of different ghrelin assays, variation in residual renal function in these patients, and possibly different clearance of ghrelin via HD versus PD among other factors (Akamizu & Kangawa, 2011). Nevertheless, ESRD appears to be associated with increases in total ghrelin levels and normal acyl ghrelin levels. This probably occurs because des-acyl ghrelin is cleared through the kidneys and accumulates with renal insufficiency leading to elevations in total ghrelin levels (Hillman et al., 2011).

In a surgical model of CKD in rats—via nephrectomy—which causes uremia and decreased accrual of lean body mass, treatment with ghrelin and GHS (BIM-28125 and BIM-28131) increased food intake and improved lean body mass by decreasing muscle protein degradation. Similar to cancer cachexia, elevated circulating cytokines have been found in ESRD cachexia. Ghrelin treatment also decreased circulating inflammatory cytokines in nephrectomized animals treated with ghrelin compared to saline (Deboer et al., 2008). Furthermore, nephrectomized rats have been shown to have impairment of skeletal muscle mitochondrial oxidative capacity (expressed by low levels of cytochrome *c* oxidase and citrate synthase). Ghrelin treatment normalizes the activity of these mitochondrial enzymes and helps preserve lean body mass in rats by stimulating AKT (PKB) phosphorylation preventing protein catabolism in muscle (Barazzoni et al., 2010).

In human trials, ghrelin has shown promising effects in CKD patients by increasing food intake in malnourished patients on peritoneal (Wynne et al., 2005) and HD (Ashby et al., 2009) after SC ghrelin injections. Since the prevalence of CKD and ESRD is predicted to increase significantly—as a result of our aging population and diabetes epidemic—cachexia resulting from chronic renal disease is likely to become more widespread. Therefore, more studies addressing the benefits and safety of ghrelin therapy in this population are needed.

11. AIDS-ASSOCIATED CACHEXIA

Cachexia has also been found in other chronic conditions such as AIDS. During the early periods of the human immune deficiency virus (HIV)/AIDS epidemic, cachexia was a common condition. This prompted significant research into possible treatments for this phenomenon and led the U.S. Food and Drug Administration to approve the use of recombinant GH therapy for HIV/AIDS wasting (Gullett, Hebbar, & Ziegler, 2010). Over the past decades, however, HIV/AIDS cachexia has become a much less common entity likely due to many factors including earlier detection of infection, more effective antiretroviral regimens leading to better control of the viral load, and more access to care for this population. For the majority of these cases, cachexia occurs usually secondary to uncontrolled HIV infection/AIDS and is often treated by optimization of antiviral therapy. To our knowledge, there are no reports of ghrelin or GHS use in this setting.

12. RA-ASSOCIATED CACHEXIA

Although RA has been affecting patients for centuries, only over the past two decades has it been recognized that in addition to joint and system-wide inflammatory damage, nearly two-thirds of all patients with RA experience a muscle wasting condition known as rheumatoid cachexia (Koca et al., 2008; Walsmith & Roubenoff, 2002). However, unlike cancer and AIDS cachexia—in which cachexia often closely precedes death–rheumatoid cachexia is not directly fatal (Roubenoff, Roubenoff, Ward, Holland, & Hellmann, 1992). RA cachexia diminishes muscle strength and functional capacity, and contributes to morbidity and reduced life expectancy in these patients (Walsmith & Roubenoff, 2002). The average loss of body cell mass (BCM) among patients with RA is between 13% and 15% or approximately one-third of the maximum survivable loss of BCM (Rall & Roubenoff, 2004). Similar to other mechanisms of cachexia, in RA, cachexia appears to be related to decreased GH/IGF-1 levels and the direct effect of the inflammatory cytokines TNF-α and IL-1β. In fact, TNF-α and IL-1β are not only responsible for inflicting joint damage in RA but also play a role in protein degradation and negative energy balance among many other cytokines: IL-6, IFN-γ, transforming growth factor-β (TGF-β_1), and the transcription factor MyoD (Rall & Roubenoff, 2004). TNF-α appears to be a central mediator of muscle wasting by acting synergistically with IL1-β and activating NF-κB (Dinarello & Roubenoff, 1996; Lecker, Solomon, Mitch, & Goldberg, 1999) to inhibit skeletal muscle differentiation by suppressing MyoD, which is essential for regulation of skeletal muscle differentiation and tissue repair, at the posttranscriptional level (Guttridge, Mayo, Madrid, Wang, & Baldwin, 2000).

To date, there are not many studies evaluating the role of ghrelin and RA. The GHS-R1a receptor is also expressed on lymphocytes, and administration of the GHS GHRP-2 in a rat model of arthritis has been shown to decrease serum levels of IL-6 and reduce signs of joint inflammation (Granado, Priego, Martin, Villanua, & Lopez-Calderon, 2005). In rat adjuvant arthritis (AA), an animal model similar to RA, cachexia is also often seen. One study evaluated NPY expression in hypothalamic arcuate nuclei (nARC) under the conditions of AA and found that decreased appetite, body mass, and epididymal fat stores positively correlated with increased ghrelin in plasma, reduced circulating and epididymal fat leptin, and decreased adiponectin. Furthermore, arcuate nucleus mRNA for the GHSR, leptin, and NPY receptor were also overexpressed in AA rats (Stofkova et al., 2009). On the other hand, another animal study found decreased ghrelin concentrations in AA rats 7 days after injection with FCA (a mycobacterium tuberculosis suspension that causes inflammation and leads to arthritis) and no difference in gastric ghrelin mRNA on days 7 and 15 between AA versus control rats (Otero et al., 2004).

In humans, Otero et al. also showed decreased ghrelin concentrations in 31 RA patients compared to 18 healthy controls (Otero et al., 2004). However, some have questioned this study; due to a heterogeneous patient population comprising males and females, only 22 of the 31 patients had active disease, and 9 patients were on TNF-α-blocking agents (Magiera et al., 2011). Similarly, a larger study of 37 patients with RA and 29 patients with Behçet's disease (BD; another chronic inflammatory condition) compared to 28 healthy controls found that total ghrelin was lower in the RA group compared to both the BD and the control group even after adjusting for age, gender, BMI, and disease duration (Koca et al., 2008). These findings may reflect the chronic nature of RA which has an indolent course and possibly reflects a net loss in muscle mass but not total weight in subjects. Ghrelin may therefore not be elevated secondary to the slow changes in body composition that occur. Interestingly, another study looked at the acute effect of infliximab (anti-TNF-α) administration on circulating ghrelin levels at baseline compared to 120 min after infusion in 33 nondiabetic patients with RA. Anti-TNF-α therapy was associated with a rapid increase in circulating ghrelin in patients with severe RA 120 min after infusion (Gonzalez-Gay et al., 2008). Patients receiving long-term infliximab therapy, however, appear to have decreased ghrelin values. For example, Magiera et al. looked at 18 NW adult women with RA and the effects of long-term infliximab and methotrexate therapy on ghrelin levels. In the absence of cachexia, ghrelin levels were higher at baseline compared to healthy individuals, and levels decreased 1 week after the first infusion, and remained low even after 1 year of infliximab treatment every 8 weeks (Magiera et al., 2011). Interestingly, ghrelin levels were different before therapy and 1 week after TNF-α blockade, but no difference was noted 1 week after treatment compared to 53 weeks after long-term therapy. This supports that TNF-α blockade has an acute effect on ghrelin levels in RA. However, both studies by Gonzalez-Gay and Magiera et al. looked at ghrelin levels in RA patients without cachexia and therefore may not be generalized to RA cachexia.

Experiments with ghrelin infusion or GHS in RA are lacking. As previous studies with ghrelin have shown, administration of supra-physiologic doses of ghrelin may be beneficial in alleviating cachexia. Ghrelin administration may decrease inflammation, improve appetite and lean body mass preservation, and decrease energy expenditure in RA-induced cachexia patients. In addition, the anti-inflammatory effects of ghrelin may not only be beneficial to combat cachexia but also play a role as a possible immunomodulatory agent to help combat disease activity in RA. Further studies are needed to see if ghrelin by itself is effective, or if it may have synergistic with other anti-inflammatory and immune-modulator therapies currently used to treat RA.

13. CONCLUSIONS

Since its discovery in 1999, ghrelin has been proposed as a treatment for sarcopenia or cachexia in many medical conditions ranging from aging to cancer cachexia, CHF and ESRD. There are a number of studies that looked at the effects of ghrelin treatment in the setting of cachexia in different animal models (Table 3.1) and also in humans (Table 3.2). Our current knowledge indicates that ghrelin may be effective at increasing appetite and body weight, and preserving lean body mass by decreasing protein degradation. In addition, ghrelin is known to affect the immune system, decreasing inflammation, and sympathetic outflow. In 13 years since its discovery, ghrelin has gone from a novel hormone to be a key player in the regulation of appetite and body weight. With several clinical trials ongoing in wasting conditions, the next decade should provide answers regarding its clinical effectiveness and safety in these settings.

ACKNOWLEDGMENTS

Dr. J. G. receives research support from the Department of Veterans Affairs (MERIT Grants: I01-BX000507 and I01 CX000174 and the NIA T32AG000183 and AG040583). Dr. B. G. is supported by a training grant from the NIA (T32AG000183).

REFERENCES

Akamizu, T., & Kangawa, K. (2011). Therapeutic applications of ghrelin to cachexia utilizing its appetite-stimulating effect. *Peptides*, *32*, 2295–2300.

Akashi, Y. J., Palus, S., Datta, R., Halem, H., Taylor, J. E., Thoene-Reineke, C., et al. (2009). No effects of human ghrelin on cardiac function despite profound effects on body composition in a rat model of heart failure. *International Journal of Cardiology*, *137*, 267–275.

Albarran-Zeckler, R. G., Sun, Y., & Smith, R. G. (2011). Physiological roles revealed by ghrelin and ghrelin receptor deficient mice. *Peptides*, *32*, 2229–2235.

Anker, S. D., Ponikowski, P., Varney, S., Chua, T. P., Clark, A. L., Webb-Peploe, K. M., et al. (1997). Wasting as independent risk factor for mortality in chronic heart failure. *Lancet*, *349*, 1050–1053.

Asakawa, A., Inui, A., Kaga, T., Yuzuriha, H., Nagata, T., Ueno, N., et al. (2001). Ghrelin is an appetite-stimulatory signal from stomach with structural resemblance to motilin. *Gastroenterology*, *120*, 337–345.

Ashby, D., Choi, P., & Bloom, S. (2008). Gut hormones and the treatment of disease cachexia. *The Proceedings of the Nutrition Society*, *67*, 263–269.

Ashby, D. R., Ford, H. E., Wynne, K. J., Wren, A. M., Murphy, K. G., Busbridge, M., et al. (2009). Sustained appetite improvement in malnourished dialysis patients by daily ghrelin treatment. *Kidney International*, *76*, 199–206.

Ashitani, J., Matsumoto, N., & Nakazato, M. (2009). Ghrelin and its therapeutic potential for cachectic patients. *Peptides*, *30*, 1951–1956.

Aygen, B., Dogukan, A., Dursun, F. E., Aydin, S., Kilic, N., Sahpaz, F., et al. (2009). Ghrelin and obestatin levels in end-stage renal disease. *The Journal of International Medical Research*, *37*, 757–765.

Babbini, M., & Davis, W. M. (1972). Time-dose relationships for locomotor activity effects of morphine after acute or repeated treatment. *British Journal of Pharmacology*, *46*, 213–224.

Bailey, J. L., Wang, X., England, B. K., Price, S. R., Ding, X., & Mitch, W. E. (1996). The acidosis of chronic renal failure activates muscle proteolysis in rats by augmenting transcription of genes encoding proteins of the ATP-dependent ubiquitin-proteasome pathway. *The Journal of Clinical Investigation*, *97*, 1447–1453.

Balasubramaniam, A., Joshi, R., Su, C., Friend, L. A., Sheriff, S., Kagan, R. J., et al. (2009). Ghrelin inhibits skeletal muscle protein breakdown in rats with thermal injury through normalizing elevated expression of E3 ubiquitin ligases MuRF1 and MAFbx. *American Journal of Physiology. Regulatory, Integrative and Comparative Physiology*, *296*, R893–R901.

Baldanzi, G., Filigheddu, N., Cutrupi, S., Catapano, F., Bonissoni, S., Fubini, A., et al. (2002). Ghrelin and des-acyl ghrelin inhibit cell death in cardiomyocytes and endothelial cells through ERK1/2 and PI 3-kinase/AKT. *The Journal of Cell Biology*, *159*, 1029–1037.

Barazzoni, R., Bosutti, A., Stebel, M., Cattin, M. R., Roder, E., Visintin, L., et al. (2005). Ghrelin regulates mitochondrial-lipid metabolism gene expression and tissue fat distribution in liver and skeletal muscle. *American Journal of Physiology. Endocrinology and Metabolism*, *288*, E228–E235.

Barazzoni, R., Zhu, X., Deboer, M., Datta, R., Culler, M. D., Zanetti, M., et al. (2010). Combined effects of ghrelin and higher food intake enhance skeletal muscle mitochondrial oxidative capacity and AKT phosphorylation in rats with chronic kidney disease. *Kidney International*, *77*, 23–28.

Bark, T. H., McNurlan, M. A., Lang, C. H., & Garlick, P. J. (1998). Increased protein synthesis after acute IGF-I or insulin infusion is localized to muscle in mice. *The American Journal of Physiology*, *275*, E118–E123.

Barsh, G. S., He, L., & Gunn, T. M. (2002). Genetic and biochemical studies of the Agouti-attractin system. *Journal of Receptor and Signal Transduction Research*, *22*, 63–77.

Barthel, A., Schmoll, D., & Unterman, T. G. (2005). FoxO proteins in insulin action and metabolism. *Trends in Endocrinology and Metabolism*, *16*, 183–189.

Bartlett, D. L., Charland, S., & Torosian, M. H. (1994). Growth hormone, insulin, and somatostatin therapy of cancer cachexia. *Cancer*, *73*, 1499–1504.

Bartlett, D. L., Stein, T. P., & Torosian, M. H. (1995). Effect of growth hormone and protein intake on tumor growth and host cachexia. *Surgery, 117*, 260–267.

Benigni, A., & Remuzzi, G. (2001). How renal cytokines and growth factors contribute to renal disease progression. *American Journal of Kidney Diseases, 37*, S21–S24.

Bodine, S. C., Stitt, T. N., Gonzalez, M., Kline, W. O., Stover, G. L., Bauerlein, R., et al. (2001). Akt/mTOR pathway is a crucial regulator of skeletal muscle hypertrophy and can prevent muscle atrophy in vivo. *Nature Cell Biology, 3*, 1014–1019.

Bologa, R. M., Levine, D. M., Parker, T. S., Cheigh, J. S., Serur, D., Stenzel, K. H., et al. (1998). Interleukin-6 predicts hypoalbuminemia, hypocholesterolemia, and mortality in hemodialysis patients. *American Journal of Kidney Diseases, 32*, 107–114.

Bowen, J., Noakes, M., & Clifton, P. M. (2007). Appetite hormones and energy intake in obese men after consumption of fructose, glucose and whey protein beverages. *International Journal of Obesity, 31*, 1696–1703.

Bowers, C. Y. (2001). Unnatural growth hormone-releasing peptide begets natural ghrelin. *The Journal of Clinical Endocrinology and Metabolism, 86*, 1464–1469.

Bowers, C. Y., Momany, F. A., Reynolds, G. A., & Hong, A. (1984). On the in vitro and in vivo activity of a new synthetic hexapeptide that acts on the pituitary to specifically release growth hormone. *Endocrinology, 114*, 1537–1545.

Bowers, C. Y., Reynolds, G. A., Chang, D., Hong, A., Chang, K., & Momany, F. (1981). A study on the regulation of growth hormone release from the pituitaries of rats in vitro. *Endocrinology, 108*, 1071–1080.

Broglio, F., Gianotti, L., Destefanis, S., Fassino, S., Abbate Daga, G., Mondelli, V., et al. (2004). The endocrine response to acute ghrelin administration is blunted in patients with anorexia nervosa, a ghrelin hypersecretory state. *Clinical Endocrinology, 60*, 592–599.

Camanni, F., Ghigo, E., & Arvat, E. (1998). Growth hormone-releasing peptides and their analogs. *Frontiers in Neuroendocrinology, 19*, 47–72.

Camina, J. P., Carreira, M. C., El Messari, S., Llorens-Cortes, C., Smith, R. G., & Casanueva, F. F. (2004). Desensitization and endocytosis mechanisms of ghrelin-activated growth hormone secretagogue receptor 1a. *Endocrinology, 145*, 930–940.

Cannata, D., Vijayakumar, A., Fierz, Y., & LeRoith, D. (2010). The GH/IGF-1 axis in growth and development: New insights derived from animal models. *Advances in Pediatrics, 57*, 331–351.

Carlsson, P., & Mahlapuu, M. (2002). Forkhead transcription factors: Key players in development and metabolism. *Developmental Biology, 250*, 1–23.

Cassoni, P., Ghe, C., Marrocco, T., Tarabra, E., Allia, E., Catapano, F., et al. (2004). Expression of ghrelin and biological activity of specific receptors for ghrelin and des-acyl ghrelin in human prostate neoplasms and related cell lines. *European Journal of Endocrinology, 150*, 173–184.

Cassoni, P., Papotti, M., Catapano, F., Ghe, C., Deghenghi, R., Ghigo, E., et al. (2000). Specific binding sites for synthetic growth hormone secretagogues in non-tumoral and neoplastic human thyroid tissue. *The Journal of Endocrinology, 165*, 139–146.

Cassoni, P., Papotti, M., Ghe, C., Catapano, F., Sapino, A., Graziani, A., et al. (2001). Identification, characterization, and biological activity of specific receptors for natural (ghrelin) and synthetic growth hormone secretagogues and analogs in human breast carcinomas and cell lines. *The Journal of Clinical Endocrinology and Metabolism, 86*, 1738–1745.

Chaiban, J. T., Bitar, F. F., & Azar, S. T. (2008). Effect of chronic hypoxia on leptin, insulin, adiponectin, and ghrelin. *Metabolism, 57*, 1019–1022.

Chen, H. Y., Trumbauer, M. E., Chen, A. S., Weingarth, D. T., Adams, J. R., Frazier, E. G., et al. (2004). Orexigenic action of peripheral ghrelin is mediated by neuropeptide Y and agouti-related protein. *Endocrinology, 145*, 2607–2612.

Chertow, G. M., Ackert, K., Lew, N. L., Lazarus, J. M., & Lowrie, E. G. (2000). Prealbumin is as important as albumin in the nutritional assessment of hemodialysis patients. *Kidney International, 58*, 2512–2517.

Chertow, G. M., Johansen, K. L., Lew, N., Lazarus, J. M., & Lowrie, E. G. (2000). Vintage, nutritional status, and survival in hemodialysis patients. *Kidney International, 57*, 1176–1181.

Clark, A. L., Knosalla, C., Birks, E., Loebe, M., Davos, C. H., Tsang, S., et al. (2007). Heart transplantation in heart failure: The prognostic importance of body mass index at time of surgery and subsequent weight changes. *European Journal of Heart Failure, 9*, 839–844.

Cowley, M. A., Smith, R. G., Diano, S., Tschop, M., Pronchuk, N., Grove, K. L., et al. (2003). The distribution and mechanism of action of ghrelin in the CNS demonstrates a novel hypothalamic circuit regulating energy homeostasis. *Neuron, 37*, 649–661.

Cruz, C. R., & Smith, R. G. (2008). The growth hormone secretagogue receptor. *Vitamins and Hormones*, 77, 47–88.

Cummings, D. E., Clement, K., Purnell, J. Q., Vaisse, C., Foster, K. E., Frayo, R. S., et al. (2002). Elevated plasma ghrelin levels in Prader Willi syndrome. *Nature Medicine, 8*, 643–644.

Cummings, D. E., & Overduin, J. (2007). Gastrointestinal regulation of food intake. *The Journal of Clinical Investigation, 117*, 13–23.

Davies, J. S., Kotokorpi, P., Eccles, S. R., Barnes, S. K., Tokarczuk, P. F., Allen, S. K., et al. (2009). Ghrelin induces abdominal obesity via GHS-R-dependent lipid retention. *Molecular Endocrinology, 23*, 914–924.

Deboer, M. D., Zhu, X., Levasseur, P. R., Inui, A., Hu, Z., Han, G., et al. (2008). Ghrelin treatment of chronic kidney disease: Improvements in lean body mass and cytokine profile. *Endocrinology, 149*, 827–835.

DeBoer, M. D., Zhu, X. X., Levasseur, P., Meguid, M. M., Suzuki, S., Inui, A., et al. (2007). Ghrelin treatment causes increased food intake and retention of lean body mass in a rat model of cancer cachexia. *Endocrinology, 148*, 3004–3012.

Dickson, S. L., Egecioglu, E., Landgren, S., Skibicka, K. P., Engel, J. A., & Jerlhag, E. (2011). The role of the central ghrelin system in reward from food and chemical drugs. *Molecular and Cellular Endocrinology, 340*, 80–87.

Dinarello, C. A., & Roubenoff, R. (1996). George Clowes' classic paper and the search for "muscle proteolysis factor" *Nutrition, 12*, 67–68.

Ding, J., List, E. O., Bower, B. D., & Kopchick, J. J. (2011). Differential effects of growth hormone versus insulin-like growth factor-I on the mouse plasma proteome. *Endocrinology, 152*, 3791–3802.

Dixit, M. P., Xu, L., Xu, H., Bai, L., Collins, J. F., & Ghishan, F. K. (2004). Effect of angiotensin-II on renal Na+/H+ exchanger-NHE3 and NHE2. *Biochimica et Biophysica Acta, 1664*, 38–44.

Dixit, V. D., Yang, H., Sun, Y., Weeraratna, A. T., Youm, Y. H., Smith, R. G., et al. (2007). Ghrelin promotes thymopoiesis during aging. *The Journal of Clinical Investigation, 117*, 2778–2790.

Dominici, F. P., Argentino, D. P., Munoz, M. C., Miquet, J. G., Sotelo, A. I., & Turyn, D. (2005). Influence of the crosstalk between growth hormone and insulin signalling on the modulation of insulin sensitivity. *Growth Hormone & IGF Research, 15*, 324–336.

Druce, M. R., Wren, A. M., Park, A. J., Milton, J. E., Patterson, M., Frost, G., et al. (2005). Ghrelin increases food intake in obese as well as lean subjects. *International Journal of Obesity, 29*, 1130–1136.

Du, J., Wang, X., Miereles, C., Bailey, J. L., Debigare, R., Zheng, B., et al. (2004). Activation of caspase-3 is an initial step triggering accelerated muscle proteolysis in catabolic conditions. *The Journal of Clinical Investigation, 113*, 115–123.

Dwyer, J. T., Larive, B., Leung, J., Rocco, M., Burrowes, J. D., Chumlea, W. C., et al. (2002). Nutritional status affects quality of life in Hemodialysis (HEMO) Study patients at baseline. *Journal of Renal Nutrition*, *12*, 213–223.

Elijah, I. E., Branski, L. K., Finnerty, C. C., & Herndon, D. N. (2011). The GH/IGF-1 system in critical illness. *Best Practice & Research. Clinical Endocrinology & Metabolism*, *25*, 759–767.

Fairburn, C. G., & Harrison, P. J. (2003). Eating disorders. *Lancet*, *361*, 407–416.

Fermoselle, C., Sanchez, F., & Barreiro, E. (2011). Reduction of muscle mass mediated by myostatin in an experimental model of pulmonary emphysema. *Archivos de Bronconeumología*, *47*, 590–598.

Filigheddu, N., Gnocchi, V. F., Coscia, M., Cappelli, M., Porporato, P. E., Taulli, R., et al. (2007). Ghrelin and des-acyl ghrelin promote differentiation and fusion of C2C12 skeletal muscle cells. *Molecular Biology of the Cell*, *18*, 986–994.

Fontana, L., Partridge, L., & Longo, V. D. (2010). Extending healthy life span—From yeast to humans. *Science*, *328*, 321–326.

Fouladiun, M., Korner, U., Bosaeus, I., Daneryd, P., Hyltander, A., & Lundholm, K. G. (2005). Body composition and time course changes in regional distribution of fat and lean tissue in unselected cancer patients on palliative care—Correlations with food intake, metabolism, exercise capacity, and hormones. *Cancer*, *103*, 2189–2198.

Fryburg, D. A. (1994). Insulin-like growth factor I exerts growth hormone- and insulin-like actions on human muscle protein metabolism. *The American Journal of Physiology*, *267*, E331–E336.

Gahete, M. D., Cordoba-Chacon, J., Hergueta-Redondo, M., Martinez-Fuentes, A. J., Kineman, R. D., Moreno-Bueno, G., et al. (2011). A novel human ghrelin variant (In1-ghrelin) and ghrelin-O-acyltransferase are overexpressed in breast cancer: Potential pathophysiological relevance. *PloS One*, *6*, e23302.

Garcia, J. M., Cata, J. P., Dougherty, P. M., & Smith, R. G. (2008). Ghrelin prevents cisplatin-induced mechanical hyperalgesia and cachexia. *Endocrinology*, *149*, 455–460.

Garcia, J. M., Garcia-Touza, M., Hijazi, R. A., Taffet, G., Epner, D., Mann, D., et al. (2005). Active ghrelin levels and active to total ghrelin ratio in cancer-induced cachexia. *The Journal of Clinical Endocrinology and Metabolism*, *90*, 2920–2926.

Garcia, J. M., Graham, C., Kumor, R., & Polvino, W. (2007). Phase II, randomized, placebo-controlled, double blind study of the efficacy and safety of RC-1291 for the treatment of cancer cachexia. *Journal of Clinical Oncology*, *25*, S25.

Garcia, J. M., & Polvino, W. J. (2007). Effect on body weight and safety of RC-1291, a novel, orally available ghrelin mimetic and growth hormone secretagogue: Results of a phase I, randomized, placebo-controlled, multiple-dose study in healthy volunteers. *The Oncologist*, *12*, 594–600.

Gianotti, L., Lanfranco, F., Ramunni, J., Destefanis, S., Ghigo, E., & Arvat, E. (2002). GH/IGF-I axis in anorexia nervosa. *Eating and Weight Disorders*, *7*, 94–105.

Giovambattista, A., Gaillard, R. C., & Spinedi, E. (2008). Ghrelin gene-related peptides modulate rat white adiposity. *Vitamins and Hormones*, *77*, 171–205.

Glauser, D. A., & Schlegel, W. (2007). The emerging role of FOXO transcription factors in pancreatic beta cells. *The Journal of Endocrinology*, *193*, 195–207.

Gnanapavan, S., Kola, B., Bustin, S. A., Morris, D. G., McGee, P., Fairclough, P., et al. (2002). The tissue distribution of the mRNA of ghrelin and subtypes of its receptor, GHS-R, in humans. *The Journal of Clinical Endocrinology and Metabolism*, *87*, 2988.

Gonzalez-Gay, M. A., Garcia-Unzueta, M. T., Berja, A., Vazquez-Rodriguez, T. R., Gonzalez-Juanatey, C., de Matias, J. M., et al. (2008). Anti-tumour necrosis factor alpha therapy modulates ghrelin in patients with severe rheumatoid arthritis. *Annals of the Rheumatic Diseases*, *67*, 1644–1646.

Gosker, H. R., Langen, R. C., Bracke, K. R., Joos, G. F., Brusselle, G. G., Steele, C., et al. (2009). Extrapulmonary manifestations of chronic obstructive pulmonary disease in a mouse model of chronic cigarette smoke exposure. *American Journal of Respiratory Cell and Molecular Biology*, *40*, 710–716.

Granado, M., Priego, T., Martin, A. I., Villanua, M. A., & Lopez-Calderon, A. (2005). Anti-inflammatory effect of the ghrelin agonist growth hormone-releasing peptide-2 (GHRP-2) in arthritic rats. *American Journal of Physiology. Endocrinology and Metabolism*, *288*, E486–E492.

Granata, R., Isgaard, J., Alloatti, G., & Ghigo, E. (2011). Cardiovascular actions of the ghrelin gene-derived peptides and growth hormone-releasing hormone. *Experimental Biology and Medicine (Maywood, NJ)*, *236*, 505–514.

Gullett, N. P., Hebbar, G., & Ziegler, T. R. (2010). Update on clinical trials of growth factors and anabolic steroids in cachexia and wasting. *The American Journal of Clinical Nutrition*, *91*, 1143S–1147S.

Guney, Y., Ozel Turkcu, U., Hicsonmez, A., Nalca Andrieu, M., & Kurtman, C. (2007). Ghrelin may reduce radiation-induced mucositis and anorexia in head-neck cancer. *Medical Hypotheses*, *68*, 538–540.

Gutierrez, J. A., Solenberg, P. J., Perkins, D. R., Willency, J. A., Knierman, M. D., Jin, Z., et al. (2008). Ghrelin octanoylation mediated by an orphan lipid transferase. *Proceedings of the National Academy of Sciences of the United States of America*, *105*, 6320–6325.

Guttridge, D. C., Mayo, M. W., Madrid, L. V., Wang, C. Y., & Baldwin, A. S., Jr. (2000). NF-kappaB-induced loss of MyoD messenger RNA: Possible role in muscle decay and cachexia. *Science*, *289*, 2363–2366.

Haentjens, P., Magaziner, J., Colon-Emeric, C. S., Vanderschueren, D., Milisen, K., Velkeniers, B., et al. (2010). Meta-analysis: Excess mortality after hip fracture among older women and men. *Annals of Internal Medicine*, *152*, 380–390.

Hahn, T. M., Breininger, J. F., Baskin, D. G., & Schwartz, M. W. (1998). Coexpression of Agrp and NPY in fasting-activated hypothalamic neurons. *Nature Neuroscience*, *1*, 271–272.

Hall, D. T., Ma, J. F., Marco, S. D., & Gallouzi, I. E. (2011). Inducible nitric oxide synthase (iNOS) in muscle wasting syndrome, sarcopenia, and cachexia. *Aging (Albany NY)*, *3*, 702–715.

Hanada, T., Toshinai, K., Date, Y., Kajimura, N., Tsukada, T., Hayashi, Y., et al. (2004). Upregulation of ghrelin expression in cachectic nude mice bearing human melanoma cells. *Metabolism*, *53*, 84–88.

Hanada, T., Toshinai, K., Kajimura, N., Nara-Ashizawa, N., Tsukada, T., Hayashi, Y., et al. (2003). Anti-cachectic effect of ghrelin in nude mice bearing human melanoma cells. *Biochemical and Biophysical Research Communications*, *301*, 275–279.

Hattori, N. (2009). Expression, regulation and biological actions of growth hormone (GH) and ghrelin in the immune system. *Growth Hormone & IGF Research*, *19*, 187–197.

Hillman, J. B., Tong, J., & Tschop, M. (2011). Ghrelin biology and its role in weight-related disorders. *Discovery Medicine*, *11*, 521–528.

Hiura, Y., Takiguchi, S., Yamamoto, K., Takahashi, T., Kurokawa, Y., Yamasaki, M., et al. (2012). Effects of ghrelin administration during chemotherapy with advanced esophageal cancer patients: A prospective, randomized, placebo-controlled phase 2 study. *Cancer*, *118*, 4785–4794.

Horvath, T. L., Diano, S., Sotonyi, P., Heiman, M., & Tschop, M. (2001). Minireview: Ghrelin and the regulation of energy balance—A hypothalamic perspective. *Endocrinology*, *142*, 4163–4169.

Hosoda, H., Kojima, M., Matsuo, H., & Kangawa, K. (2000). Ghrelin and des-acyl ghrelin: Two major forms of rat ghrelin peptide in gastrointestinal tissue. *Biochemical and Biophysical Research Communications*, *279*, 909–913.

Hotta, M., Ohwada, R., Akamizu, T., Shibasaki, T., Takano, K., & Kangawa, K. (2009). Ghrelin increases hunger and food intake in patients with restricting-type anorexia nervosa: A pilot study. *Endocrine Journal*, *56*, 1119–1128.

Howard, A. D., Feighner, S. D., Cully, D. F., Arena, J. P., Liberator, P. A., Rosenblum, C. I., et al. (1996). A receptor in pituitary and hypothalamus that functions in growth hormone release. *Science*, *273*, 974–977.

Huang, Q., Fan, Y. Z., Ge, B. J., Zhu, Q., & Tu, Z. Y. (2007). Circulating ghrelin in patients with gastric or colorectal cancer. *Digestive Diseases and Sciences*, *52*, 803–809.

Huda, M. S., Wilding, J. P., & Pinkney, J. H. (2006). Gut peptides and the regulation of appetite. *Obesity Reviews*, 7, 163–182.

Humbel, R. E. (1990). Insulin-like growth factors I and II. *European Journal of Biochemistry*, *190*, 445–462.

Iglesias, P., Diez, J. J., Fernandez-Reyes, M. J., Codoceo, R., Alvarez-Fidalgo, P., Bajo, M. A., et al. (2006). Serum ghrelin concentrations in patients with chronic renal failure undergoing dialysis. *Clinical Endocrinology*, *64*, 68–73.

Imanaka, M., Iida, K., Murawaki, A., Nishizawa, H., Fukuoka, H., Takeno, R., et al. (2008). Growth hormone stimulates mechano growth factor expression and activates myoblast transformation in C2C12 cells. *The Kobe Journal of Medical Sciences*, *54*, E46–E54.

Inui, A. (2001). Ghrelin: An orexigenic and somatotrophic signal from the stomach. *Nature Reviews. Neuroscience*, *2*, 551–560.

Isgaard, J., Carlsson, L., Isaksson, O. G., & Jansson, J. O. (1988). Pulsatile intravenous growth hormone (GH) infusion to hypophysectomized rats increases insulin-like growth factor I messenger ribonucleic acid in skeletal tissues more effectively than continuous GH infusion. *Endocrinology*, *123*, 2605–2610.

Itoh, T., Nagaya, N., Yoshikawa, M., Fukuoka, A., Takenaka, H., Shimizu, Y., et al. (2004). Elevated plasma ghrelin level in underweight patients with chronic obstructive pulmonary disease. *American Journal of Respiratory and Critical Care Medicine*, *170*, 879–882.

Jeay, S., Sonenshein, G. E., Postel-Vinay, M. C., & Baixeras, E. (2000). Growth hormone prevents apoptosis through activation of nuclear factor-kappaB in interleukin-3-dependent Ba/F3 cell line. *Molecular Endocrinology*, *14*, 650–661.

Kamegai, J., Tamura, H., Shimizu, T., Ishii, S., Sugihara, H., & Wakabayashi, I. (2001). Chronic central infusion of ghrelin increases hypothalamic neuropeptide Y and Agouti-related protein mRNA levels and body weight in rats. *Diabetes*, *50*, 2438–2443.

Kang, K., Schmahl, J., Lee, J. M., Garcia, K., Patil, K., Chen, A., et al. (2012). Mouse ghrelin-O-acyltransferase (GOAT) plays a critical role in bile acid reabsorption. *The FASEB Journal*, *26*, 259–271.

Karapanagiotou, E. M., Polyzos, A., Dilana, K. D., Gratsias, I., Boura, P., Gkiozos, I., et al. (2009). Increased serum levels of ghrelin at diagnosis mediate body weight loss in non-small cell lung cancer (NSCLC) patients. *Lung Cancer*, *66*, 393–398.

Karczewska-Kupczewska, M., Straczkowski, M., Adamska, A., Nikolajuk, A., Otziomek, E., Gorska, M., et al. (2010). Increased suppression of serum ghrelin concentration by hyperinsulinemia in women with anorexia nervosa. *European Journal of Endocrinology*, *162*, 235–239.

Kaysen, G. A., Dubin, J. A., Muller, H. G., Rosales, L., Levin, N. W., & Mitch, W. E. (2004). Inflammation and reduced albumin synthesis associated with stable decline in serum albumin in hemodialysis patients. *Kidney International*, *65*, 1408–1415.

Kemik, O., Sumer, A., Kemik, A. S., Hasirci, I., Purisa, S., Dulger, A. C., et al. (2010). The relationship among acute-phase response proteins, cytokines and hormones in cachectic patients with colon cancer. *World Journal of Surgical Oncology*, *8*, 85.

Kishimoto, M., Okimura, Y., Nakata, H., Kudo, T., Iguchi, G., Takahashi, Y., et al. (2003). Cloning and characterization of the 5(′)-flanking region of the human ghrelin gene. *Biochemical and Biophysical Research Communications*, *305*, 186–192.

Koca, S. S., Ozgen, M., Aydin, S., Dag, S., Evren, B., & Isik, A. (2008). Ghrelin and obestatin levels in rheumatoid arthritis. *Inflammation*, *31*, 329–335.

Kodama, T., Ashitani, J., Matsumoto, N., Kangawa, K., & Nakazato, M. (2008). Ghrelin treatment suppresses neutrophil-dominant inflammation in airways of patients with chronic respiratory infection. *Pulmonary Pharmacology & Therapeutics*, *21*, 774–779.

Kojima, M., Hosoda, H., Date, Y., Nakazato, M., Matsuo, H., & Kangawa, K. (1999). Ghrelin is a growth-hormone-releasing acylated peptide from stomach. *Nature*, *402*, 656–660.

Kojima, M., & Kangawa, K. (2005). Ghrelin: Structure and function. *Physiological Reviews*, *85*, 495–522.

Kopchick, J. J., & Andry, J. M. (2000). Growth hormone (GH), GH receptor, and signal transduction. *Molecular Genetics and Metabolism*, *71*, 293–314.

Korbonits, M., & Grossman, A. B. (1995). Growth hormone-releasing peptide and its analogues novel stimuli to growth hormone release. *Trends in Endocrinology and Metabolism*, *6*, 43–49.

Koyama, K. I., Yasuhara, D., Nakahara, T., Harada, T., Uehara, M., Ushikai, M., et al. (2010). Changes in acyl ghrelin, des-acyl ghrelin, and ratio of acyl ghrelin to total ghrelin with short-term refeeding in female inpatients with restricting-type anorexia nervosa. *Hormone and Metabolic Research*, *42*, 595–598.

Laviano, A., Meguid, M. M., & Rossi-Fanelli, F. (2003). Cancer anorexia: Clinical implications, pathogenesis, and therapeutic strategies. *The Lancet Oncology*, *4*, 686–694.

Lecker, S. H., Solomon, V., Mitch, W. E., & Goldberg, A. L. (1999). Muscle protein breakdown and the critical role of the ubiquitin-proteasome pathway in normal and disease states. *The Journal of Nutrition*, *129*, 227S–237S.

Lee, H. M., Wang, G., Englander, E. W., Kojima, M., & Greeley, G. H., Jr. (2002). Ghrelin, a new gastrointestinal endocrine peptide that stimulates insulin secretion: Enteric distribution, ontogeny, influence of endocrine, and dietary manipulations. *Endocrinology*, *143*, 185–190.

Legakis, I., Stathopoulos, J., Matzouridis, T., & Stathopoulos, G. P. (2009). Decreased plasma ghrelin levels in patients with advanced cancer and weight loss in comparison to healthy individuals. *Anticancer Research*, *29*, 3949–3952.

LeRoith, D., & Roberts, C. T., Jr. (1991). Insulin-like growth factor I (IGF-I): A molecular basis for endocrine versus local action? *Molecular and Cellular Endocrinology*, 77, C57–C61.

Li, W. G., Gavrila, D., Liu, X., Wang, L., Gunnlaugsson, S., Stoll, L. L., et al. (2004). Ghrelin inhibits proinflammatory responses and nuclear factor-kappaB activation in human endothelial cells. *Circulation*, *109*, 2221–2226.

Li, Y. P., & Reid, M. B. (2000). NF-kappaB mediates the protein loss induced by TNF-alpha in differentiated skeletal muscle myotubes. *American Journal of Physiology. Regulatory, Integrative and Comparative Physiology*, *279*, R1165–R1170.

Logan, C. Y., & Nusse, R. (2004). The Wnt signaling pathway in development and disease. *Annual Review of Cell and Developmental Biology*, *20*, 781–810.

Lundholm, K., Gunnebo, L., Korner, U., Iresjo, B. M., Engstrom, C., Hyltander, A., et al. (2011). Effects by daily long term provision of ghrelin to unselected weight-losing cancer patients: A randomized double-blind study. *Cancer*, *116*, 2044–2052.

Maccario, M., Grottoli, S., Procopio, M., Oleandri, S. E., Rossetto, R., Gauna, C., et al. (2000). The GH/IGF-I axis in obesity: Influence of neuro-endocrine and metabolic factors. *International Journal of Obesity and Related Metabolic Disorders*, *24*(Suppl. 2), S96–S99.

Magiera, M., Kopec-Medrek, M., Widuchowska, M., Kotulska, A., Dziewit, T., Ziaja, D., et al. (2011). Serum ghrelin in female patients with rheumatoid arthritis during treatment with infliximab. *Rheumatology International*. [Epub ahead of print].

Miljic, D., Pekic, S., Djurovic, M., Doknic, M., Milic, N., Casanueva, F. F., et al. (2006). Ghrelin has partial or no effect on appetite, growth hormone, prolactin, and cortisol release in patients with anorexia nervosa. *The Journal of Clinical Endocrinology and Metabolism, 91*, 1491–1495.

Misra, M., Miller, K. K., Kuo, K., Griffin, K., Stewart, V., Hunter, E., et al. (2005). Secretory dynamics of leptin in adolescent girls with anorexia nervosa and healthy adolescents. *American Journal of Physiology. Endocrinology and Metabolism, 289*, E373–E381.

Mitch, W. E. (2002). Malnutrition: A frequent misdiagnosis for hemodialysis patients. *The Journal of Clinical Investigation, 110*, 437–439.

Moller, N., & Jorgensen, J. O. (2009). Effects of growth hormone on glucose, lipid, and protein metabolism in human subjects. *Endocrine Reviews, 30*, 152–177.

Muccioli, G., Tschop, M., Papotti, M., Deghenghi, R., Heiman, M., & Ghigo, E. (2002). Neuroendocrine and peripheral activities of ghrelin: Implications in metabolism and obesity. *European Journal of Pharmacology, 440*, 235–254.

Muller, T. D., Tschop, M. H., Jarick, I., Ehrlich, S., Scherag, S., Herpertz-Dahlmann, B., et al. (2011). Genetic variation of the ghrelin activator gene ghrelin O-acyltransferase (GOAT) is associated with anorexia nervosa. *Journal of Psychiatric Research, 45*, 706–711.

Murphy, M. G., Plunkett, L. M., Gertz, B. J., He, W., Wittreich, J., Polvino, W. M., et al. (1998). MK-0677, an orally active growth hormone secretagogue reverses diet-induced catabolism. *The Journal of Clinical Endocrinology and Metabolism, 83*, 320–325.

Musaro, A., McCullagh, K., Paul, A., Houghton, L., Dobrowolny, G., Molinaro, M., et al. (2001). Localized Igf-1 transgene expression sustains hypertrophy and regeneration in senescent skeletal muscle. *Nature Genetics, 27*, 195–200.

Muscaritoli, M., Anker, S. D., Argiles, J., Aversa, Z., Bauer, J. M., Biolo, G., et al. (2010). Consensus definition of sarcopenia, cachexia and pre-cachexia: Joint document elaborated by Special Interest Groups (SIG) "cachexia-anorexia in chronic wasting diseases" and "nutrition in geriatrics". *Clinical Nutrition, 29*, 154–159.

Nagaya, N., Itoh, T., Murakami, S., Oya, H., Uematsu, M., Miyatake, K., et al. (2005). Treatment of cachexia with ghrelin in patients with COPD. *Chest, 128*, 1187–1193.

Nagaya, N., & Kangawa, K. (2006). Therapeutic potential of ghrelin in the treatment of heart failure. *Drugs, 66*, 439–448.

Nagaya, N., Miyatake, K., Uematsu, M., Oya, H., Shimizu, W., Hosoda, H., et al. (2001). Hemodynamic, renal, and hormonal effects of ghrelin infusion in patients with chronic heart failure. *The Journal of Clinical Endocrinology and Metabolism, 86*, 5854–5859.

Nagaya, N., Moriya, J., Yasumura, Y., Uematsu, M., Ono, F., Shimizu, W., et al. (2004). Effects of ghrelin administration on left ventricular function, exercise capacity, and muscle wasting in patients with chronic heart failure. *Circulation, 110*, 3674–3679.

Nagaya, N., Uematsu, M., Kojima, M., Date, Y., Nakazato, M., Okumura, H., et al. (2001). Elevated circulating level of ghrelin in cachexia associated with chronic heart failure: Relationships between ghrelin and anabolic/catabolic factors. *Circulation, 104*, 2034–2038.

Nagaya, N., Uematsu, M., Kojima, M., Ikeda, Y., Yoshihara, F., Shimizu, W., et al. (2001). Chronic administration of ghrelin improves left ventricular dysfunction and attenuates development of cardiac cachexia in rats with heart failure. *Circulation, 104*, 1430–1435.

Nakahara, T., Kojima, S., Tanaka, M., Yasuhara, D., Harada, T., Sagiyama, K., et al. (2007). Incomplete restoration of the secretion of ghrelin and PYY compared to insulin after food ingestion following weight gain in anorexia nervosa. *Journal of Psychiatric Research, 41*, 814–820.

Nakazato, M., Murakami, N., Date, Y., Kojima, M., Matsuo, H., Kangawa, K., et al. (2001). A role for ghrelin in the central regulation of feeding. *Nature, 409*, 194–198.

Nanjo, Y., Adachi, H., Hirai, Y., Enomoto, M., Fukami, A., Otsuka, M., et al. (2011). Factors associated with plasma ghrelin level in Japanese general population. *Clinical Endocrinology, 74*, 453–458.

Nass, R., Johannsson, G., Christiansen, J. S., Kopchick, J. J., & Thorner, M. O. (2009). The aging population—Is there a role for endocrine interventions? *Growth Hormone & IGF Research*, *19*, 89–100.

Nass, R., Pezzoli, S. S., Oliveri, M. C., Patrie, J. T., Harrell, F. E., Jr., Clasey, J. L., et al. (2008). Effects of an oral ghrelin mimetic on body composition and clinical outcomes in healthy older adults: A randomized trial. *Annals of Internal Medicine*, *149*, 601–611.

Neary, N. M., Small, C. J., Wren, A. M., Lee, J. L., Druce, M. R., Palmieri, C., et al. (2004). Ghrelin increases energy intake in cancer patients with impaired appetite: Acute, randomized, placebo-controlled trial. *The Journal of Clinical Endocrinology and Metabolism*, *89*, 2832–2836.

Nedvidkova, J., Krykorkova, I., Bartak, V., Papezova, H., Gold, P. W., Alesci, S., et al. (2003). Loss of meal-induced decrease in plasma ghrelin levels in patients with anorexia nervosa. *The Journal of Clinical Endocrinology and Metabolism*, *88*, 1678–1682.

Nogueiras, R., Lopez, M., & Dieguez, C. (2010). Regulation of lipid metabolism by energy availability: A role for the central nervous system. *Obesity Reviews*, *11*, 185–201.

Otero, M., Nogueiras, R., Lago, F., Dieguez, C., Gomez-Reino, J. J., & Gualillo, O. (2004). Chronic inflammation modulates ghrelin levels in humans and rats. *Rheumatology (Oxford, England)*, *43*, 306–310.

Otto, B., Cuntz, U., Fruehauf, E., Wawarta, R., Folwaczny, C., Riepl, R. L., et al. (2001). Weight gain decreases elevated plasma ghrelin concentrations of patients with anorexia nervosa. *European Journal of Endocrinology*, *145*, 669–673.

Palus, S., Schur, R., Akashi, Y. J., Bockmeyer, B., Datta, R., Halem, H., et al. (2011). Ghrelin and its analogues, BIM-28131 and BIM-28125, improve body weight and regulate the expression of MuRF-1 and MAFbx in a Rat heart failure model. *PloS One*, *6*, e26865.

Palyha, O. C., Feighner, S. D., Tan, C. P., McKee, K. K., Hreniuk, D. L., Gao, Y. D., et al. (2000). Ligand activation domain of human orphan growth hormone (GH) secretagogue receptor (GHS-R) conserved from Pufferfish to humans. *Molecular Endocrinology*, *14*, 160–169.

Pearse, A. G., Coulling, I., Weavers, B., & Friesen, S. (1970). The endocrine polypeptide cells of the human stomach, duodenum, and jejunum. *Gut*, *11*, 649–658.

Pickering, W. P., Price, S. R., Bircher, G., Marinovic, A. C., Mitch, W. E., & Walls, J. (2002). Nutrition in CAPD: Serum bicarbonate and the ubiquitin-proteasome system in muscle. *Kidney International*, *61*, 1286–1292.

Plata-Salaman, C. R. (2001). Cytokines and feeding. *International Journal of Obesity and Related Metabolic Disorders*, *25*(Suppl. 5), S48–S52.

Prince, A. C., Brooks, S. J., Stahl, D., & Treasure, J. (2009). Systematic review and meta-analysis of the baseline concentrations and physiologic responses of gut hormones to food in eating disorders. *The American Journal of Clinical Nutrition*, *89*, 755–765.

Rall, L. C., & Roubenoff, R. (2004). Rheumatoid cachexia: Metabolic abnormalities, mechanisms and interventions. *Rheumatology (Oxford, England)*, *43*, 1219–1223.

Reed, S. A., Sandesara, P. B., Senf, S. M., & Judge, A. R. (2012). Inhibition of FoxO transcriptional activity prevents muscle fiber atrophy during cachexia and induces hypertrophy. *The FASEB Journal*, *26*, 987–1000.

Remels, A. H., Gosker, H. R., Schrauwen, P., Hommelberg, P. P., Sliwinski, P., Polkey, M., et al. (2010). TNF-alpha impairs regulation of muscle oxidative phenotype: Implications for cachexia? *The FASEB Journal*, *24*, 5052–5062.

Rinaldi, M., Maes, K., De Vleeschauwer, S., Thomas, D., Verbeken, E. K., Decramer, M., et al. (2012). Antielastin B-cell and T-cell immunity in patients with chronic obstructive pulmonary disease. *Thorax*, *67*, 694–700. Epub ahead of print.

Rinderknecht, E., & Humbel, R. E. (1978). Primary structure of human insulin-like growth factor II. *FEBS Letters*, *89*, 283–286.

Roubenoff, R., Roubenoff, R. A., Ward, L. M., Holland, S. M., & Hellmann, D. B. (1992). Rheumatoid cachexia: Depletion of lean body mass in rheumatoid arthritis. Possible association with tumor necrosis factor. *The Journal of Rheumatology*, *19*, 1505–1510.

Rubenstein, L. Z. (2006). Falls in older people: Epidemiology, risk factors and strategies for prevention. *Age and Ageing*, *35*(Suppl. 2), ii37–ii41.

Ruegg, M. A., & Glass, D. J. (2011). Molecular mechanisms and treatment options for muscle wasting diseases. *Annual Review of Pharmacology and Toxicology*, *51*, 373–395.

Sangiao-Alvarellos, S., Vazquez, M. J., Varela, L., Nogueiras, R., Saha, A. K., Cordido, F., et al. (2009). Central ghrelin regulates peripheral lipid metabolism in a growth hormone-independent fashion. *Endocrinology*, *150*, 4562–4574.

Schols, A. M. (2002). Pulmonary cachexia. *International Journal of Cardiology*, *85*, 101–110.

Shavlakadze, T., White, J. D., Davies, M., Hoh, J. F., & Grounds, M. D. (2005). Insulin-like growth factor I slows the rate of denervation induced skeletal muscle atrophy. *Neuromuscular Disorders*, *15*, 139–146.

Shavlakadze, T., Winn, N., Rosenthal, N., & Grounds, M. D. (2005). Reconciling data from transgenic mice that overexpress IGF-I specifically in skeletal muscle. *Growth Hormone & IGF Research*, *15*, 4–18.

Shimizu, Y., Nagaya, N., Isobe, T., Imazu, M., Okumura, H., Hosoda, H., et al. (2003). Increased plasma ghrelin level in lung cancer cachexia. *Clinical Cancer Research*, *9*, 774–778.

Smith, R. G., Feighner, S., Prendergast, K., Guan, X., & Howard, A. (1999). A new orphan receptor involved in pulsatile growth hormone release. *Trends in Endocrinology and Metabolism*, *10*, 128–135.

Smith, R. G., Jiang, H., & Sun, Y. (2005). Developments in ghrelin biology and potential clinical relevance. *Trends in Endocrinology and Metabolism*, *16*, 436–442.

Smith, R. G., Van der Ploeg, L. H., Howard, A. D., Feighner, S. D., Cheng, K., Hickey, G. J., et al. (1997). Peptidomimetic regulation of growth hormone secretion. *Endocrine Reviews*, *18*, 621–645.

Soares, V. M., Garcia-Souza, E. P., Lacerda-Miranda, G., & Moura, A. S. (2012). Early life overfeeding decreases acylated ghrelin circulating levels and upregulates GHSR1a signaling pathway in white adipose tissue of obese young mice. *Regulatory Peptides*, *174*, 6–11.

Soeki, T., Kishimoto, I., Schwenke, D. O., Tokudome, T., Horio, T., Yoshida, M., et al. (2008). Ghrelin suppresses cardiac sympathetic activity and prevents early left ventricular remodeling in rats with myocardial infarction. *American Journal of Physiology. Heart and Circulatory Physiology*, *294*, H426–H432.

Solcia, E., Capella, C., Vassallo, G., & Buffa, R. (1975). Endocrine cells of the gastric mucosa. *International Review of Cytology*, *42*, 223–286.

Soriano-Guillen, L., Barrios, V., Campos-Barros, A., & Argente, J. (2004). Ghrelin levels in obesity and anorexia nervosa: Effect of weight reduction or recuperation. *The Journal of Pediatrics*, *144*, 36–42.

Stitt, T. N., Drujan, D., Clarke, B. A., Panaro, F., Timofeyva, Y., Kline, W. O., et al. (2004). The IGF-1/PI3K/Akt pathway prevents expression of muscle atrophy-induced ubiquitin ligases by inhibiting FOXO transcription factors. *Molecular Cell*, *14*, 395–403.

Stock, S., Leichner, P., Wong, A. C., Ghatei, M. A., Kieffer, T. J., Bloom, S. R., et al. (2005). Ghrelin, peptide YY, glucose-dependent insulinotropic polypeptide, and hunger responses to a mixed meal in anorexic, obese, and control female adolescents. *The Journal of Clinical Endocrinology and Metabolism*, *90*, 2161–2168.

Stofkova, A., Haluzik, M., Zelezna, B., Kiss, A., Skurlova, M., Lacinova, Z., et al. (2009). Enhanced expressions of mRNA for neuropeptide Y and interleukin 1 beta in hypothalamic arcuate nuclei during adjuvant arthritis-induced anorexia in Lewis rats. *Neuroimmunomodulation*, *16*, 377–384.

Strasser, F., Lutz, T. A., Maeder, M. T., Thuerlimann, B., Bueche, D., Tschop, M., et al. (2008). Safety, tolerability and pharmacokinetics of intravenous ghrelin for cancer-related anorexia/cachexia: A randomised, placebo-controlled, double-blind, double-crossover study. *British Journal of Cancer, 98*, 300–308.

Sun, Y., Ahmed, S., & Smith, R. G. (2003). Deletion of ghrelin impairs neither growth nor appetite. *Molecular and Cellular Biology, 23*, 7973–7981.

Sun, Y., Wang, P., Zheng, H., & Smith, R. G. (2004). Ghrelin stimulation of growth hormone release and appetite is mediated through the growth hormone secretagogue receptor. *Proceedings of the National Academy of Sciences of the United States of America, 101*, 4679–4684.

Szentirmai, E., Kapas, L., Sun, Y., Smith, R. G., & Krueger, J. M. (2009). The preproghrelin gene is required for the normal integration of thermoregulation and sleep in mice. *Proceedings of the National Academy of Sciences of the United States of America, 106*, 14069–14074.

Takada, R., Satomi, Y., Kurata, T., Ueno, N., Norioka, S., Kondoh, H., et al. (2006). Monounsaturated fatty acid modification of Wnt protein: Its role in Wnt secretion. *Developmental Cell, 11*, 791–801.

Takaya, K., Ariyasu, H., Kanamoto, N., Iwakura, H., Yoshimoto, A., Harada, M., et al. (2000). Ghrelin strongly stimulates growth hormone release in humans. *The Journal of Clinical Endocrinology and Metabolism, 85*, 4908–4911.

Tanaka, M., Naruo, T., Nagai, N., Kuroki, N., Shiiya, T., Nakazato, M., et al. (2003). Habitual binge/purge behavior influences circulating ghrelin levels in eating disorders. *Journal of Psychiatric Research, 37*, 17–22.

Tanaka, M., Naruo, T., Yasuhara, D., Tatebe, Y., Nagai, N., Shiiya, T., et al. (2003). Fasting plasma ghrelin levels in subtypes of anorexia nervosa. *Psychoneuroendocrinology, 28*, 829–835.

Tena-Sempere, M., Barreiro, M. L., Gonzalez, L. C., Gaytan, F., Zhang, F. P., Caminos, J. E., et al. (2002). Novel expression and functional role of ghrelin in rat testis. *Endocrinology, 143*, 717–725.

Terashi, M., Asakawa, A., Harada, T., Ushikai, M., Coquerel, Q., Sinno, M. H., et al. (2011). Ghrelin reactive autoantibodies in restrictive anorexia nervosa. *Nutrition, 27*, 407–413.

Theander-Carrillo, C., Wiedmer, P., Cettour-Rose, P., Nogueiras, R., Perez-Tilve, D., Pfluger, P., et al. (2006). Ghrelin action in the brain controls adipocyte metabolism. *The Journal of Clinical Investigation, 116*, 1983–1993.

Tisdale, M. J. (2002). Cachexia in cancer patients. *Nature Reviews. Cancer, 2*, 862–871.

Tschop, M., Smiley, D. L., & Heiman, M. L. (2000). Ghrelin induces adiposity in rodents. *Nature, 407*, 908–913.

Tschop, M., Weyer, C., Tataranni, P. A., Devanarayan, V., Ravussin, E., & Heiman, M. L. (2001). Circulating ghrelin levels are decreased in human obesity. *Diabetes, 50*, 707–709.

Uehara, M., Yasuhara, D., Nakahara, T., Harada, T., Koyama, K. I., Ushikai, M., et al. (2011). Increase in energy intake leads to a decrease in obestatin in restricting-type of anorexia nervosa. *Experimental and Clinical Endocrinology & Diabetes, 119*, 536–539.

Ukkola, O. (2003). Ghrelin and insulin metabolism. *European Journal of Clinical Investigation, 33*, 183–185.

Van der Lely, A. J., Tschop, M., Heiman, M. L., & Ghigo, E. (2004). Biological, physiological, pathophysiological, and pharmacological aspects of ghrelin. *Endocrine Reviews, 25*, 426–457.

Varela, L., Vazquez, M. J., Cordido, F., Nogueiras, R., Vidal-Puig, A., Dieguez, C., et al. (2011). Ghrelin and lipid metabolism: Key partners in energy balance. *Journal of Molecular Endocrinology, 46*, R43–R63.

Velloso, C. P. (2008). Regulation of muscle mass by growth hormone and IGF-I. *British Journal of Pharmacology, 154*, 557–568.

Vestergaard, E. T., Andersen, N. H., Hansen, T. K., Rasmussen, L. M., Moller, N., Sorensen, K. E., et al. (2007). Cardiovascular effects of intravenous ghrelin infusion in healthy young men. *American Journal of Physiology. Heart and Circulatory Physiology, 293*, H3020–H3026.

Vestergaard, E. T., Djurhuus, C. B., Gjedsted, J., Nielsen, S., Moller, N., Holst, J. J., et al. (2008). Acute effects of ghrelin administration on glucose and lipid metabolism. *The Journal of Clinical Endocrinology and Metabolism, 93*, 438–444.

Vogt, P. K., Jiang, H., & Aoki, M. (2005). Triple layer control: Phosphorylation, acetylation and ubiquitination of FOXO proteins. *Cell Cycle, 4*, 908–913.

Volante, M., Allia, E., Fulcheri, E., Cassoni, P., Ghigo, E., Muccioli, G., et al. (2003). Ghrelin in fetal thyroid and follicular tumors and cell lines: Expression and effects on tumor growth. *The American Journal of Pathology, 162*, 645–654.

von Haehling, S., Lainscak, M., Springer, J., & Anker, S. D. (2009). Cardiac cachexia: A systematic overview. *Pharmacology & Therapeutics, 121*, 227–252.

Walsmith, J., & Roubenoff, R. (2002). Cachexia in rheumatoid arthritis. *International Journal of Cardiology, 85*, 89–99.

Wang, L., Basa, N. R., Shaikh, A., Luckey, A., Heber, D., St-Pierre, D. H., et al. (2006). LPS inhibits fasted plasma ghrelin levels in rats: Role of IL-1 and PGs and functional implications. *American Journal of Physiology. Gastrointestinal and Liver Physiology, 291*, G611–G620.

Wang, G., Lee, H. M., Englander, E., & Greeley, G. H., Jr. (2002). Ghrelin—Not just another stomach hormone. *Regulatory Peptides, 105*, 75–81.

White, M. F. (2002). IRS proteins and the common path to diabetes. *American Journal of Physiology. Endocrinology and Metabolism, 283*, E413–E422.

Wiley, K. E., & Davenport, A. P. (2002). Comparison of vasodilators in human internal mammary artery: Ghrelin is a potent physiological antagonist of endothelin-1. *British Journal of Pharmacology, 136*, 1146–1152.

Willesen, M. G., Kristensen, P., & Romer, J. (1999). Co-localization of growth hormone secretagogue receptor and NPY mRNA in the arcuate nucleus of the rat. *Neuroendocrinology, 70*, 306–316.

Withers, D. J., Burks, D. J., Towery, H. H., Altamuro, S. L., Flint, C. L., & White, M. F. (1999). Irs-2 coordinates Igf-1 receptor-mediated beta-cell development and peripheral insulin signalling. *Nature Genetics, 23*, 32–40.

Wolf, R. F., Ng, B., Weksler, B., Burt, M., & Brennan, M. F. (1994). Effect of growth hormone on tumor and host in an animal model. *Annals of Surgical Oncology, 1*, 314–320.

Wolf, I., Sadetzki, S., Kanety, H., Kundel, Y., Pariente, C., Epstein, N., et al. (2006). Adiponectin, ghrelin, and leptin in cancer cachexia in breast and colon cancer patients. *Cancer, 106*, 966–973.

Wren, A. M., Small, C. J., Abbott, C. R., Dhillo, W. S., Seal, L. J., Cohen, M. A., et al. (2001). Ghrelin causes hyperphagia and obesity in rats. *Diabetes, 50*, 2540–2547.

Wren, A. M., Small, C. J., Ward, H. L., Murphy, K. G., Dakin, C. L., Taheri, S., et al. (2000). The novel hypothalamic peptide ghrelin stimulates food intake and growth hormone secretion. *Endocrinology, 141*, 4325–4328.

Wu, R., Dong, W., Qiang, X., Wang, H., Blau, S. A., Ravikumar, T. S., et al. (2009). Orexigenic hormone ghrelin ameliorates gut barrier dysfunction in sepsis in rats. *Critical Care Medicine, 37*, 2421–2426.

Wyke, S. M., Russell, S. T., & Tisdale, M. J. (2004). Induction of proteasome expression in skeletal muscle is attenuated by inhibitors of NF-kappaB activation. *British Journal of Cancer, 91*, 1742–1750.

Wynne, K., Giannitsopoulou, K., Small, C. J., Patterson, M., Frost, G., Ghatei, M. A., et al. (2005). Subcutaneous ghrelin enhances acute food intake in malnourished patients who receive maintenance peritoneal dialysis: A randomized, placebo-controlled trial. *Journal of the American Society of Nephrology, 16*, 2111–2118.

Xu, X. B., Pang, J. J., Cao, J. M., Ni, C., Xu, R. K., Peng, X. Z., et al. (2005). GH-releasing peptides improve cardiac dysfunction and cachexia and suppress stress-related hormones and cardiomyocyte apoptosis in rats with heart failure. *American Journal of Physiology. Heart and Circulatory Physiology, 289*, H1643–H1651.

Yang, J., Brown, M. S., Liang, G., Grishin, N. V., & Goldstein, J. L. (2008). Identification of the acyltransferase that octanoylates ghrelin, an appetite-stimulating peptide hormone. *Cell, 132*, 387–396.

Yasuda, T., Masaki, T., Kakuma, T., & Yoshimatsu, H. (2003). Centrally administered ghrelin suppresses sympathetic nerve activity in brown adipose tissue of rats. *Neuroscience Letters, 349*, 75–78.

Ying, B. W., Song, X. B., Fan, H., Wang, L. L., Li, Y. S., Cheng, Z., et al. (2008). Plasma ghrelin levels and weight loss in Chinese Uygur patients with chronic obstructive pulmonary disease. *The Journal of International Medical Research, 36*, 1371–1377.

Yoshida, T., Semprun-Prieto, L., Sukhanov, S., & Delafontaine, P. (2010). IGF-1 prevents ANG II-induced skeletal muscle atrophy via Akt- and Foxo-dependent inhibition of the ubiquitin ligase atrogin-1 expression. *American Journal of Physiology. Heart and Circulatory Physiology, 298*, H1565–H1570.

Zhu, X., Cao, Y., Voogd, K., & Steiner, D. F. (2006). On the processing of proghrelin to ghrelin. *The Journal of Biological Chemistry, 281*, 38867–38870.

Zigman, J. M., Jones, J. E., Lee, C. E., Saper, C. B., & Elmquist, J. K. (2006). Expression of ghrelin receptor mRNA in the rat and the mouse brain. *The Journal of Comparative Neurology, 494*, 528–548.

Zigman, J. M., Nakano, Y., Coppari, R., Balthasar, N., Marcus, J. N., Lee, C. E., et al. (2005). Mice lacking ghrelin receptors resist the development of diet-induced obesity. *The Journal of Clinical Investigation, 115*, 3564–3572.

CHAPTER FOUR

Ghrelin Gene Variants and Eating Disorders

Tetsuya Ando[1]
Section of Stress Research, Department of Psychosomatic Research, National Institute of Mental Health, National Center of Neurology and Psychiatry, Ogawahigashi-cho, Kodaira, Tokyo, Japan
[1]Corresponding author: e-mail address: ando-t@ncnp.go.jp

Contents

1. Introduction 108
2. Ghrelin Signaling System 108
   2.1 Ghrelin 108
   2.2 Growth hormone secretagogue receptor 109
   2.3 Ghrelin *O*-acyltransferase 109
3. Physiological Functions of Ghrelin 110
   3.1 Appetite and body weight regulation 110
   3.2 Growth hormone secretion 110
4. Ghrelin and Eating Disorders 110
5. Ghrelin Gene Variants and Eating Disorders 111
   5.1 Genetic studies of ghrelin-related genes in eating disorders 111
   5.2 Association of ghrelin polymorphisms with eating disorders 112
   5.3 Association of GHSR polymorphisms with eating disorders 115
   5.4 Association of GOAT polymorphisms with eating disorders 115
   5.5 Genome-wide studies on ghrelin-related genes and eating disorders 116
6. Association of Ghrelin Polymorphisms with Anthropometry and Eating Pathology in Young Women 116
7. Association of Ghrelin Polymorphisms with Changes in Eating Disorder Phenotypes 117
8. Conclusions 117
References 118

Abstract

Genetic factors have been implicated in playing a significant role in susceptibility to eating disorders such as anorexia nervosa (AN) and bulimia nervosa (BN). Genetic variants of ghrelin, an endogenous acylated peptide that stimulates growth hormone secretion, enhances appetite, and increases body weight, have been investigated in association with eating disorders, as changes in the ghrelin/growth hormone secretagogue receptor (GHSR)/ghrelin *O*-acyltransferase (GOAT) system have been implicated in its pathology. Although most candidate-gene association studies have not been able to identify ghrelin gene variants as being significantly associated with either AN or BN, some ghrelin variants

Vitamins and Hormones, Volume 92
ISSN 0083-6729
http://dx.doi.org/10.1016/B978-0-12-410473-0.00004-0

may be associated with BN in Japanese. Furthermore, a significant association of a *GHSR* gene variant with BN and that of a *GOAT* gene variant with AN have been found. However, there have been relatively few studies, tested variants are restricted, and sample sizes are often modest. Therefore, further studies are needed to elucidate the role of ghrelin-related gene variants in the predisposition and pathology of eating disorders.

1. INTRODUCTION

Eating disorders are characterized by severe alterations in eating behavior, body shape perception, and body weight regulation. A number of studies including familial aggregation and twin studies have suggested that genetic factors play an important role in susceptibility to eating disorders such as anorexia nervosa (AN) and bulimia nervosa (BN; Gorwood, Kipman, & Foulon, 2003; Holland, Sicotte, & Treasure, 1988; Stein et al., 1999). Many association studies have used candidate genes related to metal function, appetite control, neuro-endocrine response to stress, and energy expenditure in search of predispositions to eating disorders (Helder & Collier, 2011; Scherag, Hebebrand, & Hinney, 2010).

Ghrelin is a 28-amino acid acylated peptide first identified as an endogenous ligand for the growth hormone secretagogue receptor (GHSR; Kojima et al., 1999). Ghrelin is produced primarily by X/A-like cells in the stomach (Date et al., 2000a) and is also secreted by the hypothalamus (Sato, Fukue, Teranishi, Yoshida, & Kojima, 2005) and pancreas (Date et al., 2002a). In addition to stimulating growth hormone (GH) release, ghrelin has been further implicated in the regulation of appetite (Wren et al., 2001), secretion of gastric acid, gut motility (Masuda et al., 2000), blood pressure (Nagaya et al., 2001), and insulin secretion (Date et al., 2002b; Sato et al., 2012). The clear relationship which exists between the ghrelin signaling system and eating behavior, as well as the presence of higher plasma ghrelin levels in patients with eating disorders (Ariyasu et al., 2001; Otto et al., 2001; Prince, Brooks, Stahl, & Treasure, 2009), makes ghrelin and related substances good candidate genes for predisposing eating disorders (Liu, Garcia, & Korbonits, 2011; Yi, Heppner, & Tschöp, 2011).

2. GHRELIN SIGNALING SYSTEM

2.1. Ghrelin

Ghrelin is derived from the posttranscriptional processing of the 117-amino acid precursor peptide ghrelin/obestatin prepropeptide or pre-proghrelin (Sato et al., 2012). The human ghrelin/obestatin prepropeptide gene

(*GHRL*) is located on chromosome 3 (3p25–26) and was initially thought to consist of four exons (Wajnrajch, Ten, Gertner, & Leibel, 2000), but subsequent studies have identified additional upstream exons (Seim, Collet, Herington, & Chopin, 2007). The N-terminal 23-amino acid signal peptide of pre-proghrelin is cleaved to produce a 94-amino acid proghrelin peptide, which is further cleaved to produce a 28-amino acid ghrelin (encoded by exons 1 and 2) and a 66-amino acid C-terminal peptide C-ghrelin (Seim et al., 2007). Ghrelin undergoes *n*-octanoyl modification on its serine 3 residue to produce acyl ghrelin (Kojima et al., 1999). This is unstable so is rapidly degraded to the nonacylated form of ghrelin, des-acyl ghrelin (Date et al., 2000b; Hosoda, Kojima, Matsuo, & Kangawa, 2000). The *n*-octanoylation at serine 3 is thought to be essential for GHSR binding and performing its activity (Kojima et al., 1999).

Des-acyl ghrelin has recently been reported to play a role in the stimulation of food intake and the inhibition of isoproterenol-induced lipolysis in rodents (Toshinai et al., 2006). However, its effects on energy balance are controversial and remain to be clarified (Inhoff et al., 2008). C-ghrelin contains a 23-amino acid sequence known as obestatin, which was shown by Zhang et al., 2005 to reduce food intake, oppose ghrelin-induced weight gain, and inhibit gastric emptying. However, these findings could not be reproduced by several groups and remain controversial (Gourcerol et al., 2007; Holst et al., 2007).

2.2. Growth hormone secretagogue receptor

GHSR is a G-protein-coupled seven-transmembrane receptor. The GHSR gene (*GHSR*) is located at chromosome 3q26.31 and consists of two exons and one intron. Two types of GHSR mRNA, GHSR-1a and GHSR-1b, are produced through alternative splicing (Howard et al., 1996). GHSR-1a contains all seven-transmembrane domains and possesses high affinity binding to ghrelin (McKee et al., 1997). GHSR-1b mRNA is encoded by exon 1 and the intronic region, and it is physiologically inactive. The highest expression levels of GHSR-1a are found in the central nervous system (CNS) and in the pituitary gland, while lower expression is detected in other peripheral organs, including adrenal glands, the heart, thyroid glands, and adipose tissue (Gnanapavan et al., 2002).

2.3. Ghrelin *O*-acyltransferase

The ability of ghrelin to bind and activate GHSR-1a depends on posttranslational acylation at the serine 3 residue by ghrelin *O*-acyltransferase (GOAT; Gutierrez et al., 2008; Yang, Brown, Liang, Grishin, &

Goldstein, 2008). GOAT is considered to be the only enzyme capable of acylating ghrelin *in vivo* (Gutierrez et al., 2008), which utilizes orally ingested medium-chain fatty acids (Nishi et al., 2005).

The GOAT gene (*MBOAT4*) is located on chromosome 8p12 and consists of three exons (Liu et al., 2011). GOAT mRNA is expressed mainly in the stomach and pancreas (Gutierrez et al., 2008). The activity of GOAT may be more important than ghrelin synthesis in the determination of the ghrelin signal (Liu et al., 2011).

3. PHYSIOLOGICAL FUNCTIONS OF GHRELIN

3.1. Appetite and body weight regulation

Ghrelin is secreted primarily from the stomach in response to hunger and starvation and serves as a peripheral signal that stimulates appetite and promotes feeding and adiposity in rodents and humans (Nakazato et al., 2001; Tschop, Smiley, & Heiman, 2000; Wren et al., 2001). Ghrelin secretion is upregulated under conditions of negative energy balance, such as emaciation, and is downregulated under conditions of positive energy balance, such as obesity (Hansen et al., 2002; Otto et al., 2001; Tschop et al., 2001). Plasma levels of ghrelin rise during fasting and fall quickly after consumption of a meal or oral glucose administration (Shiiya et al., 2002). Thus, ghrelin plays a role in both long-term and short-term regulation of feeding. In the CNS, ghrelin activates hypothalamic neuropeptide Y and agouti-related protein-expressing neurons involved in appetite regulation (Nakazato et al., 2001).

3.2. Growth hormone secretion

Ghrelin has strong GH-releasing activity in both human and rats (Arvat et al., 2000; Kojima et al., 1999). The maximum stimulation of GH affected by ghrelin is greater than that of GHRH, which peaks about 5–15 min after intravenous ghrelin injection (Arvat et al., 2000; Arvat et al., 2001). Ghrelin stimulates GH release from primary pituitary cells (Kojima et al., 1999). In addition to the direct action on pituitary, ghrelin-mediated stimulation of GH release has been shown to involve the hypothalamus and the vagus nerve (Date et al., 2002).

4. GHRELIN AND EATING DISORDERS

The possible role of ghrelin in the pathogenesis of eating disorders has been extensively investigated because ghrelin is a potential regulator of food intake and body weight. Plasma levels of total and acyl ghrelin are elevated in patients with AN compared with normal-weight control subjects and these raised concentrations return to normal after weight gain (Ariyasu et al., 2001; Misra et al., 2004; Otto et al., 2001; Prince et al., 2009; Tanaka et al., 2003).

High levels of ghrelin in underweight AN patients could be the result of a compensatory mechanism to stimulate feeding. Alternatively, loss of function within the ghrelin system may contribute toward caloric restriction in AN. However, Hotta et al., 2009 demonstrated that intravenous administration of ghrelin to AN patients decreased gastrointestinal symptoms while increasing sensations of hunger and daily energy intake, suggesting that AN patients are able to respond to ghrelin. Postprandial suppression of ghrelin in AN has not been reported to differ from that in controls (Misra et al., 2004; Otto et al., 2001; Stock et al., 2005; Tanaka et al., 2003).

AN patients also have an impaired GH/insulin-like growth factor 1 (IGF-1) axis. Fasting serum GH and insulin-like growth factor binding protein 1 (IGFBP-1) and IGFBP-2 levels were increased, while IGF-1 levels were decreased in underweight AN patients, suggesting that AN patients exhibit GH resistance (Counts, Gwirtsman, Carlsson, Lesem, & Cutler, 1992; Misra et al., 2003).

Basal ghrelin concentrations in BN patients were found to vary between studies (Kojima et al., 2005; Monteleone, Martiadis, Fabrazzo, Serritella, & Maj, 2003; Monteleone et al., 2005). However, some research has demonstrated that the postprandial suppression of ghrelin is attenuated in BN, suggesting that ghrelin is involved in its pathogenesis through the promotion of binge eating behavior (Kojima et al., 2005; Monteleone et al., 2003; Monteleone et al., 2005).

5. GHRELIN GENE VARIANTS AND EATING DISORDERS

5.1. Genetic studies of ghrelin-related genes in eating disorders

The involvement of genetic factors in the etiology of eating disorders has been demonstrated in family and twin studies (Fichter & Noegel, 1990; Gorwood et al., 2003; Holland et al., 1988; Stein et al., 1999; Treasure & Holland, 1989), the latter of which estimated the contribution of genetic factors in AN to be 33–84% (Wade, Bulik, Neale, & Kendler, 2000) and that in BN to be 28–83% (Bulik, Sullivan, Wade, & Kendler, 2000). Genetic association studies using ghrelin-related genes as candidates have also been conducted for eating disorders. Case–control association studies are the most widely performed in which significant differences in allele frequency between cases and controls are used as evidence of an allele being involved in disease susceptibility (Liu et al., 2011). An observed association indicates one of three following situations: the allele itself may be functional and may contribute directly to the phenotype; the allele may be in linkage disequilibrium (LD) with an allele at another locus that directly affects the phenotype; or the association may be due to chance or artifact (Silverman & Palmer, 2000).

Family-based association studies can avoid false-positive findings created by population stratification using methods such as the transmission-disequilibrium test (TDT; Cardon & Palmer, 2003). However, such studies are less powerful than case–control association studies for the detection of weak genetic effects (Liu et al., 2011; Risch & Teng, 1998).

5.2. Association of ghrelin polymorphisms with eating disorders

Three nonsynonymous polymorphisms in the *GHRL* have been reported: Arg51Gln (rs34911341), Leu72Met (rs696217), and Gln90Leu SNPs (rs4684677). The Arg51Gln single-nucleotide polymorphism (SNP) changes the amino acid sequence of the ghrelin peptide COOH terminal-processing site within its precursor protein from Pro-Arg to Pro-Gln, preventing the normal cleavage necessary to produce mature ghrelin. Arg51Gln has been associated with lower levels of ghrelin and IGF-1, which is an indicator of serum GH levels (Poykko, Ukkola, Kauma, Savolainen, & Kesaniemi, 2003; Ukkola et al., 2002). The more common Leu72Met is outside the coding region of the mature ghrelin but within the prepro-ghrelin C-terminal tail, and Vivenza et al., 2004 showed that obese Caucasian carriers of the 72Met allele possess higher IGF-1 levels than subjects homozygous for the 72Leu allele. The Gln90Leu SNP lies in the region coding for obestatin and changes its amino acid sequence, though its function has not been reported.

Monteleone, Tortorella, Castaldo, Di Filippo, & Maj, 2006 investigated the Arg51Gln SNP and Leu72Met SNP in 59 AN, 114 BN, and 119 healthy controls. The minor allele frequency of the Arg51Gln SNP was very low (0.003), while no significant differences were found in the frequencies of the Leu72Met SNP among AN and BN patients or controls. Moreover, no significant differences were observed between patients with and without the minor 72Met allele in terms of eating-related psychopathology as assessed by the Eating Disorder Inventory-2 (EDI-2) and Bulimia Investigation Test Edinburgh (BITE), body mass index, age of illness onset, and weekly frequency of binge eating and vomiting (Monteleone et al., 2006). Kindler et al., 2011 also reported no significant difference in Arg51Gln, Leu72Met, and Gln90Leu SNPs in a small case–control study of 114 eating disorders (46 AN, 30 BN, and 36 binge eating disorders) and 164 controls. However, Ando et al., 2006 found that both the Leu72Met and 3056 T > C (rs2075356) SNP in intron 2, which were found in LD, were significantly associated with BN-P in a case–control association study of 336 eating disorder patients (131 AN restricting type (AN-R), 97 AN binge-purging type (AN-BP), and 108 BN purging type (BN-P)) and 300 controls. In addition, they observed a significant increase in the frequency of the Met72-3056C haplotype in BN-P patients. These findings together suggest that the Leu72Met and 3056 T > C SNPs of the pre-proghrelin gene are associated with susceptibility to BN-P in the Japanese population (Ando et al., 2006). Monteleone, Tortorella, Castaldo, Di Filippo, & Maj, 2007 examined whether the Arg51Gln and Leu72Met SNPs were associated with binge eating disorders (BED) in 90 women patients and 119 controls and showed that women with BED exhibited a statistically significant higher prevalence of heterozygote for Leu72Met than controls.

In a large case–control study of patients recruited from seven European countries (Italy, Spain, Germany, Slovenia, France, Austria, and the United Kingdom), the three nonsynonymous *GHRL* SNPs were studied in 692 Caucasian cases (366 AN and 326 BN) and in 529 AN and BN trios (patients and both parents; Cellini et al., 2006). The combined analysis of all populations revealed no significant genotype- or allele-wise association with the three SNPs for the AN or BN groups. Similarly, the family-based analysis provided no evidence for transmission distortion of any of the ghrelin SNPs. However, preferential transmission of the Gln90Leu72Arg51 haplotype and a reduction of the Gln90Met72Arg51 allelic combination to the BN offspring was observed, suggesting possible involvement of this allelic combination in the etiology of BN (Cellini et al., 2006). Dardennes et al., 2007 carried out TDT analysis of Gln90Leu and Leu72Met SNPs as well as *BDNF* Val66Met and *AGRP* Ala67Thr SNPs in 114 probands with AN and both their parents. This family-based analysis provided evidence for the preferential transmission of the Leu72Met variant with an excess of Gln90Leu72 haplotype transmission in AN patients. Preferential transmission and association of the Met72 allele was also observed with the AN-BP subtype compared with the AN-R subtype (Dardennes et al., 2007).

Based on these studies, it appears unlikely that *GHRL* polymorphisms contribute significantly to AN or BN risk in Caucasians, although a significant relationship may be present with BN in the Japanese population (Table 4.1). However, these studies have a number of limitations. First,

Table 4.1 Summary of frequencies of ghrelin Leu72Met polymorphism in eating disorders

					Genotype-wise			Allele-wise				
Author	**Year**	**Population**	**Group**	***N***	**Leu72Leu**	**Leu72Met**	**Met72Met**	**Leu**	**Met**	**Leu (%)**	**Met (%)**	***P***
Monteleone	2006	Caucasian	Con	119	109	10	0	228	10	0.96	0.04	
			AN	59	52	7	0	111	7	0.94	0.06	0.47
			BN	114	103	11	0	217	11	0.95	0.05	0.74
Cellini	2006	Caucasian	Con	342				622	62	0.91	0.09	
			AN	366				671	61	0.92	0.08	0.63
			BN	326				611	41	0.94	0.06	0.057
Kindler	2011	Caucasian	Con	164	147	16	1	310	18	0.95	0.05	
			AN	46	41	5	0	87	5	0.95	0.05	0.98
			BN	30	25	4	1	54	6	0.90	0.10	0.18
Overall of studies in Caucasian			Con	625	256	26	1	1160	90	0.93	0.07	
			AN	471	93	12	0	869	73	0.92	0.08	0.63
			BN	470	128	15	1	882	58	0.94	0.06	0.34
Ando	2006	Japanese	Con	300	205	84	11	494	106	0.82	0.18	
			AN	228	142	77	9	361	95	0.79	0.21	0.19
			BN	108	56	52	0	164	52	0.76	0.24	0.041*

AN, anorexia nervosa; BN, bulimia nervosa; Con, control.

because minor allele frequencies of Arg51Gln and Gln90Leu SNPs are so small, a larger sample is necessary to detect any SNP association. Second, only some ghrelin gene polymorphisms have been examined. Ghrelin promoter variants have been shown to alter promoter activity and are linked to different postprandial responses of the anorexic hormone PYY and perceived levels of hunger (den Hoed et al., 2008). Studies covering promoter variations as well as coding regions of ghrelin in larger populations are therefore needed to derive clear conclusions.

5.3. Association of GHSR polymorphisms with eating disorders

To date, only one study searching for an association between *GHSR* polymorphisms and eating disorders has been carried out by Miyasaka et al., 2006. They examined the 171 T > C SNP of *GHSR* (rs495225) in 228 Japanese eating disorder patients and 284 age- and gender-matched unrelated controls. The eating disorder group contained 96 AN (47 AN-R, 49 AN-BP), 116 BN (91 BN-P, 25 BN-NP), and 16 eating disorder not otherwise specified. The 171CC genotype was found to be more frequently present in BN patients (14.7%) compared with controls (7.7%) but was not associated with AN subtypes or all eating disorders (Miyasaka et al., 2006). The function of 171 T > C SNP is unknown, but the 171 T allele was previously reported to be more prevalent in obese than lean young German subjects (Wang et al., 2004). Larger studies are recommended to verify this result.

5.4. Association of GOAT polymorphisms with eating disorders

Müller et al., 2011 recently reported that GOAT gene polymorphisms may influence AN risk. They studied the association between six tagging SNPs (rs1355412, rs10096097, rs16876504, rs3735989, rs13272159, and rs4733400) in 543 AN patients and 612 healthy controls in Germany. The SNPs were predicted to cover 96% of the GOAT coding region and 50 kb of the 5′ and 3′ flanking regions. An association of the G/G genotype was observed at SNP rs10096097 (located 24.981 bp upstream of the GOAT translation start codon (ATG)), but the implication of the SNP for AN remains unknown (Müller et al., 2011). Gain-of-function mutations in GOAT might account for the observed higher plasma levels of acyl ghrelin in patients with AN, which can lead to the development of ghrelin resistance. Alternatively, loss-of-function GOAT mutations might cause decreased appetite and food intake (Müller et al., 2011).

5.5. Genome-wide studies on ghrelin-related genes and eating disorders

A genome-wide association analysis was performed by Nakabayashi et al., 2009 using microsatellite markers for AN in a Japanese population. They reported that two loci, 1q41 and 11q22, were significantly associated with AN, but ghrelin, GHRS and GOAT loci were not identified. Linkage studies for AN have detected significant linkage at two regions on chromosome 1 (Grice et al., 2002) and suggestive linkage at a number of additional loci (Bacanu et al., 2005; Devlin et al., 2002). Linkage analysis of a BN cohort also detected significant linkage at 10p13 and suggestive linkage at 14q22.2–23.1.16 (Bulik et al., 2003), but regions containing ghrelin-related genes were again not identified. Pinheiro et al., 2010 conducted an association study of 182 candidate genes including *GHRL* and *GHRS* in 1085 AN cases and 677 individuals. After accounting for multiple comparisons, there were no statistically significant associations for any individual SNP or haplotype block with any definition of illness (Pinheiro et al., 2010).

6. ASSOCIATION OF GHRELIN POLYMORPHISMS WITH ANTHROPOMETRY AND EATING PATHOLOGY IN YOUNG WOMEN

In addition to susceptibility to eating disorders, psychopathologies relevant to eating disorders, such as drive for thinness and body dissatisfaction, along with body mass index, in healthy individuals are known to have a considerable genetic component (Keski-Rahkonen et al., 2005; Rutherford, McGuffin, Katz, & Murray, 1993).

Ando, Ichimaru, Konjiki, Shoji, & Komaki, 2007 conducted a cross-sectional study comparing eating disorder-related phenotypic and anthropometry measures between *GHRL* Leu72Met and 3056 T > C SNP genotypes in 264 female Japanese volunteers. The 3056C allele was significantly associated with higher acyl ghrelin concentration, body weight, body mass index, fat mass, waist circumference, thickness of skin folds, and lower HDL-cholesterol concentration. Interestingly, the 3056C allele was related to elevated scores in the Drive for Thinness-Body Dissatisfaction subscale of the EDI-2. These findings suggest that the 3056 T > C SNP is associated with changes in basal ghrelin concentrations and physical and psychological variables related to eating disorders (Ando et al., 2007).

7. ASSOCIATION OF GHRELIN POLYMORPHISMS WITH CHANGES IN EATING DISORDER PHENOTYPES

AN and BN share common pathologies such as the intense fear of gaining weight and the excessive consideration of body weight and shape during self-evaluation, but characteristics specific to each category of eating disorder also exist. A substantial number of patients with eating disorder crossover from one diagnosis or subtype to another during the clinical course of their illness (Fairburn & Harrison, 2003; Milos, Spindler, Schnyder, & Fairburn, 2005). AN-R patients often develop bulimic symptoms and 62% of patients are reported to crossover to AN-BP(Eddy et al., 2002), while 21–36% change to BN (Strober, Freeman, & Morrell, 1997; Tozzi et al., 2005) during the course of their illness.

Ando et al., 2010 investigated the relationship between the 3056 T > C SNP pre-proghrelin variant and the rate of change from AN-R to other eating disorder phenotypes (Ando et al., 2010). Patients with the TT genotype at 3056 T > C had a higher probability and hazard ratio for recovery of normal weight, but there was no relationship with onset of binge eating. These findings suggest that the 3056 T > C SNP is related to the probability and rate of recovery of normal body weight from AN-R. Although the retrospective nature of the report and marginally significant results after correction for multiple comparisons are study limitations, the observed association with weight recovery indicates that individual biological differences may impact on weight restoration in AN (Ando et al., 2010).

8. CONCLUSIONS

The possible role of ghrelin, GHSR, and GOAT gene variants in the pathogenesis of eating disorders has been extensively investigated as the ghrelin system is a potential regulator of food intake, body weight, and GH secretion (Table 4.2). Although most candidate-gene association studies have not been able to identify ghrelin variants as being significantly associated with either AN or BN in Caucasian populations, they may be significantly associated with BN in the Japanese population. However, only three nonsynonymous SNPs and one intronic SNP among many known ghrelin gene variants have thus far been examined, but the statistical powers of the studies are limited. Moreover, only one candidate-gene study each is available for GHSR and GOAT. A significant association of GHSR with

Table 4.2 Summary of genetic studies on ghrelin, GHRS, and GOAT genes in eating disorders

		Candidate gene studies		
Association		Ghrelin	GHSR	GOAT
AN	Yes	Dardennes et al. (2007)		Müller et al. (2011)
	No	Monteleone et al. (2006) Kindler et al. (2011) Cellini et al. (2006) Ando et al. (2006) Pinheiro et al. (2010)	Miyasaka et al. (2006) Pinheiro et al. (2010)	
BN	Yes	Ando et al. (2006)	Miyasaka et al. (2006)	
	No	Monteleone et al. (2006) Kindler et al. (2011) Cellini et al. (2006)		

GHRS, growth hormone secretagogue receptor; GOAT, growth hormone secretagogue receptor; AN, anorexia nervosa; BN, bulimia nervosa.

BN and GOAT with AN was found, but these findings need to be replicated by others to rule out false positives. Nevertheless, ghrelin-related genes remain important and relevant candidates, but further studies are needed to elucidate their role in predisposition to eating disorders.

REFERENCES

Ando, T., Komaki, G., Naruo, T., Okabe, K., Takii, M., Kawai, K., et al. (2006). Possible role of preproghrelin gene polymorphisms in susceptibility to bulimia nervosa. *American Journal of Medical Genetics. Part B, Neuropsychiatric Genetics*, *141B*, 929–934.

Ando, T., Ichimaru, Y., Konjiki, F., Shoji, M., & Komaki, G. (2007). Variations in the preproghrelin gene correlate with higher body mass index, fat mass, and body dissatisfaction in young Japanese women. *The American Journal of Clinical Nutrition*, *86*, 25–32.

Ando, T., Komaki, G., Nishimura, H., Naruo, T., Okabe, K., Kawai, K., et al. (2010). A ghrelin gene variant may predict crossover rate from restricting-type anorexia nervosa to other phenotypes of eating disorders: A retrospective survival analysis. *Psychiatric Genetics*, *20*, 153–159.

Ariyasu, H., Takaya, K., Tagami, T., Ogawa, Y., Hosoda, K., Akamizu, T., et al. (2001). Stomach is a major source of circulating ghrelin, and feeding state determines plasma ghrelin-like immunoreactivity levels in humans. *The Journal of Clinical Endocrinology and Metabolism*, *86*, 4753–4758.

Arvat, E., Di Vito, L., Broglio, F., Papotti, M., Muccioli, G., Dieguez, C., et al. (2000). Preliminary evidence that ghrelin, the natural GH secretagogue (GHS)-receptor ligand, strongly stimulates GH secretion in humans. *Journal of Endocrinological Investigation*, *23*, 493–495.

Arvat, E., Maccario, M., Di Vito, L., Broglio, F., Benso, A., Gottero, C., et al. (2001). Endocrine activities of ghrelin, a natural growth hormone secretagogue (GHS), in humans: Comparison and interactions with hexarelin, a nonnatural peptidyl GHS, and GH-releasing hormone. *The Journal of Clinical Endocrinology and Metabolism*, *86*, 1169–1174.

Bacanu, S. A., Bulik, C. M., Klump, K. L., Fichter, M. M., Halmi, K. A., Keel, P., et al. (2005). Linkage analysis of anorexia and bulimia nervosa cohorts using selected behavioral phenotypes as quantitative traits or covariates. *American Journal of Medical Genetics. Part B, Neuropsychiatric Genetics*, *139*, 61–68.

Bulik, C. M., Sullivan, P. F., Wade, T. D., & Kendler, K. S. (2000). Twin studies of eating disorders: A review. *The International Journal of Eating Disorders*, *27*, 1–20.

Bulik, C. M., Devlin, S., Bacanu, S. A., Thornton, L., Klump, K. L., Fichter, M. M., et al. (2003). Significant linkage on chromosome 10p in families with bulimia nervosa. *American Journal of Human Genetics*, *72*, 200–207.

Cardon, L. R., & Palmer, L. J. (2003). Population stratification and spurious allelic association. *Lancet*, *361*, 598–604.

Cellini, E., Nacmias, B., Brecelj-Anderluh, M., Badia-Casanovas, A., Bellodi, L., Boni, C., et al. (2006). Case-control and combined family trios analysis of three polymorphisms in the ghrelin gene in European patients with anorexia and bulimia nervosa. *Psychiatric Genetics*, *16*, 51–52.

Counts, D. R., Gwirtsman, H., Carlsson, L. M., Lesem, M., & Cutler, G. B., Jr. (1992). The effect of anorexia nervosa and refeeding on growth hormone-binding protein, the insulin-like growth factors (IGFs), and the IGF-binding proteins. *The Journal of Clinical Endocrinology and Metabolism*, *75*, 762–767.

Dardennes, R. M., Zizzari, P., Tolle, V., Foulon, C., Kipman, A., Romo, L., et al. (2007). Family trios analysis of common polymorphisms in the obestatin/ghrelin, BDNF and AGRP genes in patients with Anorexia nervosa: Association with subtype, body-mass index, severity and age of onset. *Psychoneuroendocrinology*, *32*, 106–113.

Date, Y., Kojima, M., Hosoda, H., Sawaguchi, A., Mondal, M. S., Suganuma, T., et al. (2000a). Ghrelin, a novel growth hormone-releasing acylated peptide, is synthesized in a distinct endocrine cell type in the gastrointestinal tracts of rats and humans. *Endocrinology*, *141*, 4255–4261.

Date, Y., Murakami, N., Kojima, M., Kroiwa, T., Matsukura, S., Kangawa, K., et al. (2000b). Central effects of a novel acylated peptides, ghrelin, on growth hormone release in rats. *Biochemical and Biophysical Research Communications*, *275*, 477–480.

Date, Y., Murakami, N., Toshinai, K., Matsukura, S., Niijima, A., Matsuo, H., et al. (2002a). The role of the gastric afferent vagal nerve in ghrelin-induced feeding and growth hormone secretion in rats. *Gastroenterology*, *123*, 1120–1128.

Date, Y., Nakazato, M., Hashiguchi, S., Dezaki, K., Mondal, M. S., Hosoda, H., et al. (2002b). Ghrelin is present in pancreatic alpha-cells of humans and rats and stimulates insulin secretion. *Diabetes*, *51*, 124–129.

den Hoed, M., Smeets, A. J., Veldhorst, M. A. B., Nieuwenhuizen, A. G., Bouwman, F. G., Heidema, A. G., et al. (2008). SNP analyses of postprandial responses in (an)orexigenic hormones and feelings of hunger reveal long-term physiological adaptations to facilitate homeostasis. *International Journal of Obesity*, *32*, 1790–1798.

Devlin, B., Bacanu, S. A., Klump, K. L., Bulik, C. M., Fichter, M. M., Halmi, K. A., et al. (2002). Linkage analysis of anorexia nervosa incorporating behavioral covariates. *Human Molecular Genetics*, *11*, 689–696.

Eddy, K. T., Keel, P. K., Dorer, D. J., Delinsky, S. S., Franko, D. L., & Herzog, D. B. (2002). Longitudinal comparison of anorexia nervosa subtypes. *The International Journal of Eating Disorders*, *31*, 191–201.

Fairburn, C. G., & Harrison, P. J. (2003). Eating disorders. *Lancet*, *361*, 407–416.

Fichter, M., & Noegel, R. (1990). Concordance for bulimia nervosa in twins. *The International Journal of Eating Disorders*, *9*, 255–263.

Gnanapavan, S., Kola, B., Bustin, S. A., Morris, D. G., McGee, P., Fairclough, P., et al. (2002). The tissue distribution of the mRNA of ghrelin and subtypes of its receptor, GHS-R, in humans. *The Journal of Clinical Endocrinology and Metabolism*, *87*, 2988–2991.

Gorwood, P., Kipman, A., & Foulon, C. (2003). The human genetics of anorexia nervosa. *European Journal of Pharmacology*, *480*, 163–170.

Gourcerol, G., Coskun, T., Craft, L. S., Mayer, J. P., Heiman, M. L., & Wang, L. (2007). Preproghrelin-derived peptide, obestatin, fails to influence food intake in lean or obese rodents. *Obesity (Silver Spring)*, *15*, 2643–2652.

Grice, D. E., Halmi, K. A., Fichter, M. M., Strober, M., Woodside, D. B., Treasure, J. T., et al. (2002). Evidence for a susceptibility gene for anorexia nervosa on chromosome 1. *American Journal of Human Genetics*, *70*, 787–792.

Gutierrez, J. A., Solenberg, P. J., Perkins, D. R., Willency, J. A., Knierman, M. D., Jin, J., et al. (2008). Ghrelin octanoylation mediated by an orphan lipid transferase. *Proceedings of the National Academy of Sciences of the United States of America*, *105*, 6320–6325.

Hansen, T. K., Dall, R., Hosoda, H., Kojima, M., Kangawa, K., Christiansen, J. S., et al. (2002). Weight loss increases circulating levels of ghrelin in human obesity. *Clinical Endocrinology*, *56*, 203–206.

Helder, S. G., & Collier, D. A. (2011). The genetics of eating disorders. *Current Topics in Behavioral Neurosciences*, *6*, 157–175.

Holland, A. J., Sicotte, N., & Treasure, J. (1988). Anorexia nervosa: Evidence for a genetic basis. *Journal of Psychosomatic Research*, *32*, 561–571.

Holst, B., Egerod, K. L., Schild, E., Vickers, S. P., Cheetham, S., Gerlach, L. O., et al. (2007). GPR39 signaling is stimulated by zinc ions but not by obestatin. *Endocrinology*, *148*, 13–20.

Hosoda, H., Kojima, M., Matsuo, H., & Kangawa, K. (2000). Ghrelin and des-acyl ghrelin: Two major forms of rat ghrelin peptide in gastrointestinal tissue. *Biochemical and Biophysical Research Communications*, *279*, 909–913.

Hotta, M., Ohwada, R., Akamizu, T., Shibasaki, T., Takano, K., & Kangawa, K. (2009). Ghrelin increases hunger and food intake in patients with restricting-type anorexia nervosa: A pilot study. *Endocrine Journal*, *56*, 1119–1128.

Howard, A. D., Feighner, S. D., Cully, D. F., Arena, J. P., Liberator, P. A., Rosenblum, C. I., et al. (1996). A receptor in pituitary and hypothalamus that functions in growth hormone release. *Science*, *273*, 974–977.

Inhoff, T., Mönnikes, H., Noetzel, S., Stengel, A., Goebel, M., Dinh, Q. T., et al. (2008). Desacyl ghrelin inhibits the orexigenic effect of peripherally injected ghrelin in rats. *Peptides*, *29*, 2159–2168.

Keski-Rahkonen, A., Bulik, C. M., Neale, B. M., Rose, R. J., Rissanen, A., & Kaprio, J. (2005). Body dissatisfaction and drive for thinness in young adult twins. *The International Journal of Eating Disorders*, *37*, 188–199.

Kindler, J., Bailer, U., deZwaan, M., Fuchs, K., Leisch, F., Grun, B., et al. (2011). No association of the neuropeptide Y (Leu7Pro) and ghrelin gene (Arg51Gln, Leu72Met, Gln90Leu) single nucleotide polymorphisms with eating disorders. *Nordic Journal of Psychiatry*, *65*, 203–207.

Kojima, M., Hosoda, H., Date, Y., Nakazato, M., Matsuo, H., & Kangawa, K. (1999). Ghrelin is a growth-hormone-releasing acylated peptide from stomach. *Nature*, *402*, 656–660.

Kojima, S., Nakahara, T., Nagai, N., Muranaga, T., Tanaka, M., Yasuhara, D., et al. (2005). Altered ghrelin and peptide YY responses to meals in bulimia nervosa. *Clinical Endocrinology*, *62*, 74–78.

Liu, B., Garcia, E. A., & Korbonits, M. (2011). Genetic studies on the ghrelin, growth hormone secretagogue receptor (GHSR) and ghrelin O-acyl transferase (GOAT) genes. *Peptides*, *32*, 2191–2207.

Masuda, Y., Tanaka, T., Inomata, N., Ohnuma, N., Tanaka, S., Itoh, Z., et al. (2000). Ghrelin stimulates gastric acid secretion and motility in rats. *Biochemical and Biophysical Research Communications*, *276*, 905–908.

McKee, K. K., Palyha, O. C., Feighner, S. D., Hreniuk, D. L., Tan, C. P., Phillips, M. S., et al. (1997). Molecular analysis of rat pituitary and hypothalamic growth hormone secretagogue receptors. *Molecular Endocrinology, 11*, 415–423.

Milos, G., Spindler, A., Schnyder, U., & Fairburn, C. G. (2005). Instability of eating disorder diagnoses: Prospective study. *The British Journal of Psychiatry, 187*, 573–578.

Misra, M., Miller, K. K., Bjornson, J., Hackman, A., Aggarwal, A., Chung, J., et al. (2003). Alterations in growth hormone secretory dynamics in adolescent girls with anorexia nervosa and effects on bone metabolism. *The Journal of Clinical Endocrinology and Metabolism, 88*, 5615–5623.

Misra, M., Miller, K. K., Herzog, D. B., Ramaswamy, K., Aggarwal, A., Almazan, C., et al. (2004). Growth hormone and ghrelin responses to an oral glucose load in adolescent girls with anorexia nervosa and controls. *The Journal of Clinical Endocrinology and Metabolism, 89*, 1605–1612.

Miyasaka, K., Hosoya, H., Sekime, A., Ohta, M., Amono, H., Matsushita, S., et al. (2006). Association of ghrelin receptor gene polymorphism with bulimia nervosa in a Japanese population. *Journal of Neural Transmission, 113*, 1279–1285.

Monteleone, P., Martiadis, V., Fabrazzo, M., Serritella, C., & Maj, M. (2003). Ghrelin and leptin responses to food ingestion in bulimia nervosa: Implications for binge-eating and compensatory behaviours. *Psychological Medicine, 33*, 1387–1394.

Monteleone, P., Martiadis, V., Rigamonti, A. E., Fabrazzo, M., Giordani, C., Muller, E. E., et al. (2005). Investigation of peptide YY and ghrelin responses to a test meal in bulimia nervosa. *Biological Psychiatry, 57*, 926–931.

Monteleone, P., Tortorella, A., Castaldo, E., Di Filippo, C., & Maj, M. (2006). No association of the Arg51Gln and Leu72Met polymorphisms of the ghrelin gene with anorexia nervosa or bulimia nervosa. *Neuroscience Letters, 398*, 325–327.

Monteleone, P., Tortorella, A., Castaldo, E., Di Filippo, C., & Maj, M. (2007). The Leu72Met polymorphism of the ghrelin gene is significantly associated with binge eating disorder. *Psychiatric Genetics, 17*, 13–16.

Müller, T. D., Tschöp, M. H., Jarick, I., Ehrlich, S., Scherag, S., Herpertz-Dahlmann, B., et al. (2011). Genetic variation of the ghrelin activator gene ghrelin O-acyltransferase (GOAT) is associated with anorexia nervosa. *Journal of Psychiatric Research, 45*, 706–711.

Nagaya, N., Kojima, M., Uematsu, M., Yamagishi, M., Hosoda, H., Oya, H., et al. (2001). Hemodynamic and hormonal effects of human ghrelin in healthy volunteers. *American Journal of Physiology. Regulatory, Integrative and Comparative Physiology, 280*, R1483–R1487.

Nakabayashi, K., Komaki, G., Tajima, A., Ando, T., Ishikawa, M., Nomoto, J., et al. (2009). Identification of novel candidate loci for anorexia nervosa at 1q41 and 11q22 in Japanese by a genome-wide association analysis with microsatellite markers. *Journal of Human Genetics, 54*, 531–537.

Nakazato, M., Murakami, N., Date, Y., Kojima, M., Matsuo, H., Kangawa, K., et al. (2001). A role for ghrelin in the central regulation of feeding. *Nature, 409*, 194–198.

Nishi, Y., Hiejima, H., Hosoda, H., Kaiya, H., Mori, K., Fukue, Y., et al. (2005). Ingested medium-chain fatty acids are directly utilized for the acyl modification of ghrelin. *Endocrinology, 146*, 2255–2264.

Otto, B., Cuntz, U., Fruehauf, E., Wawarta, R., Folwaczny, C., Riepl, R. L., et al. (2001). Weight gain decreases elevated plasma ghrelin concentrations of patients with anorexia nervosa. *European Journal of Endocrinology, 145*, 669–673.

Pinheiro, A. P., Bulik, C. M., Thornton, L. M., Sullivan, P. F., Root, T. L., Bloss, C. S., et al. (2010). Association Study of 182 Candidate Genes in Anorexia Nervosa. *American Journal of Medical Genetics. Part B, Neuropsychiatric Genetics, 153B*, 1070–1080.

Poykko, S., Ukkola, O., Kauma, H., Savolainen, M. J., & Kesaniemi, Y. A. (2003). Ghrelin Arg51Gln mutation is a risk factor for Type 2 diabetes and hypertension in a random sample of middle-aged subjects. *Diabetologia, 46*, 455–458.

Prince, A. C., Brooks, S. J., Stahl, D., & Treasure, J. (2009). Systematic review and meta-analysis of the baseline concentrations and physiologic responses of gut hormones to food in eating disorders. *The American Journal of Clinical Nutrition, 89*, 755–765.

Risch, N., & Teng, J. (1998). The relative power of family-based and case–control designs for linkage disequilibrium studies of complex human diseases—I. DNA pooling. *Genome Research, 8*, 1273–1288.

Rutherford, J., McGuffin, P., Katz, R. J., & Murray, R. M. (1993). Genetic influences on eating attitudes in a normal female twin population. *Psychological Medicine, 23*, 425–436.

Sato, T., Fukue, Y., Teranishi, H., Yoshida, Y., & Kojima, M. (2005). Molecular forms of hypothalamic ghrelin and its regulation by fasting and 2-deoxy-d-glucose administration. *Endocrinology, 146*, 2510–2516.

Sato, T., Nakamura, Y., Shiimura, Y., Ohgusu, H., Kangawa, K., & Kojima, M. (2012). Structure, regulation and function of ghrelin. *Journal of Biochemistry, 151*, 119–128.

Scherag, S., Hebebrand, J., & Hinney, A. (2010). Eating disorders: The current status of molecular genetic research. *European Child & Adolescent Psychiatry, 19*, 211–226.

Seim, I., Collet, C., Herington, A. C., & Chopin, L. K. (2007). Revised genomic structure of the human ghrelin gene and identification of novel exons, alternative splice variants and natural antisense transcripts. *BMC Genomics, 8*, 298.

Shiiya, T., Nakazato, M., Mizuta, M., Date, Y., Mondal, M. S., Tanaka, M., et al. (2002). Plasma ghrelin levels in lean and obese humans and the effect of glucose on ghrelin secretion. *The Journal of Clinical Endocrinology and Metabolism, 87*, 240–244.

Silverman, E. K., & Palmer, L. J. (2000). Case–control association studies for the genetics of complex respiratory diseases. *American Journal of Respiratory Cell and Molecular Biology, 22*, 645–648.

Stein, D., Lilenfeld, L. R., Plotnicov, K., Pollice, C., Rao, R., Strober, M., et al. (1999). Familial aggregation of eating disorders: Results from a controlled family study of bulimia nervosa. *The International Journal of Eating Disorders, 26*, 211–215.

Stock, S., Leichner, P., Wong, A. C. K., Ghatei, M. A., Kieffer, T. J., Bloom, S. R., et al. (2005). Ghrelin, peptide YY, glucose-dependent insulinotropic polypeptide, and hunger responses to a mixed meal in anorexic, obese, and control female adolescents. *The Journal of Clinical Endocrinology and Metabolism, 90*, 2161–2168.

Strober, M., Freeman, R., & Morrell, W. (1997). The long-term course of severe anorexia nervosa in adolescents: Survival analysis of recovery, relapse, and outcome predictors over 10-15 years in a prospective study. *The International Journal of Eating Disorders, 22*, 339–360.

Tanaka, M., Tatebe, Y., Nakahara, T., Yasuhara, D., Sagiyama, K., Muranaga, T., et al. (2003). Eating pattern and the effect of oral glucose on ghrelin and insulin secretion in patients with anorexia nervosa. *Clinical Endocrinology, 59*, 574–579.

Toshinai, K., Yamaguchi, H., Sun, Y., Smith, R. G., Yamanaka, A., Sakurai, T., et al. (2006). Des-acyl ghrelin induces food intake by a mechanism independent of the growth hormone secretagogue receptor. *Endocrinology, 147*, 2306–2314.

Tozzi, F., Thornton, L. M., Klump, K. L., Fichter, M. M., Halmi, K. A., Kaplan, A. S., et al. (2005). Symptom fluctuation in eating disorders: Correlates of diagnostic crossover. *The American Journal of Psychiatry, 162*, 732–740.

Treasure, J., & Holland, A. (1989). Genetic vulnerability to eating disorders: Evidence from twin studies. In H. Remschmidt & M. Schmidt (Eds.), *Child and youth psychiatry: European perspectives* (pp. 59–68). New York: Hogrefe and Huber.

Tschop, M., Weyer, C., Tataranni, P. A., Devanarayan, V., Ravussin, E., & Heiman, M. L. (2001). Circulating ghrelin levels are decreased in human obesity. *Diabetes, 50*, 707–709.

Tschop, M., Smiley, D., & Heiman, M. (2000). Ghrelin induces adiposity in rodents. *Nature, 407*, 908–913.

Ukkola, O., Ravussin, E., Jacobson, P., Perusse, L., Rankinen, T., Tschop, M., et al. (2002). Role of ghrelin polymorphisms in obesity based on three different studies. *Obesity Research, 10*, 782–791.

Vivenza, D., Rapa, A., Castellino, N., Bellone, S., Petri, A., Vacca, G., et al. (2004). Ghrelin gene polymorphisms and ghrelin, insulin, IGF-I, leptin and anthropometric data in children and adolescents. *European Journal of Endocrinology, 151*, 127–133.

Wade, T. D., Bulik, C. M., Neale, M., & Kendler, K. S. (2000). Anorexia nervosa and major depression: Shared genetic and environmental risk factors. *The American Journal of Psychiatry, 157*, 469–471.

Wajnrajch, M. P., Ten, I. S., Gertner, J. M., & Leibel, R. L. (2000). Genomic organization of the human ghrelin gene. *The Journal of Endocrine Genetics, 1*, 231–233.

Wang, H. J., Geller, F., Dempfle, A., Schäuble, N., Friedel, S., Lichtner, P., et al. (2004). Ghrelin receptor gene: Identification of several sequence variants in extremely obese children and adolescents, healthy normal-weight and underweight students, and children with short normal stature. *The Journal of Clinical Endocrinology and Metabolism, 89*, 157–162.

Wren, A., Seal, L. J., Cohen, M. A., Brynes, A. E., Frost, G. S., Murphy, K. G., et al. (2001). Ghrelin enhances appetite and increases food intake in humans. *The Journal of Clinical Endocrinology and Metabolism, 86*, 5992–5995.

Yang, J., Brown, M. S., Liang, G., Grishin, N. V., & Goldstein, J. L. (2008). Identification of the acyltransferase that octanoylates ghrelin, an appetite-stimulating peptide hormone. *Cell, 132*, 387–396.

Yi, C.-X., Heppner, K., & Tschöp, M. H. (2011). Ghrelin in eating disorders. *Molecular and Cellular Endocrinology, 340*, 29–34.

Zhang, J. V., Ren, P.-G., Avsian-Kretchmer, O., Luo, C.-W., Rauch, R., Klein, C., et al. (2005). Obestatin, a peptide encoded by the ghrelin gene, opposes ghrelin's effects on food intake. *Science, 310*, 996–999.

CHAPTER FIVE

Steroid Metabolism and Excretion in Anorexia Nervosa

Wassif Samuel Wassif*,[1], Andrew Rashad Ross†
*Department of Clinical Biochemistry, Bedford Hospital NHS Trust, Kempston Road, MK42 9DJ Bedford, United Kingdom
†Department of Ophthalmology, University Hospital, Assiut, Egypt
[1]Corresponding author: e-mail address: ws.wassif@bedfordhospital.nhs.uk

Contents

1. Introduction 125
2. Steroid Metabolism in Health 126
   2.1 Steroidogenesis 126
   2.2 Basic structure of steroids 127
   2.3 Regulation of steroid synthesis 128
3. Steroid Metabolism in AN 129
4. Steroid Excretion in AN 130
5. Effects of Refeeding 136
6. Conclusions 137
Acknowledgments 138
References 138

Abstract

Few organ systems are spared the progressive deterioration seen in critically ill patients with anorexia nervosa. Most of the endocrine disturbances discussed are due to starvation and represent appropriate metabolic adaptation of the body to food restriction and negative energy balance. In a starving patient, a lowered metabolic rate, increased cortisol and growth hormone level and reduced fertility are all appropriate adaptations to an abnormal and highly stressful state. Most metabolic abnormalities can be reversed with a well-planned refeeding program and nutritional recovery.

1. INTRODUCTION

Among the plethora of physical problems and metabolic disturbances associated with anorexia nervosa (AN), endocrine manifestations have received relatively large attention. The extreme weight loss produced by

Vitamins and Hormones, Volume 92
ISSN 0083-6729
http://dx.doi.org/10.1016/B978-0-12-410473-0.00005-2

self-imposed dietary restriction in AN is obviously the cause of a profound whole-body metabolic disturbance. Few organ systems are spared the progressive deterioration seen in severely ill patients with AN. Most of the metabolic complications of AN are due to starvation and represent appropriate adjustment of the body to reduced energy intake.

Denial is a prominent feature of AN, and patients resist evaluation and treatment. In the "restricting" form of AN, patients lose weight by self-induced starvation. Compulsive exercising increases calorie debt even further. Most of the medical conditions associated with AN are found in uncomplicated starvation and are reversed by a return to normal healthy diet and weight, but there are important differences between AN and simple starvation in those elements of diet that are deficient. In AN, protein intake is usually adequate, but carbohydrates, fat, and therefore calories are lacking. Vitamin deficiencies are uncommon.

The endocrine manifestations of AN essentially reflect the body's appropriate adaptation to starvation rather than a primary disorder of hypothalamic–pituitary function, and in many respects, these alterations reflect the endocrinology of reduced energy intake.

AN is one of the best examples of providing an insight into not only disorder-associated endocrinopathies but also into disease reversibility on successful refeeding and restoration of body weight.

2. STEROID METABOLISM IN HEALTH

2.1. Steroidogenesis

Steroids are synthesized in the adrenal cortex from cholesterol by a sequence of enzyme-catalyzed reactions. Three major groups of steroids are produced: mineralocorticoids by outer cortical zona glomerulosa, glucocorticoids by the intermediate zona fasciculata, and adrenal androgens by inner zona reticularis.

Mineralocorticoids (primarily aldosterone) regulate blood pressure, vascular volume, and electrolyte transport across epithelial surfaces and are essential in renal conservation of sodium in exchange for potassium. Glucocorticoids (primarily cortisol) promote and inhibit gene transcription in many cells. Other functions of glucocorticoids include modulation of intermediary metabolism and immune responses, prominent anti-inflammatory effects, as well as stimulating hepatic gluconeogenesis. Adrenal androgen precursors are converted in the gonads and target peripheral cells to sex steroids that work through nuclear androgen and estrogen receptors.

Androgens (primarily dehydroepiandrosterone, DHEA, and androstenedione) are responsible for secondary sexual characteristics (in females) after conversion to testosterone and dihydrotestosterone.

2.2. Basic structure of steroids

All steroid hormones are derived from the cyclopentanoperhydrophenanthrene structure: three cyclohexane rings (designated as rings A–C) and a single cyclopentane ring (the D ring). Steroids are built upon a specific arrangement of these four rings that are joined to each other (Fig. 5.1). The carbon atoms are numbered in a sequence beginning with ring A. Steroids vary by the functional groups attached to this four ring core and by the oxidation state of the rings. Adrenal steroids contain either 19 or 21 carbon atoms. The C_{19} steroids with methyl groups at positions C-18 and C-19 have primarily androgenic activity. 17-Ketosteroids have a ketone group at C-17 of C_{19} steroids. The C_{21} steroids have a 2-carbon side chain (C-20 and C-21) attached at position 17 and methyl groups at C-18 and C-19; C_{21} steroids with a hydroxyl group at position 17 are termed *17-hydroxycorticosteroids*. The C_{21} steroids have either glucocorticoid or mineralocorticoid properties.

Cholesterol, derived from the diet and from endogenous synthesis, is the substrate for steroidogenesis. Adrenocorticotropic hormone (ACTH), also known as corticotropin, stimulation is required for the initiation of steroidogenesis. The initial rate-limiting step in steroidogenesis in the normal subject is the conversion of cholesterol to pregnenolone, where ACTH has a major action. Uptake of cholesterol by the adrenal cortex is mediated by the

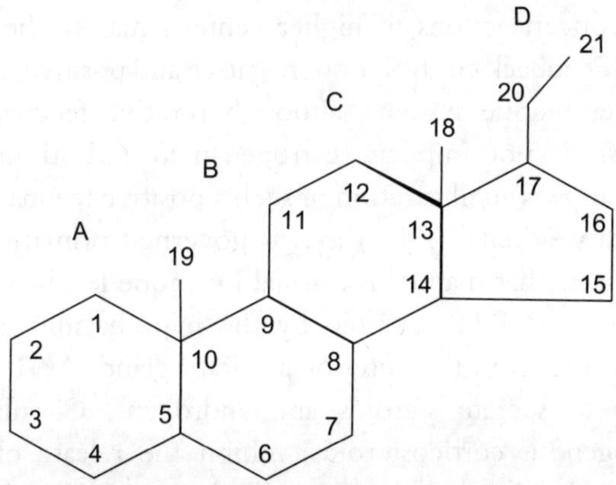

Figure 5.1 The cyclopentanoperhydrophenanthrene structure of steroid hormones; three cyclohexane rings (A–C) and a single cyclopentane ring (the D ring).

low-density lipoprotein (LDL) receptor. Stimulation of the adrenal cortex by ACTH increases the number of LDL receptors. This is a mitochondrial step and is mediated, like the majority of steroidogenic enzymes, by one of the many cytochrome p450 oxygenase enzymes which are located either in the mitochondrion or in the endoplasmic reticulum membrane within steroidogenic pathways. The ACTH receptor MC2R (melanocortin 2 receptor) interacts with the MC2R-accessory protein (MRAP), and the complex is transported to the adrenocortical cell membrane, where it binds to ACTH. The MRAP is one of a growing number of G protein-coupled receptor accessory proteins that add control and complexity to G protein-coupled receptor functional expression and signal transduction. It interacts directly with MC2R and is necessary for its trafficking from the endoplasmic reticulum to the cell surface, where it acts as the receptor for the pituitary hormone ACTH. In addition, MRAP2, a recently described homolog of MRAP, is also able to support the cell surface expression of MC2R. It appears that both MRAP and MRAP2 have a role in the regulation of other melanocortin receptors. Stimulation of ACTH by the MC2R and MRAP complex generates cyclic AMP, which upregulates the protein kinase A signaling pathway. Steroidogenic acute regulatory protein initiates the transfer of cholesterol into the mitochondrion and shuttles it from the outer to the inner mitochondrial membrane, an important step required in all steroidogenic pathways.

2.3. Regulation of steroid synthesis

Steroid hormone concentrations are maintained within a relatively narrow range by the concert actions of higher centers, mainly the pituitary and hypothalamus. Feedback control, both negative and positive, is a fundamental feature of endocrine systems, although positive feedback control of steroid synthesis is not implicit. Estrogen-mediated stimulation of the mid-cycle LH surge is an illustration of such a positive feedback. The hypothalamic–pituitary–adrenal (HPA) axis is governed primarily by negative feedback, a process that maintains normal hormone levels. Corticotropin-releasing hormone (CRH) secreted by the hypothalamus stimulates the secretion of ACTH from the anterior pituitary gland. ACTH induces the adrenal cortex to secrete steroids and androgens. Circulating steroids (including exogenous corticosteroids) inhibit the release of ACTH and CRH by a negative feedback control. Without ACTH stimulation, the adrenal cortex atrophies and steroid synthesis virtually ceases.

3. STEROID METABOLISM IN AN

The eating disorder, AN, is an important and often under-recognized cause of a wide range of abnormalities in steroid metabolism. Many endocrine aberrations occur in AN patients, including hypogonadotropic hypogonadism and hypercortisolemia, and these mediate some of the clinical manifestations of this disease (Lawson & Klibanski, 2008). Although in many respects the endocrine changes in AN represent physiologic adaptation of the body to starvation, some of these changes can persist after recovery and may contribute to the susceptibility to AN recurrence (Lawson & Klibanski, 2008). The endocrinopathies associated with AN are complex and involve multiple endocrine systems and pathogenesis that are designed to conserve energy necessary to safeguard essential organs. Most of the endocrine disorders associated with AN are due to the adaptation to hunger. These include a lowered metabolic rate, increased cortisol concentration, and reduced fertility. The hypothalamus has a central role in mediating these adaptive mechanisms to protect these vital organs in need of significant energy, such as the adrenal glands and the reproductive system. The hypothalamus therefore appears to have a vital role in organizing signals that control weight and food intake and is involved in compound and complex pathways that mediate these adaptive changes (Warren, 2011).

Patients with AN have elevated cortisol concentrations in serum and urine but no Cushingoid-like features are present. Altered cortisol metabolism may explain the diminished cortisol metabolic clearance rate in AN. While secretory patterns show normal cortisol production, cortisol half-life is prolonged and metabolic clearance rate is decreased (Boyar et al., 1977). Though conjugation status is unchanged (Vierhapper et al., 1990), 5α-reduction and 11-dehydrogenation are diminished (Vanluchene, Aertsens, & Vandekerckhove, 1979). Rodin, Thakkar, Taylor, and Clayton (1993) have demonstrated, however, that oxidoreduction at C11 may be a more influential determinant of clearance rate. Cortisol circadian rhythm is preserved in AN patients, although at a new higher set point. Raised CRH concentrations have also been shown in cerebral spinal fluid, indicating a centrally induced mechanism for the hypercortisolemia noted in AN patients (Hotta et al., 1986). Other factors which can influence cortisol levels, such as cortisol-binding globulin and ACTH, are similar in AN and normal weight subjects (Gwirtsman et al., 1989). Nonetheless, in AN subjects, urinary cortisol excretion in response to ACTH stimulation is diminished compared to normal weight subjects (Cooke, James, Landon, & Wynn, 1964) and dexamethasone fails to fully suppress cortisol, suggesting an impaired feedback mechanism and/or an altered set point. Impaired urinary cortisol excretion following ACTH stimulation has also been shown in malnourished patients (Russell, 1967). AN subjects do not develop the common clinical features of hypercortisolemia, and it may be that paucity of metabolic substrates accounts for the lack of Cushingoid features in AN (Invitti, Redaelli, Baldi, & Cavagnini, 1999). Recently, however, Estour et al. (2010) have demonstrated hormonal profile heterogeneity and documented two types of hormonal responses in AN patients, those with hormonal disorders including increased cortisol concentration as a normal adaptation to starvation and those with blunted hormonal responses. Whether such blunted response accounts for an abnormal response to starvation or due to resistance to undernutrition is currently been debated. Interestingly, a recent study indicated a genetic influence on hormonal set point in different subjects (Panicker et al., 2008). The balance of evidence suggests that an altered hormonal set point in a subset of AN patients is responsible for such diverse hormonal response noted in anorexia nervosa (Warren, 2011).

Although an alteration in steroid metabolism appears to be directly associated with weight loss, Hotta et al. (1986) have shown that body mass index (BMI) accounted only partly for the variation in cortisol concentration and Lawson et al. (2011) confirmed that higher levels of cortisol were associated with AN independent of BMI in women across the weight spectrum. Derangements of steroid metabolism appear to become more evident as the disease progresses and becomes more severe. Although most medical complications of AN can be reversed with a well-planned refeeding program, weight recovery does not appear to fully normalize HPA axis.

4. STEROID EXCRETION IN AN

Capillary gas chromatography (GC) is the method of choice for obtaining detailed urinary steroid profile (Shackleton and Honour, 1976). Because of its high specificity and resolution, GC can clearly identify urinary cardinal steroid metabolites. However, a number of preparatory steps are required prior to GC analysis including extraction of conjugated steroids, hydrolysis of glucuronide/sulfate conjugates, and reextraction. Internal standards are then added, and a purification step is included to remove water-soluble material that may interfere with the derivatization process. Following derivatization, steroid identity is checked by gas chromatography–mass spectrometry. Metabolites are quantified by relating peak heights with those of the internal standards (Bevan et al., 1986). The concentration of steroid present in the original urine sample is calculated according to the following formula:

$$\frac{\text{Unknown peak height} \times \mu\text{g standard in derivative}}{\text{Standard peak height} \times \text{fraction of extract used for derivative} \times \text{fraction of 24-h urine volume analyzed}}.$$

The principal urinary metabolites of cortisol measured by GC are shown in Fig. 5.2. Steroid metabolites are typically analyzed in 24 h collections of urine, and steroid profile is used to obtain direct assessments of daily production rates of androgen metabolites (AM, androsterone and etiocholanolone) and cortisol metabolites (CM, tetrahydrocortisone, 5α- and 5β-tetrahydrocortisol, 20α- and 20β-cortolone, and 20α- and 20β-cortol). Urine metabolites are sensitive indicators of suppression of adrenal steroidogenesis (Fink et al., 2002). Ratios of urine metabolites provide indices of activity of the major routes of peripheral phase 1 metabolism as follows: 5α- compared with 5β-reduction: androsterone (5α)/etiocholanolone (5β) and 5α-/5β-tetrahydrocortisol; 11-oxidoreduction compared with 11-dehydrogenation:tetrahydrocortisols (11-OH)/tetrahydrocortisone (11-oxo); 20-oxidoreduction compared with 20-dehydrogenation:cortols + cortolones (20-OH)/tetrahydrocortisone +tetrahydrocortisols (20-oxo); and 20α- compared with 20β-reduction: 20α-cortolone + 20α-cortol/20β-cortolone + 20β-cortol. The biosynthesis and origin of urinary steroid metabolites are described in Fig. 5.3 and a typical chromatogram is shown in Fig. 5.4.

Underweight AN patients tend to have relatively lower concentrations of urinary excretion of total CM and total AM. In untreated patients, urinary androsterone, 5α-tetrahydrocortisol (5α-THF), α-cortolone, and α-cortol are low (Table 5.1). Before refeeding, anorexic patients have reduced 5α- and 5β-reductases activities: both of the androsterone/etiocholanolone

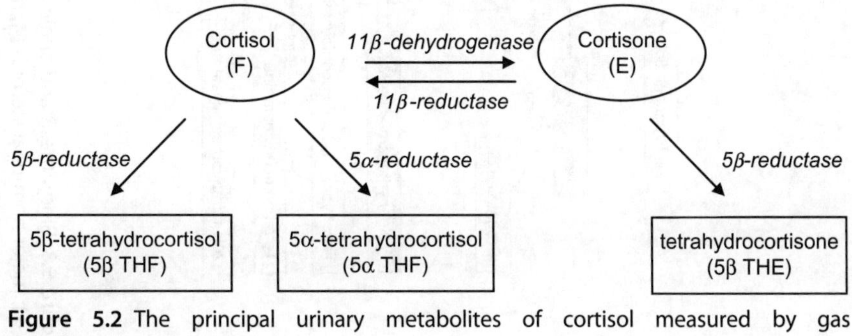

Figure 5.2 The principal urinary metabolites of cortisol measured by gas chromatography.

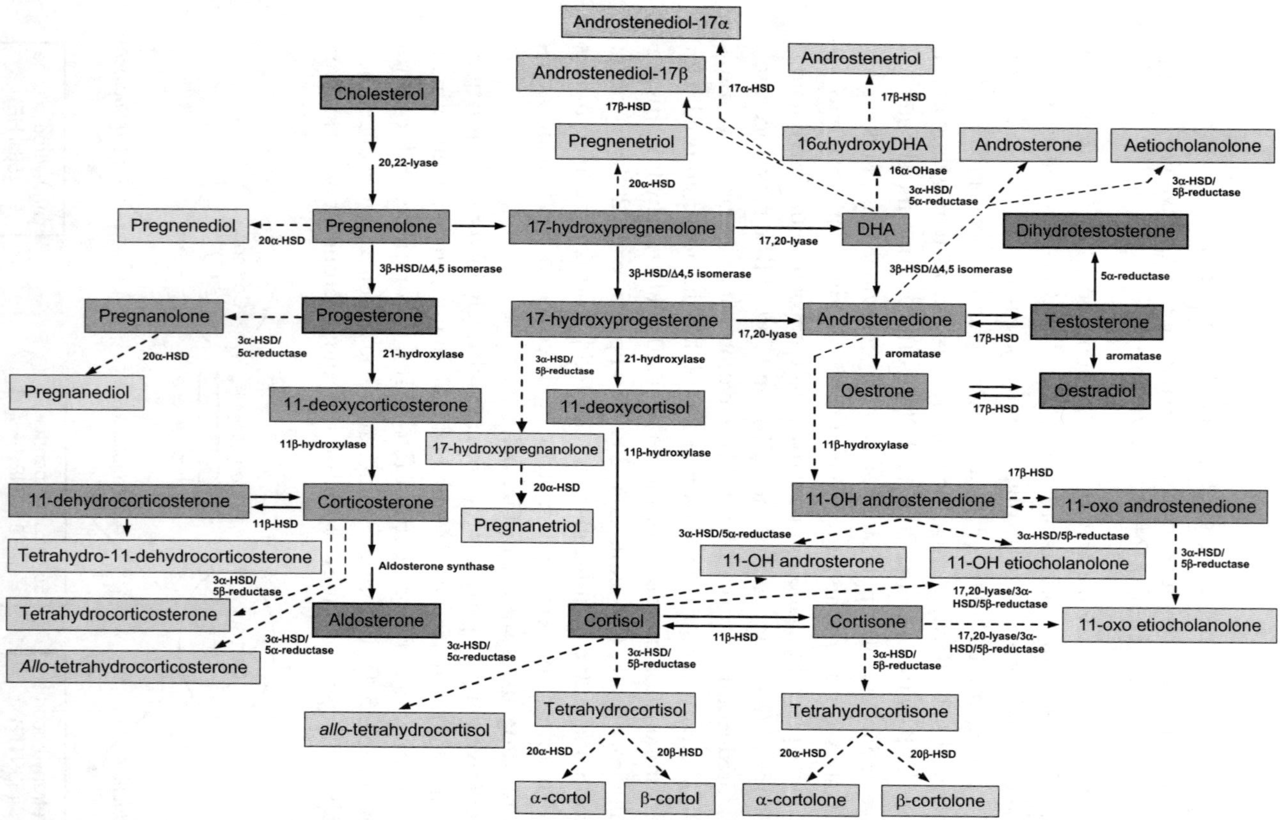

Figure 5.3 Biosynthesis and origin of urinary steroid metabolites. Anabolic pathways are represented by a solid arrow (⟶); catabolic pathways (- - ->); major hormonal steroids ■; major urinary metabolites □; intermediates ■. DHA represents dehydroepiandrosterone; HSD, hydroxy dehydrogenase (courtesy of Dr. N. Taylor). (See Color Insert.)

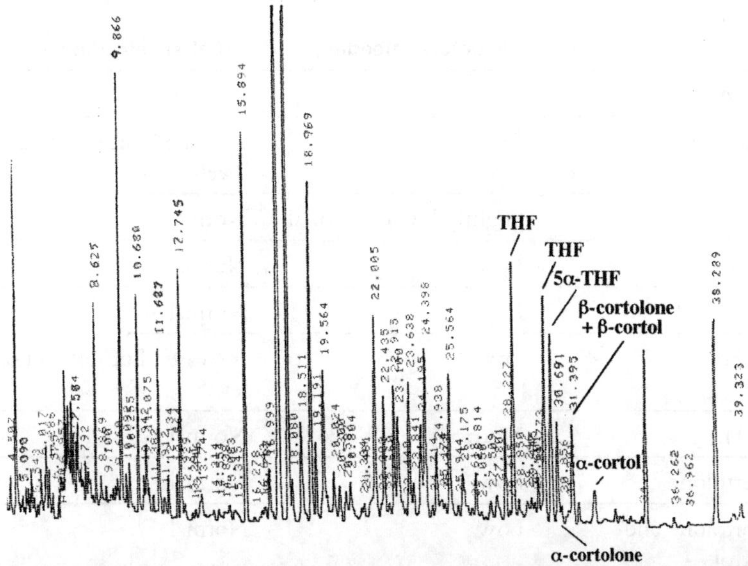

Figure 5.4 A typical chromatogram of urinary steroid profile. THE, tetrahydrocortisone; THF, tetrahydrocortisol (courtesy of Dr. N. Taylor).

(andro/etio) ratio as well the 5α-/5β-THF ratio are significantly low (Wassif et al., 2011). The andro/etio and 5α-/5β-THF ratios reflect relative activities of the same 5-reductase enzymes. Changes in these ratios are accounted for by the 5α-reduced component, since androsterone and 5α-THF are reduced, while the 5β-epimers are not different from normal. In contrast, the 5β-reduced components (etiocholanolone, 5β-THF) are comparable to normal weight subjects (Bradlow, Boyar, O'Connor, Zumoff, & Hellman, 1976; Wassif et al., 2011). Low ratios mimic findings in patients with 5α-reductase deficiency and during treatment with the 5α-reductase inhibitor finasteride. In 5α-reductase deficiency, the 5α-reductase II enzyme is deficient, and both ratios are very low. Steroid metabolic changes in AN are similar to those in hypothyroidism (Bradlow et al., 1976). The 5α-/5β-THF ratio and andro/etio ratio are significantly higher in hyperthyroid patients and significantly lower in hypothyroid patients compared to normal subjects (Hoshiro, Ohno, Masaki, Iwase, & Aoki, 2006). This may be explained by anorexics being essentially hypothyroid due to metabolic adaptation that lowers the resting energy expenditure during chronic starvation (Usdan, Khaodhiar, & Apovian, 2008).

Similarly, starving AN patients have abnormal 20α- and 20β-hydroxysteroid dehydrogenase (HSD) activities and the 20-OH/20-oxo

Table 5.1 Steroid metabolites in patients with anorexia nervosa during starvation and after refeeding

	AN before refeeding	**AN after refeeding**
Total AM	Low	Normal
Andro	Low	Increased but not to normal levels
Etio	Slightly low or normal	Normal
Total CM	Low	Normal
THE	Low	Normal
5α-THF	Low	Increased but not to normal levels
5β-THF	Normal	Normal
α-Cortolone	Low	Normal
β-Cortolone and β-cortol	Low	Normal
α-Cortol	Low	Normal
5α- and 5β-reductase activities		
Andro/etio	Low	Normal
5α/5β-THF	Low	Normal
11β-HSD activities		
THFs/THE	High	Normal
20α- and 20β-HSD activities		
20-OH/20-oxo	Low	Normal
α/β-cortolone and cortol	Low	Normal

Abbreviations: Total AM, androgen metabolites (androsterone (5α) + etiocholanolone (5β)); andro, androsterone; etio, etiocholanolone; total CM, cortisol metabolites; THE, tetrahydrocortisone; 5α-T-HF, 5α-tetrahydrocortisol; 5β-THF, 5β-tetrahydrocortisol; 5α/5β THF, 5α/5β tetrahydrocortisol; THFs/THE, (5α-THF + 5β-THF)/tetrahydrocortisone; 20-OH/20-oxo, 20-hydroxycorticosteroid (cortolone + cortol)/20-oxocorticosteroid (THE + THFs); 20α/20β, 20α/20β-reduced cortisol metabolites (cortols and cortolones); HSD, hydroxysteroid dehydrogenase; α/β cortolone and cortol, 20α-cortolone + 20α-cortol/20β-cortolone + 20β-cortol; AN, anorexia nervosa.

[20-hydroxycorticosteroid (cortolone + cortol)/20-oxocorticosteroid (THE + THFs)] metabolite ratio is reduced before refeeding (Table 5.1). However, the 20α-cortol + α-cortolone/20β-cortol + β-cortolone ratio, which examines 20α- versus 20β-reduction, is not altered in AN patients. Anorexic patients also appear to have reduced 11β-HSD activity (reflected by higher ratio of tetrahydrocortisols/tetrahydrocortisone; THFs/THE). There are two main 11β-HSD enzymes: type-1 is predominant in the liver and acts as a reductase (converting cortisone to cortisol) while type-2 is predominantly renal and acts as a dehydrogenase (converting cortisol to cortisone) (Fig. 5.3). Cortisol metabolic clearance rate is greatly influenced by 11β-HSD activity. In most conditions in which the ratio of cortisol:cortisone metabolites changes (apart from specific enzyme deficiencies), such as differences of fat deposits and growth hormone status, it is the type-1 enzyme activity which is changed (Gelding et al., 1998). Increased activity results in a lower clearance rate, while decreased activity (or increased 11β-HSD 2 activity) results in a higher clearance rate (Boyar et al., 1977; Müssig et al., 2008). Studies of steroid excretion in AN have indicated reduced activity of the 11-oxidation component of 11β-HSD (Lawson & Klibanski, 2008; Wassif et al., 2011). This is supported by the finding of higher ratios of THFs/THE. As in the situation with 5α-reductase, changes in 11β-HSD activity are similar to those in hypothyroidism with a THFs/THE ratio that is lower in hyperthyroid patients and higher in hypothyroid patients compared to normal subjects (Hoshiro et al., 2006). In specific type-2 enzyme deficiency (apparent mineralocorticoid excess), the THFs/THE ratio is very high, but the 5α-reduced steroids are also relatively increased and this is evidently a secondary phenomenon. In AN, increase in the THFs/THE ratio is accompanied by decrease in 5α-reduction, so the latter clearly has another origin.

In contrast to AN patients, overweight individuals show enhanced androgen and cortisol metabolite excretion and increased net 5α-reductase and 11-oxidation activities (Boyar et al., 1977; Vassiliadi et al., 2009). Adipose tissue samples taken from obese subjects show increased expression of 11β-HSD1 (Rask et al., 2001) which would be expected to lead to a stimulated conversion of cortisone to cortisol and subsequently increased intracellular glucocorticoid reactivation and activity (Svendsen, Madsbad, Nilas, Paulsen, & Pedersen, 2009).

Weight-reducing diets for obese subjects are associated with an increased 11β-HSD1 and diminished 5-reductase activities (Svendsen et al., 2009). Wassif et al. (2011) have shown that a high-calorie diet in AN patients achieves the opposite changes, with decrease of THFs/THE. Previous studies have demonstrated that weight loss (Engeli et al., 2004) and a low-carbohydrate diet (Stimson et al., 2007) are not associated with changes in 5α-reductase and 11β-HSD1 activities in adipose tissue. Hence, these changes are likely to occur predominantly in the liver.

A novel finding in AN patients of reduced 20-OH/20-oxo ratio, indicating decreased 20-reduction over 20-dehydrogenation, has been recently reported (Wassif et al., 2011). This phenomenon is likely to be responsible for decreased cortisol metabolic clearance rate.

5. EFFECTS OF REFEEDING

Significant changes in urinary cortisol metabolites, androgen metabolites, and metabolite ratios are apparent in starved AN patients; these changes are reversible with successful refeeding and return to normal healthy diet (Wassif et al., 2011). For cortisol, these are decrease of 5α-/5β-tetrahydrocortisol and 20-OH/20-oxo metabolites, and for androgen, decrease of andro/etio.

On refeeding, fat gain is primarily responsible for most (77%) of the weight increase in recovering AN patients (Russell & Mezey, 1962). Fat gain in women preserves the gynoid fat distribution pattern, with no preferential deposition in central regions (Orphanidou, McCargar, Birmingham, & Belzberg, 1997). Deposition of fat and lean tissue during weight recovery in healthy subjects is determined mainly by individual variations in percentage of body fat before weight loss (Dulloo, Jacquet, & Girardier, 1996) and the same may apply to AN patients (Mika, Herpertz-Dahlmann, Heer, & Holtkamp, 2004).

In men, obesity is associated with a higher ratio of THFs/THE; the ratio is also higher in women than in men. This ratio represents the whole-body equilibrium between cortisol and cortisone, as determined by the balance of activities of 11β-dehydrogenase (the product of 11β-HSD type 2 gene) and 11β-reductase (the product of 11β-HSD type 1 gene). In the kidney and other mineralocorticoid target tissues, 11β-HSD2 converts cortisol to cortisone; in that way it protects mineralocorticoid receptors from inappropriate activation by cortisol. Impaired 11β-HSD2 is associated therefore with increased urinary free cortisol/cortisone ratio. It appears that 11β-HSD2 is not related to obesity or fat gain as the increased ratio of THFs/THE observed in women and obese men was not associated with increased urinary cortisol/cortisone ratio (Andrew, Phillips, & Walker, 1998). Upregulation of 11β-HSD1 results in enhanced reactivation of cortisol from cortisone in the liver, fat, and other glucocorticoid target tissues by 11β-reductase in obese men and in women generally. Studies in rats indicate that 11β-HSD1 expression is downregulated by insulin (Jamieson, Chapman,

Edwards, & Seckl, 1995) and estrogen (Low et al., 1994). As such, in obese men, upregulation of enzyme activity in visceral fat may be secondary to resistance to the normal inhibition of insulin on 11β-HSD1, due to insulin resistance, altered growth hormone profile, and increased number of adipocytes expressing 11β-HSD1 activities. In postmenopausal women, estrogen deficiency is likely to be responsible (Andrew et al., 1998).

The ratio of urinary 11-OH/11-oxo steroids reflects the net activities of oxidation and reduction. Some researchers favor the THFs/THE ratio, but this ratio only looks at the A ring-reduced metabolites of cortisol and cortisone, whereas the 11-OH/11-oxo ratio looks at all the major products of cortisol and cortisone. They generally give just the same information. The 11-OH/11-oxo ratio reflects 11β-HSD activity and the ratio decreases with increasing fat mass (Weaver, Taylor, Monson, Wood, & Kelly, 1998). Thus, a decrease of this ratio, as observed in patients with AN after refeeding, can probably be ascribed to an increase in fat mass. When emaciated, no relationships between steroid metabolism and body indices were observed. However, after refeeding, a significant correlation was noted between 5α-/5β-THF ratio and BMI. Interestingly, changes in 5α-/5β-THF before and after refeeding were significantly correlated with that in both body weight and BMI (Wassif et al., 2011).

Impaired urinary cortisol excretion after corticotropin stimulation has been shown in malnourished patients, and this normalized with improvement in their nutritional status (Russell, 1967). Refeeding also corrected 20-OH/20-oxo ratio. Although this ratio does not change in many clinical states, it is increased in alcoholic liver disease. Zumoff and colleagues (1967) have ascribed this to increased liver activity of 20-reductases. As 20-reduction is decreased while 11-reduction is increased in patients with AN, these changes therefore are not due to a generalized change in the status of steroid oxidation versus reduction. After successful refeeding, all other abnormalities in steroid metabolites are reversed and are comparable to normal weight subjects, although androsterone and 5α-THF do not fully normalize.

6. CONCLUSIONS

The endocrine manifestations of AN essentially reflect the body's appropriate adaptation to starvation rather than a primary disorder of hypothalamic–pituitary function, and in many respects, these alterations reflect the endocrinology of reduced energy intake. Such metabolic adjustments are designed to conserve energy in order to protect vital organs. In a starving patient, a lowered metabolic rate, decreased thyroid hormones, increased cortisol and growth hormone levels (promoting gluconeogenesis and reducing peripheral use of glucose), and reduced fertility are all necessary and appropriate adaptations to an abnormal and highly stressful state.

Numerous endocrine abnormalities occur in AN, and few organ systems are spared the progressive deterioration seen in seriously ill patients. Most of the medical complications associated with AN represent appropriate metabolic adjustments of the body to food restriction and negative energy balance, and are found in uncomplicated starvation. Most of these complications are reversed with a well-planned refeeding program and return to normal healthy diet and weight. Altered cortisol and androgen metabolism (but not in production rate) occur on starvation. Such changes are apparent in urine steroid metabolite excretion and in activities of the enzymes 5α-reductase, 11β-HSD 1, and 20α- and 20β-HSD, and are due to chronic starvation. These changes are reversible with nutritional rehabilitation and correlate with weight gain (Wassif et al., 2011).

ACKNOWLEDGMENTS

We are grateful to Miss Amy Wassif for technical computer assistance. Figures 5.3 and 5.4 were provided with permission, courtesy of Dr. Norman Taylor, director of Steroid Supra Regional Assay Laboratory at King's College, London. The cooperation of patients and contribution of many collaborators, in particular, Prof. Declan McLoughlin, Dr. Norman Taylor, Prof. Gerald Russell, and Dr. Royce Vincent, are acknowledged.

REFERENCES

Andrew, R., Phillips, D., & Walker, B. (1998). Obesity and gender influence cortisol secretion and metabolism in man. *The Journal of Clinical Endocrinology and Metabolism*, *83*, 1806–1809.

Bevan, B. R., Savvas, M., Jenkins, J. M., Baker, K., Pennington, G., & Taylor, N. F. (1986). Abnormal steroid excretion in gestational trophoblastic disease complicated by ovarian theca-lutein cysts. *Journal of Clinical Pathology*, *39*, 627–634.

Boyar, R. M., Hellman, L. D., Roffwarg, H., Katz, J., Zumoff, B., O'Connor, J., et al. (1977). Cortisol secretion and metabolism in anorexia nervosa. *The New England Journal of Medicine*, *296*, 190–193.

Bradlow, H. L., Boyar, R. M., O'Connor, J., Zumoff, B. J., & Hellman, L. D. (1976). Hypothyroid-like alterations in testosterone metabolism in anorexia nervosa. *The Journal of Clinical Endocrinology and Metabolism*, *43*, 571–574.

Cooke, J. N., James, V. H., Landon, J., & Wynn, V. (1964). Adrenocortical function in chronic malnutrition. *British Medical Journal*, *1*, 662–666.

Dulloo, A. G., Jacquet, J., & Girardier, L. (1996). Autoregulation of body composition during weight recovery in human: The Minnesota Experiment revisited. *International Journal of Obesity and Related Metabolic Disorders*, *20*, 393–405.

Engeli, S., Bohnke, J., Feldpausch, M., Gorzelniak, K., Heintze, U., Janke, J., et al. (2004). Regulation of 11β-HSD genes in human adipose tissue: Influence of central obesity and weight loss. *Obesity Research*, *12*, 9–17.

Estour, B., Germain, N., Diconne, E., Frere, D., Cottet-Emard, J. M., Carrot, G., et al. (2010). Hormonal profile heterogeneity and short-term physical risk in restrictive anorexia nervosa. *The Journal of Clinical Endocrinology and Metabolism*, *95*, 2203–2210.

Fink, R. S., Pierre, L. N., Daley-Yates, P. T., Richards, D. H., Gibson, A., & Honour, J. W. (2002). Hypothalamic-pituitary-adrenal axis function after inhaled corticosteroids: Unreliability of urinary free cortisol estimation. *The Journal of Clinical Endocrinology and Metabolism*, *87*, 4541–4546.

Gelding, S. V., Taylor, N. F., Wood, P. J., Noonan, K., Weaver, J. U., Wood, D. F., et al. (1998). The effect of growth hormone replacement therapy on cortisol–cortisone interconversion in hypopituitary adults: Evidence for growth hormone modulation of extrarenal 11β-hydroxysteroid dehydrogenase activity. *Clinical Endocrinology*, *48*, 153–162.

Gwirtsman, H. E., Kaye, W. H., George, D. T., Jimerson, D. C., Ebert, M. H., & Gold, P. (1989). Central and peripheral ACTH and cortisol levels in anorexia nervosa and bulimia. *Archives of General Psychiatry*, *46*, 61–69.

Hoshiro, M., Ohno, Y., Masaki, H., Iwase, H., & Aoki, N. (2006). Comprehensive study of urinary cortisol metabolites in hyperthyroid and hypothyroid patients. *Clinical Endocrinology*, *64*, 37–45.

Hotta, M., Shibasaki, T., Masuda, A., Imaki, T., Demura, H., Ling, N., et al. (1986). The responses of plasma adrenocorticotropin and cortisol to corticotropin-releasing hormone (CRH) and cerebrospinal fluid immunoreactive CRH in anorexia nervosa patients. *The Journal of Clinical Endocrinology and Metabolism*, *62*, 319–324.

Invitti, C., Redaelli, G., Baldi, G., & Cavagnini, F. (1999). Glucocorticoid receptors in anorexia nervosa and Cushing's disease. *Biological Psychiatry*, *45*, 1467–1471.

Jamieson, P. M., Chapman, K. E., Edwards, C. R., & Seckl, J. R. (1995). 11 beta-Hydroxysteroid dehydrogenase is an exclusive 11 beta-reductase in primary cultures of rat hepatocytes: Effect of physicochemical and hormonal manipulations. *Endocrinology*, *136*, 4754–4761.

Lawson, E. A., Eddy, K. T., Donoho, D., Misra, M., Miller, K. K., Meenaghan, E., et al. (2011). Appetite-regulating hormones cortisol and peptide YY are associated with disordered eating psychopathology, independent of body mass index. *European Journal of Endocrinology*, *164*(2), 253–261.

Lawson, E. A., & Klibanski, A. (2008). Endocrine abnormalities in anorexia nervosa. *Nature Clinical Practice Endocrinology & Metabolism*, *4*, 407–414.

Low, S. C., Chapman, K. E., Edwards, C. R., Wells, T., Robinson, I. C., & Seckl, J. R. (1994). Sexual dimorphism of hepatic 11 beta-hydroxysteroid dehydrogenase in the rat: The role of growth hormone patterns. *Journal of Endocrinology*, *143*, 541–548.

Mika, C., Herpertz-Dahlmann, B., Heer, M., & Holtkamp, K. (2004). Improvement of nutritional status as assessed by multifrequency BIA during 15 weeks of refeeding in adolescent girls with anorexia nervosa. *The Journal of Nutrition*, *134*, 3026–3030.

Müssig, K., Remer, T., Haupt, A., Gallwitz, B., Fritsche, A., Häring, H. U., et al. (2008). 11 beta-Hydroxysteroid dehydrogenase 2 activity is elevated in severe obesity and negatively associated with insulin sensitivity. *Obesity (Silver Spring)*, *16*, 1256–1260.

Orphanidou, C. I., McCargar, L. J., Birmingham, C. L., & Belzberg, A. S. (1997). Changes in body composition and fat distribution after short-term weight gain in patients with anorexia nervosa. *The American Journal of Clinical Nutrition*, *65*, 1034–1041.

Panicker, V., Wilson, S. G., Spector, T. D., Brown, S. J., Kato, B. S., Reed, P. W., et al. (2008). Genetic loci linked to pituitary-thyroid axis set points: A genome-wide scan of a large twin cohort. *The Journal of Clinical Endocrinology and Metabolism*, *93*, 3519–3523.

Rask, E., Olsson, T., Söderberg, S., Andrew, R., Livingstone, D. E., Johnson, O., et al. (2001). Tissue-specific dysregulation of cortisol metabolism in human obesity. *The Journal of Clinical Endocrinology and Metabolism, 86*, 1418–1421.

Rodin, D. A., Thakkar, H., Taylor, N. F., & Clayton, R. N. (1993). Hyperandrogenism in polycystic ovary syndrome. Evidence for dysregulation of 11B-hydroxysteroid dehydrogenase. *The New England Journal of Medicine, 330*, 460–465.

Russell, G. F. M. (1967). The nutritional disorder in anorexia nervosa. *Journal of Psychiatric Research, 11*, 141–149.

Russell, G. F. M., & Mezey, A. G. (1962). An analysis of weight gain in patients with anorexia nervosa treated with high calorie diets. *Clinical Science, 23*, 449–461.

Shackleton, C. H., & Honour, J. W. (1976). Simultaneous estimation of urinary steroids by semi-automated gas chromatography. Investigation of neo-natal infants and children with abnormal steroid synthesis. *Clinica chimica acta, 69*, 267–283.

Stimson, R. H., Johnstone, A. M., Homer, N. Z., Wake, D. J., Morton, N. M., Andrew, R., et al. (2007). Dietary macronutrient content alters cortisol metabolism independently of body weight changes in obese men. *The Journal of Clinical Endocrinology and Metabolism, 92*, 4480–4484.

Svendsen, P. F., Madsbad, S., Nilas, L., Paulsen, S. K., & Pedersen, S. B. (2009). Expression of 11beta-hydroxysteroid dehydrogenase 1 and 2 in subcutaneous adipose tissue of lean and obese women with and without polycystic ovary syndrome. *International Journal of Obesity, 33*, 1249–1256.

Usdan, L. S., Khaodhiar, L., & Apovian, C. M. (2008). The endocrinopathies of anorexia nervosa. *Endocrine Practice, 14*, 1055–1063.

Vanluchene, E., Aertsens, W., & Vandekerckhove, D. V. (1979). Steroid excretion in anorexia nervosa patients. *Acta Endocrinologica, 90*, 133–138.

Vassiliadi, D. A., Barber, T. M., Hughes, B. A., McCarthy, M. I., Wass, J. A., Franks, S., et al. (2009). Increased 5 alphareductase activity and adrenocortical drive in women with polycystic ovary syndrome. *The Journal of Clinical Endocrinology and Metabolism, 94*, 3558–3566.

Vierhapper, H., Kisss, A., Novotny, P., Wiesnagrotski, S., Monder, C., & Waldehäusl, W. (1990). Metabolism of cortisol in anorexia nervosa. *Acta Endocrinologica (Copenhagen), 122*, 753–758.

Warren, M. P. (2011). Endocrine manifestations of eating disorders. *The Journal of Clinical Endocrinology and Metabolism, 96*, 333–343.

Wassif, W. S., McLoughlin, D., Vincent, R., Conroy, S., Russell, G. F. M., & Taylor, N. (2011). Steroid metabolism and excretion in severe anorexia nervosa: Effects of refeeding. *The American Journal of Clinical Nutrition, 93*(5), 911–917.

Weaver, J. U., Taylor, N. F., Monson, J. P., Wood, P. J., & Kelly, W. F. (1998). Sexual dimorphism in 11β hydroxysteroid dehydrogenase activity and its relation to fat distribution and insulin sensitivity: A study in hypopituitary subjects. *Clinical Endocrinology, 49*, 13–20.

Zumoff, B., Bradlow, H. L., Gallagher, T. F., & Hellman, L. (1967). Cortisol metabolism in cirrhosis. *Journal of Clinical Investigation, 46*, 1735–1743.

CHAPTER SIX

Anorexia Nervosa and Estrogen Receptors

Nicolas Ramoz*[,1], Audrey Versini*, Philip Gorwood*[,†]
*INSERM UMR894, Centre de Psychiatrie et Neurosciences, Paris, France
†CMME, Sainte-Anne Hospital, Paris Descartes University, Paris, France
[1]Corresponding author: e-mail address: nicolas.ramoz@inserm.fr

Contents

1. Introduction 142
2. Anorexia Nervosa 142
3. Estrogens and Estrogen Receptors and Pathways 145
4. Estrogen and Anorexia 147
   4.1 Animal models, estrogen pathway, and anorexia 147
   4.2 Estrogens and food intake in brain 148
   4.3 Sexual hormones, estrogens, in AN patients 150
   4.4 Hypoestrogenism in anorexia nervosa 150
5. Human Genetics of Estrogen Pathway in Anorexia Nervosa 151
6. Conclusions 155
References 156

Abstract

Anorexia nervosa (AN) is a chronic psychiatric disorder with a high prevalence of 0.6% and the highest mortality rates among psychiatric diseases, around 10%, mostly due to undernutrition and suicide. AN is characterized by physiological features with a body mass index less than 17.5 kg/m^2, low bone mineral density and amenorrhea, psychological symptoms with a distortion of image body, and behavioral abnormalities. Estrogen molecules and estrogen biological pathway are clearly involved in food intake and body weight in animals and humans. Further, hypoestrogenism has been demonstrated in AN patients and convergent evidence involves the estrogen pathway in the development of AN. AN presents a high heritability and polymorphisms in genes coding the estrogen receptors alpha and beta have been found significantly associated with the disorder. This chapter shows the implication of estrogens in AN and suggests investigation to develop future pharmacological treatments for anorexia.

Vitamins and Hormones, Volume 92
ISSN 0083-6729
http://dx.doi.org/10.1016/B978-0-12-410473-0.00006-4

1. INTRODUCTION

Anorexia nervosa (AN) is characterized by an eating restriction, repeated and obsessive fears of being fat, and the voluntary pursuit of leanness (Bulik, Reba, Siega-Riz, & Reichborn-Kjennerud, 2005). It is a chronic disorder with a prevalence of 0.3–0.6% (Hoek & Van Hoeken, 2003; Hudson, Hiripi, Pope, & Kessler, 2007). AN represents one of the highest mortality rates among psychiatric diseases, around 10% per decade, mostly due to undernutrition and suicide (Birmingham, Su, Hlynsky, Goldner, & Gao, 2005; Millar et al., 2005). The mortality rate was recently reevaluated in a meta-analysis and the study found a rate close to 6/1000 AN deaths per year, with 20% due to suicide (Arcelus, Mitchell, Wales, & Nielsen, 2011). Thus, AN represents a major problem of public health. Further, osteoporosis is an important comorbid condition in 40% of AN patients, and an osteopenia is observed in 92% of cases (Mehler, Cleary, & Gaudiani, 2011). Reported low bone mineral density in AN patients could be the result of multiple factors. One of these contributors might be the level of estrogen, which has been found to be severely lower in AN patients compared to controls (Brambilla et al., 2003; Estour et al., 2010; Ohwada, Hotta, Sato, Shibasaki, & Takano, 2007). However, estrogen replacements have yielded disappointing effects to restore a normal bone mineral density in AN patients. In contrast, recent observations in animal models and molecular biology suggest that the estrogen receptor alpha could play a central role in AN. AN presents a high heritability, and genetic analysis, in AN families and in case–control studies, also supports an involvement of estrogen pathway in vulnerability to AN (Hinney, Scherag, & Hebebrand, 2010; Ramoz, Versini, & Gorwood, 2007; Rask-Andersen, Olszewski, Levine, & Schiöth, 2010; Versini et al., 2010). The hypothesis of the involvement of estrogen in the control of food intake and in AN has been discussed for a long time (Butera, 2010; Young, 1991, 2010). This chapter focuses on the biological pathway of estrogen receptors and their potential role in the development of AN.

2. ANOREXIA NERVOSA

AN represents one of the three major eating disorders (EDs) with bulimia nervosa (BN) and eating disorders not otherwise specified (EDNOS), including binge eating disorder (BED). EDs are complex and multifactorial psychiatric diseases characterized by severe disturbances in eating behavior, leading to pathophysiological effects. Anorexia and bulimia are the most studied EDs because of their dramatic consequences on the physical health of patients, such as undernutrition, somatic complications, and mental disorders.

According to the Diagnostic and Statistical Manual for Mental Disorders IV (DSM-IV) and the International Classification of Diseases 10 (ICD-10), the diagnostic criteria of AN are based on three domains: (1) physical features, the weight being lower than 85% of the ideal body weight (corresponding to a body mass index [BMI] less than 17.5 kg/m^2); (2) psychological symptoms with a distortion of image body, the fear of gaining weight or becoming fat; and (3) behavioral abnormalities leading to inappropriate weight loss by reducing food intake and/or purging processes (American Psychiatric Association, 1999; Hebebrand & Bulik, 2011). According to the DSM-IV, AN patients are divided into two categories: (1) a restricting type of AN (RAN), where patients restrict their food intake; and (2) a binge eating/purging AN subtype (BPAN), where patients restrict their food intake or alternate between binge eating (eating an unusually large amount of food in a short period of time and feeling out of control) and self-induced vomiting, laxative, or diuretic abuses. Patients in RAN and BPAN subtypes can be distinguished by specific clinical features. Thus, BMI of RAN patients is significantly lower than in BPAN patients (Eddy et al., 2002). An increased impulsivity and a higher rate of self-harm and suicide were reported in BPAN than RAN (Eddy et al., 2002; Foulon et al., 2007; Milos, Spindler, Hepp, & Schnyder, 2004).

The average prevalence of AN has been reported to be 0.3% with a ratio of nine women affected for one man (Hoek, 2006; Hoek & Van Hoeken, 2003). A recent epidemiology study performed in 9000 adults reported an estimation of lifetime prevalence of AN of 0.6%, with a ratio of three men for every nine women affected (Hudson et al., 2007). The incidence of AN is over 8 per 100,000 persons, with a peak of onset in young adulthood, between 15 and 19 years of age (Favaro, Caregaro, Tenconi, Bosello, & Santonastaso, 2009; Hoek, 2006; Hudson et al., 2007). More than two-third of AN patients present a remission (Keel & Brown, 2010; Keski-Rahkonen, Hoek, Sihvola, Rissanen, & Kaprio, 2007). However, the outcome of AN patients is dependent on the protocol of the remission used and the follow-up of the patients. Remission status is not stable in the time with relapse and remission phases during a mean period of 5 years, and full recovery and cure of AN remain challenges (Keski-Rahkonen et al., 2007; Kordy et al., 2002; Ramoz et al., 2007). Epidemiological studies have reported one of the highest mortality rates among psychiatric diseases for AN, with a rate of about 10% per decade, mostly due to undernutrition and suicide (Birmingham et al., 2005; Millar et al., 2005). A meta-analysis recently reevaluated the rate of mortality as 5.86 deaths in 1000 AN patients per year, with 20% due to suicide (Arcelus et al., 2011). Comorbid conditions are associated with AN, along with lower bone mineral density and amenorrhea (Attia & Roberto, 2009). Thus, about 40% of patients show signs of osteoporosis and 92% of osteopenia (Mehler et al., 2011). A reduction in body weight often leads to amenorrhea, but amenorrhea appears also prior to reduction in body weight in 20% of AN patients and could persist after weight gain (Brambilla et al., 2003; Falk & Halmi, 1982). Due to the dramatic consequences of AN, the disorder represents a major problem of public health.

The etiology of AN remains unknown, which renders the treatment to this disorder difficult. Thus, the treatment of AN, and EDs in general, is a complex process that combines the treatment of the medical complications, psychological therapies, pharmacological treatments, and nutritional counseling. The aim of the therapy is double: restoring weight to the normal and correcting the disturbance of the body image of the patient. The results of the pharmacological treatments were limited in terms of clinical benefits and appeared inconsistent due to the discrepancies observed in the results of the investigations (Aigner, Treasure, Kaye, & Kasper, 2011; Ramoz et al., 2007). Thus, drug therapies are more focused on the medical complications developed during the disease, such as mood and anxiety disorders, and physical and psychological comorbidities. Recently, three psychotherapies, cognitive behavior therapy, interpersonal psychotherapy, with or without a control condition, and specialist supportive clinical management, were assessed in AN (Carter et al., 2011). Significant patterns of benefits were identified across time, but the treatment response was modest in patients. Efficient treatment of AN continues to be restoration of nutritional status and somatic health, with psychological support offered to the patient and the family. The identification of the factors involved in AN at the neurobiological, psychological, and sociocultural levels is required to design effective therapies, including medication . This strategy has been applied to target some treatments specific to comorbidities, such as low bone mineral density Sand estrogen replacement.

While AN etiology remains unkown, convergent evidence support the involvement of genetic factors in the development of the AN disorder. Thus, several studies have observed a familial aggregation for EDs, and AN in particular. This higher frequency of AN in relatives of the patients compared to relatives of controls allows the estimation of genetic factors with a heritability value of 70% (Gorwood, Kipman, & Foulon, 2003; Hinney et al., 2010). Further, concordance between monozygotic twins, who share the same genome, and concordance between dizygotyic twins allowed researchers to estimate the heritability of AN to be about 90% (Bulik, Sullivan, & Kendler, 1998; Gorwood et al., 2003; Hinney et al., 2010). Several approaches of molecular genetic methods were performed to identify the genes involved in the vulnerability to AN, including linkage analysis, candidate gene association study, and recently, genome-wide association study (GWAS) (Hinney et al., 2010; Ramoz et al., 2007; Rask-Andersen et al., 2010; Wang et al., 2011). These studies were carried out on AN families to analyze the transmission and segregation between markers and the disorder and in case versus control analysis to observe the difference in the distribution of the allelic frequencies. Candidate genes, such as the *BDNF* gene that encodes for the brain-derived neurotrophic factor, were found associated with AN in several studies (Hinney et al., 2010; Ramoz et al., 2007; Rask-Andersen et al., 2010). Polymorphisms located in genes involved in estrogen biological pathway have also been found to be associated with AN and are discussed in Section 5 (Hinney et al., 2010; Ramoz et al., 2007; Rask-Andersen et al., 2010; Versini et al., 2010).

3. ESTROGENS AND ESTROGEN RECEPTORS AND PATHWAYS

Estrogen molecules, which include estradiol (the most commonly named estrogen), estrone, and estriol, have the ability to bind to estrogen receptors (ERs). Estrogens are steroids derived from progesterone. Two enzymes participate in the synthesis of estrogens, the aromatase and the 17-beta hydroxysteroid dehydrogenase. The aromatase enzyme is encoded by *CYP19* gene, while the 17-beta hydroxysteroid dehydrogenase presents several isoforms encoded by several genes, mainly *HSD17B1* and *HSD17B2* genes. It is important to note that another enzyme that could be important for the limited synthesis of progesterone is the hydroxy-delta-5-steroid dehydrogenase, encoded by the *HSD3B1* gene. Then, estrogens could be metabolized by cytochrome P450 members, encoded by *CYP1A1*, *CYP1A2*, *CYP17A1*, *CYP19A1*, *CYP1B1*, and *CYP3A4* genes.

Two isoforms of ERs, ER alpha and ER beta, are respectively encoded by *ESR1* and *ESR2* genes. ERs have steroid-binding domains and DNA-binding domains. By fixing on ERs, estrogens trigger gene activation leading to pleiotropic effects in the human body.

Thus, estrogens stimulate synthesis of the main growth factors (transforming growth factor beta, bone morphogenetic protein 6, and insulin-like growth factor 1 (IGF-1)), inhibit RANKL (receptor activator of nuclear factor kappa B ligand) production, increase osteoprotegerin gene expression (inhibitor of osteoclasts formation), and decrease proresorptive cytokine synthesis (Taes et al., 2009). For these reasons, estrogen replacement was used to restore bone metabolism in AN patients. However, this approach of estrogen replacement, added with calcium and vitamin D supplementation, yielded disappointing results in the increase of bone mineral density of AN patients, with a beneficient effect on the lowest bone densities (Grinspoon et al., 2000; Klibanski, Biller, Schoenfeld, Herzog, & Saxe, 1995). Further, no bone density increase was observed with an estrogen–progesterone combination treatment (Golden et al., 2002; Munoz et al., 2002). However, a recent study suggests that a physiological dose of estrogen, at least in adolescent AN patients, provides a beneficient effect by increasing the bone mineral density (Misra et al., 2011). Renutrition helps to restore the bone health of AN patients. Estrogen is one of the molecules that contribute to the recovery of bone density, but it is not the only one deficient in AN patients because IGF-1 also leads to beneficient effects. Another reason is that the deficit of estrogen is more global to this biological pathway and could affect also the receptors. By their effect on the regulation of transcription of target genes of the human genome, ERs also affect the feeding regulation, as it has been showed in animal models and human as discussed in Section 4.2. (Geary, Asarian, Korach, Pfaff, & Ogawa, 2001; Liang et al., 2002; Santollo, Katzenellenbogen, Katzenellenbogen, & Eckel, 2010; Santollo, Wiley, & Eckel, 2007; Yu, Geary, & Corwin, 2011). Further, estradiol has been shown to bind to a membrane receptor in the hypothalamus that can transduce to multiple downstream actions in the brain (Qiu et al., 2006; Roepke, Qiu, Bosch, Rønnekleiv, & Kelly, 2009).

The estrogen alpha and beta receptors are expressed in nonoverlapping brain regions (Osterlund, Gustafsson, Keller, & Hurd, 2000; Osterlund & Hurd, 2001). At least, expression of estrogen alpha receptors and their sensitivity for estrogen are modulated by oxytocin (Perry, Paramadilok, & Cushing, 2009). They colocalize with corticotropin-releasing factor and modulate its expression (Bao, Hestiantoro, Van Someren, Swaab, & Zhou, 2005; Dagnault & Richard, 1997). ERs and the corticotropin-releasing hormone participate in the regulation of the hypothalamic–pituitary–adrenal (HPA) axis (Licinio, Wong, & Gold, 1996). The HPA axis has been reported altered in AN (Van de Stolpe et al., 2004). One hypothesis is that this disruption could result in the modification of the estrogen pathway in AN patients.

4. ESTROGEN AND ANOREXIA

4.1. Animal models, estrogen pathway, and anorexia

The effects of estrogens on food intake in animal models have been known for a long time. In normal rats, food intake decreased after a continuous administration of estradiol (Wade & Gray, 1979). This effect appeared for a week and then animals returned to normal food intake despite reduced body weight. Further, low prepubertal levels of estrogens that do not affect the function of reproductive organs could also modify the regulation of feeding. A 4-day cycle of food intake is observed in prepubertal rats before the vaginal opening, and the synchronicity of these cycles is critical for the postpubertal cycles in food intake (Nance, 1983; Sieck, Nance, Ramaley, Taylor, & Gorski, 1977). The anorexic effect of high estrogen levels was also found in mouse models (Couse & Korach, 1999). In ovariectomized rodents, the absence of estrogen and effect on food intake can be modulated by treatment (Asarian & Geary, 2006; Butera, 2010; Yu et al., 2011). Thus, ovariectomy in adult female rats led to an increase in food intake and body weight. Treatment with estradiol reduced food intake in ovariectomized rats (Gray & Wade, 1981). Further, cyclic treatment by estradiol, corresponding to physiological concentration as in normal rats, normalized the body weight of ovariectomized rats (Asarian & Geary, 2002; Geary & Asarian, 1999). These studies on rodents suggest that the ovarian estrogens have a direct impact on anorexic behavior. On one hand, this effect seems central and requires the involvement of the biological pathway of estrogen. On the other hand, it has been shown in rodents that estrogen induces taste aversion (Ganesan & Simpkins, 1991; Ossenkopp, Rabi, & Eckel, 1996). However, this hypothesis was not confirmed by recent studies (Flanagan-Cato, Grigson, & King, 2001). In primates also, the anorexigenic effect of estradiol has been observed. In that case, the reduction of body weight is induced by estrogen, but it is also influenced by environmental and psychosocial stressors, such as the social status for primates (Michopoulos & Wilson, 2011). Thus, environmental, social, and psychological factors could also act directly on the food intake and body weight or via the axis of stress to impact the biological pathway of estrogens.

Mice invalidated for gene encoding, respectively, the ER alpha or beta, usually named knock-out (KO) mice, have been bred for more than 15 years. Female KO mice for ER alpha exhibited an increased body weight compared to their wild-type littermates, at 4 and 8 months of age (Couse & Korach, 1999; Vidal et al., 1999). Further, diet enriched with the phytoestrogen genistein helped to reduce the body weight of the ER alpha KO mice compared to ER alpha KO mice without enriched diet. Sexually mature mice knock out for ER beta gene did not exhibit significant differences in body weight for both sexes (Couse & Korach, 1999). Convergent studies have reported that ER alpha is necessary for normal responsivity of food intake and body weight, but ER beta was not sufficient for these effects (Couse & Korach, 1999; Geary et al., 2001). One explanation for the difference in the body weight observed in ER alpha but not in ER beta KO mice is that the regulation of skeletal growth and maturation is modulated by estrogen, exclusively via ER alpha (Vidal et al., 2000). Recent strategy using interference RNA to block the expression of a candidate gene also demonstrates the involvement of the estrogen alpha receptor in the regulation of food intake and eating behavior in mouse models (Musatov, Chen, Pfaff, Kaplitt, & Ogawa, 2006; Musatov et al., 2007). Further, pharmacological treatment of ovariectomized rats by acute administration of a selective ER alpha agonist provokes a decrease in daily food intake and body weight (Santollo et al., 2007). In contrast, ER alpha antagonist treatment failed to reduce food intake decrease in ovariectomized rats (Santollo & Eckel, 2009). In female mice, treatments by agonists of ER receptors led also to the development of different effects on social learning of food preferences compared to nontreated mice (Clipperton, Spinato, Chernets, Pfaff, & Choleris, 2008). Finally, it has been shown in rodents that the anorexigenic effect of estradiol is dependent on the activation of the ER alpha (Santollo et al., 2010).

4.2. Estrogens and food intake in brain

In women, when levels of estrogen are elevated during the days of the menstrual cycle, a reduction of the caloric intake by about 10% has been observed (Asarian & Geary, 2006). However, this phenomenon has not been clearly investigated. Again, an aversion to tastes may occur during the estrogenic phase, leading to a reduction in food intake. However, this is not supported by recent work, which reported no effect of the menstrual cycle phase and oral contraception on caloric intake or hedonic food effect (Tucci, Murphy, Boyland, Dye, & Halford, 2010). Another hypothesis is that the major modification of hormonal levels during this period confers mood changes that reduce the appetite and/or starvation. In premenstrual dysphoric disorder, women have increased food cravings and food intake (Reed, Levin, & Evans, 2008). This disorder can be regulated by treatment with specific serotonin reuptake inhibitors. The anorexigenic effect of estradiol is mediated by serotonin neurotransmitter and receptor 2C at least (Rivera, Santollo, Nikonova, & Eckel, 2012). Thus, reduced appetite in human is directly impacted by brain regulation via hormones, neurotransmitters, neuropeptides, and receptors.

In fact, estrogens have multiple effects via the hypothalamus by regulating several homeostatic functions such as reproduction, temperature, and energy balance (Kelly & Qiu, 2010; Roepke et al., 2010; Roepke, Ronnekleiv, & Kelly, 2011). The activation of ERs in the mediobasal hypothalamus or in the dorsal medulla appears necessary for the anorexigenic effect of estrogens (Musatov et al., 2007; Thammacharoen, Geary, Lutz, Ogawa, & Asarian, 2009; Thammacharoen, Lutz, Geary, & Asarian, 2008). These brain regions contain numerous neurotransmitters and neuropeptides and receptors that play a role in the regulation of food intake, appetite, and starvation (Barsh & Schwartz, 2002; Kaye, 2008; Kaye, Fudge, & Paulus, 2009; Schwartz, Woods, Porte, Seeley, & Baskin, 2000). Several studies have involved these molecules in the genetic vulnerability for AN (Hinney et al., 2010; Ramoz et al., 2007; Rask-Andersen et al., 2010). Neurons that control the food intake via the expression of neuropeptide Y and proopiomelanocortin as neurotransmitters are modulated by estrogens (Blutstein et al., 2006; Blutstein, Baab, Zielke, & Mong, 2009; Kelly & Qiu, 2010; Roepke et al., 2008). Gene expression induced by estrogen has been studied in different tissues, including the brain (Roepke et al., 2008; Watanabe et al., 2002). Thus, it has been reported that the expression of 241 genes is modulated after the stimulation of a membrane-associated form of ER (Roepke et al., 2011, 2008). Estrogen molecules can also have a direct impact on the sensitivity of the brain to satiety factors such as leptin, ghrelin glucose transporter, insulin factors, and cholecystokinin (Butera, Xiong, Davis, & Platania, 1996; Cheng, Cohen, Wang, & Bondy, 2001; Clegg, Brown, Woods, & Benoit, 2006; Clegg et al., 2007; Gao et al., 2007; Thammacharoen et al., 2009, 2008). Defaults or modification on the expression of the possible targets of estrogens could lead to AN or predispose to AN vulnerability. Thus, hypoestrogenism is observed in AN patients (see subsequent sections 4.4). Neuroendocrine consequences of AN have also been reported, such as high levels of ghrelin and low levels of leptin and insulin (Misra & Klibanski, 2011; Ramoz et al., 2007; Rask-Andersen et al., 2010).

4.3. Sexual hormones, estrogens, in AN patients

In AN, sexual hormones have been poorly investigated. However, the biological pathway of estrogens could be involved in the disorder and there is evidence to support this hypothesis. First, AN patients are mainly women, with a ratio of 9 females to 1–3 men (Hudson et al., 2007; Ramoz et al., 2007). Second, among the psychiatric disorders, AN occurs during puberty or in young women, with an age at onset between 15 and 19 years (Favaro et al., 2009; Hoek, 2006; Hudson et al., 2007). This onset of the disease corresponds to the presence of estrogenic peaks. Also, sex-specific effects of puberty on genetic risk for EDs have been reported, which provide indirect evidence for the role of ovarian hormones and/or other female-specific factors (Klump et al., 2012). Third, as recently shown in a study, sex hormone, such as prenatal hormone, exposure could play a role in the risk of EDs (Culbert, Breedlove, Burt, & Klump, 2008), but this observation has not been replicated by other authors (Baker et al., 2009; Coyle, 2008; Raevuori et al., 2008). Fourth, as clearly shown in animal models, estrogen molecules appear also to activate mesolimbic dopaminergic reward systems in women (Dreher et al., 2007). Thus, an increase of activity of the reward system is observed during the peak of estrogen at the midfollicular phase. Also, in AN patients and recovery cases, compulsivity and absence of differential activity in response to positive and negative stimuli suggest an alteration in the reward system (Keating, Tilbrook, Rossell, Enticott, & Fitzgerald, 2012; Wagner et al., 2007). These defects of dopamine pathway in the reward system of AN patients are likely more traits rather than a state of the disorder (Kaye et al., 2009). Thus, dopamine dysfunction could be the result of an alteration of the gonadal steroid hormones, in particular, the estrogens, which regulate the mesolimbic dopamine systems. Finally (fifth), abnormal cognitive function and brain structure modifications have been reported in AN patients compared to healthy controls (Chui et al., 2008; Kaye et al., 2009).

4.4. Hypoestrogenism in anorexia nervosa

Numerous studies have demonstrated that estradiol levels were lower in anorexia patients than in controls (Brambilla et al., 2003; Estour et al., 2010; Galderisi et al., 2003; Misra et al., 2006; Ohwada et al., 2007). Twenty-two AN patients versus twenty controls at age 23.4 years showed a significant lower concentration of 17-beta estradiol in AN (46.1 ± 31.9 ng/L) compared to controls (82.7 ± 61.4 ng/L) (Brambilla et al., 2003). In Galderisi et al., 2003, 14 AN patients presented a lower concentration of estrogen (17.5 ± 17.9 ng/L) compared to 45 healthy comparison subjects (79.8 ± 46.6 ng/L). Significant lower concentration of 17-beta estradiol was also reported in 22 adolescent AN patients (16.7 ± 6.6 ng/L) versus 21 matched-age controls (21.9 ± 8.8 ng/L) (Misra et al., 2006). Dosage of 17-beta estradiol was performed in 26 AN patients, including 19 RAN and 7 BPAN, and 7 controls in Ohwada's work. This study found a significant decrease of 17-beta estradiol in AN (12.5 ± 2.8 ng/L) compared to controls (50.6 ± 10.5 ng/L), with a hypo-estrogenism in RAN patients (8.6 ± 2.1 ng/L) compared to BPAN (21.7 ± 7.2 ng/L) and controls (Ohwada et al., 2007). Estour and colleagues reported a significantly lower concentration of 17-beta estradiol with a mean of 14.8 ng/L for a total of 210 restrictive AN patients, compared to 57.8 ng/L in a total of 42 healthy controls (Estour et al., 2010). If estrogen level is important, then it should also play a role in male AN patients. This level of estrogens in males is less than three-fourth of the values seen in females (Brambilla, Matsumoto, Araujo, & McKinlay, 2009). However, significant metabolic effects are mediated by estrogens in men, even with small amounts of estrogens (Prossnitz & Barton, 2011). These levels of estrogen and the estrogen pathway participate in health and disease (Prossnitz & Barton, 2011; Vandenput & Ohlsson, 2009). Further, disordered eating attitudes and behaviors and salivary estradiol level were measured in 198 female twins and showed a genetic influence on disordered eating attitudes and a high level of estradiol (Klump, Keel, Sisk, & Burt, 2010).

All these convergent observations, sustained by other evidence, including molecular genetic cues (see subsequent section 5), suggest that during puberty, estrogens could lead to an abnormal response in the brain that predisposes to the physiopathology of AN (Butera, 2010; Klump et al., 2012, 2010; Qiu et al., 2006; Young, 2010). In contrast, during AN disorder, patients present a lower level of estrogen compared to normal and amenorrhea symptoms (Audi et al., 2002). Further, administration of luteinizing hormone–releasing hormone that restores ovarian function and menstruation in anorexics has no effect on their weight gain and food intake. These observations suggest that the implication of estrogen in AN is not focused on the estradiol molecule alone but is more dependent of the whole biological pathway, including the ERs.

5. HUMAN GENETICS OF ESTROGEN PATHWAY IN ANOREXIA NERVOSA

The sex steroid-related candidate genes, including *ESR1* and *ESR2* human genes that encode ER alpha and ER beta, respectively, have been investigated in psychiatric disorders, in particular, in EDs and AN (Westberg & Eriksson, 2008).

The human gene *ESR2* was the first screened gene for mutation analysis in EDs and AN (Rosenkranz et al., 1998). The *ESR2* gene is located on chromosome 14q23.2 and is composed of nine exons with alternative splices. In 1998, Rosenkranz and colleagues reported five variants in a total cohort of 201 sequenced subjects. Two variants corresponding to two common single nucleotide polymorphisms (SNPs) at position 1730 (G1730A, rs4986938) and 1082 (G1082A, rs1256049) were identified in a population of 50 AN patients (Rosenkranz et al., 1998). A nominal significant difference in the distribution of frequencies was observed for rs1256049 between AN and other groups of subjects (BN or obese and underweight cases). Another group also screened these two SNPs in 170 AN patients and 152 female controls (Eastwood, Brown, Markovic, & Pieri, 2002). A significant difference for rs1256049 was also observed with an excess of heterozygote in AN compared to controls and no difference was reported with rs4986938 (Eastwood et al., 2002). In contrast, significant association was found with rs4986938 and rs928554, and no association with rs1256049, in BN and EDs not otherwise specified (Nilsson et al., 2004). We genotyped four SNPs encompassing *ESR2* gene (rs8006145, rs4986938, rs17766755 and rs17179740) in 321 AN families, including 153 RAN and 154 BPAN subset families (Versini et al., 2010). Our four SNPs are in linkage disequilibrium ($D' > 0.9$) with the rs1256049 and rs4986938, and the *ESR2* gene spread on 112 kb and it is represented by only one haplotype block according to the database. No association was observed between our four SNPs and AN, RAN, or BPAN subgroups of patients (Versini et al., 2010). To date, close to 2000 SNPs have been identified across the *ESR2* gene. Additional genotyping for novel polymorphisms could be investigated in a larger group of AN cases.

The human *ESR1* gene is located on 6q25.1 and is composed of 11 exons covering 296 kb of the genome. Eastwood and colleagues screened two SNPs (IVS1–397T/C; rs2234693 and IVS1–351 A/C; rs9340799) in intronic regions of *ESR1* gene in 170 AN patients and 152 female controls but failed to identify an association (Eastwood et al., 2002). We genotyped 13 SNPs, including rs11155819 in complete linkage disequilibrium with rs2234693 and rs9340799, in 321 AN families (Versini et al., 2010). We identified two SNPs (rs726281 and rs2295193) in significant excess of transmission in AN patients. Further, three SNPs were significantly associated with the subgroup of RAN patients and four SNPs were found in excess of transmission with the paternal transmission, suggesting an imprinting effect on the ESR1 gene (Versini et al., 2010). Finally, a significant overtransmission of an haplotype block of eight SNPs was found with RAN patients and with the paternal transmission. We also reported that one associated SNP (rs726281) was also found in excess of transmission in an independent cohort of 41 RAN families, and another SNP (rs3798577) was observed associated with EDs (Versini et al., 2010). The haplotype block of eight SNPs associated with AN encompasses the C-terminal E/F region of the ER alpha protein , which corresponds to the fixation domain of the ligand of the nuclear receptor. So, we speculated that variants of *ESR1* gene may lead to changes of ligand binding domain of ER alpha in RAN patients. Functional analysis of the polymorphisms in the *ESR1* gene is needed to clarify its role in AN. Recent study has found a dysregulation of *ESR1* gene expression in the hypothalamus of depressive patients compared to controls (Wang, Kamphuis, Huitinga, Zhou, & Swaab, 2008). An increase of ESR1 mRNA level in seven depressive patients, compared to the level of seven controls, was reported but no correlation with polymorphisms in the *ESR1* gene was investigated (Wang et al., 2008). In obesity, one polymorphism of the *ESR1* gene (rs532010) appears to be associated with lipolytic sensitivity to noradrenaline showing the putative functional role of ESR1 variants (Nilsson et al., 2007).

To date, no genetic study has been performed on the *CYP19* gene, which encodes the aromatase enzyme, nor on the *HSD17B1* and *HSD17B2* genes, which encode the 17-beta hydroxysteroid dehydrogenase, or on the *CYP1A1*, *CYP1A2*, *CYP17A1*, *CYP19A1*, *CYP1B1*, and *CYP3A4* genes, which encode the estrogen metabolizer cytochrome P450 members. These genes present numerous polymorphisms reported in databases and screened in other diseases, including breast cancer and osteoporosis (Mendoza et al., 2012; Reding et al., 2012). Variants in these enzymes could modulate the levels of estrogens or affect the synthesis of neurosteroids within the brain itself (Dunning et al., 2004; Micevych, Soma, & Sinchak, 2008). Thus, polymorphisms in these genes have been found to directly impact the estrogen levels and could play a role in AN (Olson, Bandera, & Orlow, 2007). However, recently, a GWAS and a screening of 182 candidate genes have been performed on AN versus control studies (Pinheiro et al., 2010; Wang et al., 2011). In these two cases, more than a thousand AN patients were genotyped with thousands of SNPs. Among these SNPs, some were located across the *ESR1* or *ESR2* genes, and close to or across the other putative candidate genes. However, none of the top associated SNPs were mapped on a gene of the estrogen biological pathway (Pinheiro et al., 2010; Wang et al., 2011). Nevertheless, our colleagues and we contributed to the largest consortium on the genetics of AN, and a GWAS was carried out on more than 4000 AN patients and several thousands of controls. The genotyping of SNP among the whole genome, with no *a priori* candidate gene(s) involved, is important because estrogen biological pathway modulates the expression of target genes but it is also affected by other molecules encoded by genes (Klinge, 2001). Thus, the stimulation and regulation of transcription of ERs is dependent on proteins that modulate the role of ER, cofactors which activate or repress ERs (Klinge, 2000). At least 19 cofactors specific to the ER alpha have been identified and some of them increase specifically the transcriptional activity of ER alpha but not that of ER beta (Klinge, 2000; Suen et al., 1998). The role of these cofactors has been investigated in breast cancer but remains unknown in AN. It should be very interesting to focus on them in AN because these coactivators have an important action on estrogen in the brain, including the hypothalamus, leading to modulation in behaviors (Tetel, 2009; Tetel & Pfaff, 2010). A product of the *AGRP* gene is the hypothalamic peptide Agouti-related protein that plays a crucial role in the regulation of food intake and body weight and also in the modulation of the responsiveness of the hypothalamus to estrogen (Schioth, Kakizaki, Kohsaka, Suda, & Watanobe, 2001). And, AGRP, but also NPY neurons are request to observe the anorexigenic effect of estrogen (Olofsson, Pierce, & Xu, 2009). The *AGRP* and *NPY* genes were studied in AN, and associations have been reported between polymorphisms and anorexia disorder (Rask-Andersen et al., 2010). Numerous genes have been investigated as candidates for AN and replicative studies are poor, except for the *BDNF* gene. This neurotrophic factor has been found associated with AN in family study and case–control analysis (Rask-Andersen et al., 2010). Further, other neurotrophic factors have recently been associated with AN (Gratacòs et al., 2010; Mercader et al., 2008; Rask-Andersen et al., 2010). Interestingly, estrogen response elements are present in the *BDNF* gene, and estrogen and the neurotrophins act in concert and reciprocally (Scharfman & MacLusky, 2006; Toran-Allerand, 1996). This interplay underlines the complexity of the genetics of AN and reinforces the importance of analyzing the whole genome of patients to decipher the gene–gene interactions that could play a role in the mediation of the anorexigenic effect of estrogen.

6. CONCLUSIONS

The link between the genetic factor and the pathophysiological effects of estrogen pathway abnormality need to be further demonstrated for AN. In particular, to date, no study has shown that the lower level of estrogen in AN patients is a cause or a consequence of the disorder. Further, additional studies are needed in AN patients to correlate the hypoestrogenism and polymorphisms in genes of the estrogen biological pathway.

However, the estrogen hypothesis of AN may not be exclusive (Kaye, 2008). Other hormonal and neurochemical pathways might also be involved in this psychiatric disorder (Lawson & Klibanski, 2008; Miller, 2011). The control of appetite by the central nervous system and peripheral organs is an important regulatory network that is altered in AN (Kaye, 2008). At least, it is known that the anorexigenic effect of estrogen is mediated by the AGRP and NPY neurons. But estrogens act also on neurotrophic factors such as BDNF, whose *BDNF* gene is associated with AN, and reciprocally neurotrophic factors play a role on estrogen pathway.

One main difficulty in studying AN pathogenesis is that AN starts when a patient reduces food intake and the lower intake of nutrients clearly impacts the physiology and brain homeostasia of the subject (Kishi & Elmquistn, 2005). The consequences of denutrition and starvation are psychological features observed in anorexia, such as mood, compulsivity, perfectionism, and preoccupation with body image (Ioakimidis et al., 2011; Södersten, Nergårdh, Bergh, Zandian, & Scheurink, 2008). Study of remission in AN cases should help in the understanding the physiopathogenesis and the involvement of estrogens.

AN is also considered an addictive behavior caused by fasting. Lower caloric intake can activate reward circuits of the mesolimbic dopaminergic system (Kaye et al., 2009; Keating et al., 2012). Again, the pleiotropic effect of estrogens in the brain mediates the effect on reward circuits. Translational researches, including animal models and clinical investigations, combining domains of addiction, neuroendocrine, and steroid studies will help in understanding the biological mechanisms involved.

Genetic studies on estrogens in AN are at the beginning stages, and large cohorts of AN patients and families are needed. Thus, an international consortium such as GCAN is welcome to screen polymorphisms in the whole human genome. But others mechanisms and factors in molecular biology also play a role in the heritability of AN. Thus, micro RNAs have been recently isolated and shown to play a crucial role in the regulation of gene expression. Many micro RNAs that have estrogen effects have been identified and are known to play a role in breast cancer (Klinge, 2012). These molecules need to be analyzed in studying AN.

To conclude, an understanding of the complex roles of estrogens in the vulnerability to AN will provide novel tools of treatment to patients. Already, estrogen therapy may be of help in the remission of some AN cases (Keating, Tilbrook, & Kulkarni, 2011; Misra et al., 2011). Future directions to cure anorexia will be combinations of several pharmacological treatments, including estrogen medication and psychological therapies.

REFERENCES

Aigner, M., Treasure, J., Kaye, W., & Kasper, S. WFSBP Task Force On Eating Disorders. (2011). World Federation of Societies of Biological Psychiatry (WFSBP) guidelines for the pharmacological treatment of eating disorders. *The World Journal of Biological Psychiatry*, *12*(6), 400–443.

American Psychiatric Association, (1999). *DSM-IV: Diagnostic and statistical manual of mental disorders*. (4th ed.). Washington, DC: American Psychiatric Association.

Arcelus, J., Mitchell, A. J., Wales, J., & Nielsen, S. (2011). Mortality rates in patients with anorexia nervosa and other eating disorders. A meta-analysis of 36 studies. *Archives of General Psychiatry*, *68*(7), 724–731.

Asarian, L., & Geary, N. (2002). Cyclic estradiol treatment normalizes body weight and restores physiological patterns of spontaneous feeding and sexual receptivity in ovariectomized rats. *Hormones and Behavior*, *42*(4), 461–471.

Asarian, L., & Geary, N. (2006). Modulation of appetite by gonadal steroid hormones. *Philosophical Transactions of the Royal Society of London. Series B: Biological Sciences*, *361*(1471), 1251–1263.

Attia, E., & Roberto, C. A. (2009). Should amenorrhea be a diagnostic criterion for anorexia nervosa? *The International Journal of Eating Disorders*, *42*(7), 581–589.

Audi, L., Vargas, D. M., Gussinyé, M., Yeste, D., Martí, G., & Carrascosa, A. (2002). Clinical and biochemical determinants of bone metabolism and bone mass in adolescent female patients with anorexia nervosa. *Pediatric Research*, *51*(4), 497–504.

Baker, J. H., Maes, H. H., Lissner, L., Aggen, S. H., Lichtenstein, P., & Kendler, K. S. (2009). Genetic risk factors for disordered eating in adolescent males and females. *Journal of Abnormal Psychology*, *118*(3), 576–586.

Bao, A. M., Hestiantoro, A., Van Someren, E. J., Swaab, D. F., & Zhou, J. N. (2005). Colocalization of corticotropin-releasing hormone and oestrogen receptor-alpha in the paraventricular nucleus of the hypothalamus in mood disorders. *Brain*, *128*(Pt 6), 1301–1313.

Barsh, G. S., & Schwartz, M. W. (2002). Genetic approaches to studying energy balance: Perception and integration. *Nature Reviews. Genetics*, *3*(8), 589–600.

Birmingham, C. L., Su, J., Hlynsky, J. A., Goldner, E. M., & Gao, M. (2005). The mortality rate from anorexia nervosa. *The International Journal of Eating Disorders*, *38*(2), 143–146.

Blutstein, T., Baab, P. J., Zielke, H. R., & Mong, J. A. (2009). Hormonal modulation of amino acid neurotransmitter metabolism in the arcuate nucleus of the adult female rat: A novel action of estradiol. *Endocrinology*, *150*(7), 3237–3244.

Blutstein, T., Devidze, N., Choleris, E., Jasnow, A. M., Pfaff, D. W., & Mong, J. A. (2006). Oestradiol up-regulates glutamine synthetase mRNA and protein expression in the hypothalamus and hippocampus: Implications for a role of hormonally responsive glia in amino acid neurotransmission. *Journal of Neuroendocrinology*, *18*(9), 692–702.

Brambilla, D. J., Matsumoto, A. M., Araujo, A. B., & McKinlay, J. B. (2009). The effect of diurnal variation on clinical measurement of serum testosterone and other sex hormone levels in men. *The Journal of Clinical Endocrinology and Metabolism, 94*(3), 907–913.

Brambilla, F., Monteleone, P., Bortolotti, F., Dalle Grave, R., Todisco, P., & Favaro, A. (2003). Persistent amenorrhoea in weight recovered anorexics: Psychological and biological aspects. *Psychiatry Research, 118*(3), 249–257.

Bulik, C. M., Reba, L., Siega-Riz, A. M., & Reichborn-Kjennerud, T. (2005). Anorexia nervosa: Definition, epidemiology, and cycle of risk. *The International Journal of Eating Disorders, 37*, S2–S9.

Bulik, C. M., Sullivan, P. F., & Kendler, K. S. (1998). Heritability of binge-eating and broadly defined bulimia nervosa. *Biological Psychiatry, 44*(12), 1210–1218.

Butera, P. C. (2010). Estradiol and the control of food intake. *Physiology & Behavior, 99*(2), 175–180.

Butera, P. C., Xiong, M., Davis, R. J., & Platania, S. P. (1996). Central implants of dilute estradiol enhance the satiety effect of CCK-8. *Behavioral Neuroscience, 110*(4), 823–830.

Carter, F. A., Jordan, J., McIntosh, V. V., Luty, S. E., McKenzie, J. M., Frampton, C. M., et al. (2011). The long-term efficacy of three psychotherapies for anorexia nervosa: A randomized, controlled trial. *The International Journal of Eating Disorders, 44*(7), 647–654.

Cheng, C. M., Cohen, M., Wang, J., & Bondy, C. A. (2001). Estrogen augments glucose transporter and IGF1 expression in primate cerebral cortex. *The FASEB Journal, 15*(6), 907–915.

Chui, H. T., Christensen, B. K., Zipursky, R. B., Richards, B. A., Hanratty, M. K., Kabani, N. J., et al. (2008). Cognitive function and brain structure in females with a history of adolescent-onset anorexia nervosa. *Pediatrics, 122*(2), e426–e437.

Clegg, D. J., Brown, L. M., Woods, S. C., & Benoit, S. C. (2006). Gonadal hormones determine sensitivity to central leptin and insulin. *Diabetes, 55*(4), 978–987.

Clegg, D. J., Brown, L. M., Zigman, J. M., Kemp, C. J., Strader, A. D., Benoit, S. C., et al. (2007). Estradiol-dependent decrease in the orexigenic potency of ghrelin in female rats. *Diabetes, 56*(4), 1051–1058.

Clipperton, A. E., Spinato, J. M., Chernets, C., Pfaff, D. W., & Choleris, E. (2008). Differential effects of estrogen receptor alpha and beta specific agonists on social learning of food preferences in female mice. *Neuropsychopharmacology, 33*(10), 2362–2375.

Couse, J. F., & Korach, K. S. (1999). Estrogen receptor null mice: What have we learned and where will they lead us? *Endocrine Reviews, 205*(3), 358–417.

Coyle, J. T. (2008). Erratum: "Prevalence, Heritability, and Prospective Risk Factors for Anorexia Nervosa" (2006;63[3]:305–312). *Archives of General Psychiatry, 65*(9), 994.

Culbert, K. M., Breedlove, S. M., Burt, S. A., & Klump, K. L. (2008). Prenatal hormone exposure and risk for eating disorders: A comparison of opposite-sex and same-sex twins. *Archives of General Psychiatry, 65*(3), 329–336.

Dagnault, A., & Richard, D. (1997). Involvement of the medial preoptic area in the anorectic action of estrogens. *The American Journal of Physiology, 272*(1 Pt 2), R311–R317.

Dreher, J. C., Schmidt, P. J., Kohn, P., Furman, D., Rubinow, D., & Berman, K. F. (2007). Menstrual cycle phase modulates reward-related neural function in women. *Proceedings of the National Academy of Sciences of the United States of America, 104*(7), 2465–2470.

Dunning, A. M., Dowsett, M., Healey, C. S., Tee, L., Luben, R. N., Folkerd, E., et al. (2004). Polymorphisms associated with circulating sex hormone levels in postmenopausal women. *Journal of the National Cancer Institute, 96*(12), 936–945.

Eastwood, H., Brown, K. M., Markovic, D., & Pieri, L. F. (2002). Variation in the ESR1 and ESR2 genes and genetic susceptibility to anorexia nervosa. *Molecular Psychiatry, 7*(1), 86–89.

Eddy, K. T., Keel, P. K., Dorer, D. J., Delinsky, S. S., Franko, D. L., & Herzog, D. B. (2002). Longitudinal comparison of anorexia nervosa subtypes. *The International Journal of Eating Disorders, 31*(2), 191–201.

Estour, B., Germain, N., Diconne, E., Frere, D., Cottet-Emard, J. M., Carrot, G., et al. (2010). Hormonal profile heterogeneity and short-term physical risk in restrictive anorexia nervosa. *The Journal of Clinical Endocrinology and Metabolism*, *95*(5), 2203–2210.

Falk, J. R., & Halmi, K. A. (1982). Amenorrhea in anorexia nervosa: Examination of the critical body weight hypothesis. *Biological Psychiatry*, *17*(7), 799–806.

Favaro, A., Caregaro, L., Tenconi, E., Bosello, R., & Santonastaso, P. (2009). Time trends in age at onset of anorexia nervosa and bulimia nervosa. *The Journal of Clinical Psychiatry*, *70*(12), 1715–1721.

Flanagan-Cato, L. M., Grigson, P. S., & King, J. L. (2001). Estrogen-induced suppression of intake is not mediated by taste aversion in female rats. *Physiology & Behavior*, *72*(4), 549–558.

Foulon, C., Guelfi, J. D., Kipman, A., Adès, J., Romo, L., Houdeyer, K., et al. (2007). Switching to the bingeing/purging subtype of anorexia nervosa is frequently associated with suicidal attempts. *European Psychiatry*, *22*(8), 513–519.

Galderisi, S., Mucci, A., Monteleone, P., Sorrentino, D., Piegari, G., & Maj, M. (2003). Neurocognitive functioning in subjects with eating disorders: The influence of neuroactive steroids. *Biological Psychiatry*, *53*(10), 921–927.

Ganesan, R., & Simpkins, J. W. (1991). Conditioned taste aversion induced by estradiol pellets. *Physiology & Behavior*, *50*(4), 849–852.

Gao, Q., Mezei, G., Nie, Y., Rao, Y., Choi, C. S., Bechmann, I., et al. (2007). Anorectic estrogen mimics leptin's effect on the rewiring of melanocortin cells and Stat3 signaling in obese animals. *Nature Medicine*, *13*(1), 89–94.

Geary, N., & Asarian, L. (1999). Cyclic estradiol treatment normalizes body weight and test meal size in ovariectomized rats. *Physiology & Behavior*, *67*(1), 141–147.

Geary, N., Asarian, L., Korach, K. S., Pfaff, D. W., & Ogawa, S. (2001). Deficits in E2-dependent control of feeding, weight gain, and cholecystokinin satiation in ER-alpha null mice. *Endocrinology*, *142*(11), 4751–4757.

Golden, N. H., Lanzkowsky, L., Schebendach, J., Palestro, C. J., Jacobson, M. S., & Shenker, I. R. (2002). The effect of estrogen–progestin treatment on bone mineral density in anorexia nervosa. *Journal of Pediatric and Adolescent Gynecology*, *15*(3), 135–143.

Gorwood, P., Kipman, A., & Foulon, C. (2003). The human genetics of anorexia nervosa. *European Journal of Pharmacology*, *480*(1–3), 163–170.

Gratacòs, M., Escaramís, G., Bustamante, M., Saus, E., Agüera, Z., Bayés, M., et al. (2010). Role of the neurotrophin network in eating disorders' subphenotypes: Body mass index and age at onset of the disease. *Journal of Psychiatric Research*, *44*(13), 834–840.

Gray, J. N., & Wade, G. N. (1981). Food intake, body weight, and adiposity in female rats: Actions and interactions of progestins and antiestrogens. *The American Journal of Physiology*, *240*(5), E474–E481.

Grinspoon, S., Thomas, E., Pitts, S., Gross, E., Mickley, D., Miller, K., et al. (2000). Prevalence and predictive factors for regional osteopenia in women with anorexia nervosa. *Annals of Internal Medicine*, *133*(10), 790–794.

Hebebrand, J., & Bulik, C. M. (2011). Critical appraisal of the provisional DSM-5 criteria for anorexia nervosa and an alternative proposal. *The International Journal of Eating Disorders*, *44*(8), 665–678.

Hinney, A., Scherag, S., & Hebebrand, J. (2010). Genetic findings in anorexia and bulimia nervosa. *Progress in Molecular Biology and Translational Science*, *94*, 241–270.

Hoek, H. W. (2006). Incidence, prevalence and mortality of anorexia nervosa and other eating disorders. *Current Opinion in Psychiatry*, *19*(4), 389–394.

Hoek, H. W., & Van Hoeken, D. (2003). Review of the prevalence and incidence of eating disorders. *The International Journal of Eating Disorders*, *34*(4), 383–396.

Hudson, J. I., Hiripi, E., Pope, H. G. Jr., & Kessler, R. C. (2007). The prevalence and correlates of eating disorders in the national comorbidity survey replication. *Biological Psychiatry*, *61*(3), 348–358.

Ioakimidis, I., Zandian, M., Ulbl, F., Bergh, C., Leon, M., & Södersten, P. (2011). How eating affects mood. *Physiology & Behavior*, *103*(3–4), 290–294.

Kaye, W. (2008). Neurobiology of anorexia and bulimia nervosa. *Physiology & Behavior*, *94*(1), 121–135.

Kaye, W. H., Fudge, J. L., & Paulus, M. (2009). New insights into symptoms and neurocircuit function of anorexia nervosa. *Nature Reviews. Neuroscience*, *10*(8), 573–584.

Keating, C., Tilbrook, A., & Kulkarni, J. (2011). Oestrogen: An overlooked mediator in the neuropsychopharmacology of treatment response? *The International Journal of Neuropsychopharmacology*, *14*(4), 553–566.

Keating, C., Tilbrook, A. J., Rossell, S. L., Enticott, P. G., & Fitzgerald, P. B. (2012). Reward processing in anorexia nervosa. *Neuropsychologia*, *50*(5), 567–575.

Keel, P. K., & Brown, T. A. (2010). Update on course and outcome in eating disorders. *The International Journal of Eating Disorders*, *43*(3), 195–204.

Kelly, M. J., & Qiu, J. (2010). Estrogen signaling in hypothalamic circuits controlling reproduction. *Brain Research*, *1364*, 44–52.

Keski-Rahkonen, A., Hoek, H. W., Sihvola, E., Rissanen, A., & Kaprio, J. (2007). Epidemiology and course of anorexia nervosa in the community. *The American Journal of Psychiatry*, *164*(8), 1259–1265.

Kishi, T., & Elmquistn, J. K. (2005). Body weight is regulated by the brain: A link between feeding and emotion. *Molecular Psychiatry*, *10*(2), 132–146.

Klibanski, A., Biller, B., Schoenfeld, D. A., Herzog, D. B., & Saxe, V. C. (1995). The effects of estrogen administration on trabecular bone loss in young women with anorexia nervosa. *The Journal of Clinical Endocrinology and Metabolism*, *80*(3), 898–904.

Klinge, C. M. (2000). Estrogen receptor interaction with co-activators and co-repressors. *Steroids*, *65*(5), 227–251.

Klinge, C. M. (2001). Estrogen receptor interaction with estrogen response elements. *Nucleic Acids Research*, *29*(14), 2905–2919.

Klinge, C. M. (2012). miRNAs and estrogen action. *Trends in Endocrinology and Metabolism*, *23*(5), 223–233.

Klump, K. L., Culbert, K. M., Slane, J. D., Burt, S. A., Sisk, C. L., & Nigg, J. T. (2012). The effects of puberty on genetic risk for disordered eating: Evidence for a sex difference. *Psychological Medicine*, *42*(3), 627–637.

Klump, K. L., Keel, P. K., Sisk, C., & Burt, S. A. (2010). Preliminary evidence that estradiol moderates genetic influences on disordered eating attitudes and behaviors during puberty. *Psychological Medicine*, *40*(10), 1745–1753.

Kordy, H., Krämer, B., Palmer, R. L., Papezova, H., Pellet, J., Richard, M., et al. (2002). Remission, recovery, relapse, and recurrence in eating disorders: Conceptualization and illustration of a validation strategy. *Journal of Clinical Psychology*, *58*(7), 833–846.

Lawson, E. A., & Klibanski, A. (2008). Endocrine abnormalities in anorexia nervosa. *Nature Clinical Practice. Endocrinology & Metabolism*, *4*(7), 407–414.

Liang, Y. Q., Akishita, M., Kim, S., Ako, J., Hashimoto, M., Iijima, K., et al. (2002). Estrogen receptor beta is involved in the anorectic action of estrogen. *International Journal of Obesity and Related Metabolic Disorders*, *26*(8), 1103–1109.

Licinio, J., Wong, M. L., & Gold, P. W. (1996). The hypothalamic-pituitary-adrenal axis in anorexia nervosa. *Psychiatry Research*, *62*(1), 75–83.

Mehler, P. S., Cleary, B. S., & Gaudiani, J. L. (2011). Osteoporosis in anorexia nervosa. *Eating Disorders*, *19*(2), 194–202.

Mendoza, N., Quereda, F., Presa, J., Salamanca, A., Sánchez-Borrego, R., Vázquez, F., et al. (2012). Estrogen-related genes and postmenopausal osteoporosis risk. *Climacteric, 15*(6), 587–593.

Mercader, J. M., Saus, E., Agüera, Z., Bayés, M., Boni, C., Carreras, A., et al. (2008). Association of NTRK3 and its interaction with NGF suggest an altered cross-regulation of the neurotrophin signaling pathway in eating disorders. *Human Molecular Genetics, 17*(9), 1234–1244.

Micevych, P., Soma, K. K., & Sinchak, K. (2008). Neuroprogesterone: Key to estrogen positive feedback? *Brain Research Reviews, 57*(2), 470–480.

Michopoulos, V., & Wilson, M. E. (2011). Body weight decreases induced by estradiol in female rhesus monkeys are dependent upon social status. *Physiology & Behavior, 102* (3–4), 382–388.

Millar, H. R., Wardell, F., Vyvyan, J. P., Naji, S. A., Prescott, G. J., & Eagles, J. M. (2005). Anorexia nervosa mortality in Northeast Scotland, 1965–1999. *The American Journal of Psychiatry, 162*(4), 753–757.

Miller, K. K. (2011). Endocrine dysregulation in anorexia nervosa update. *The Journal of Clinical Endocrinology and Metabolism, 96*(10), 2939–2949.

Milos, G., Spindler, A., Hepp, U., & Schnyder, U. (2004). Suicide attempts and suicidal ideation: Links with psychiatric comorbidity in eating disorder subjects. *General Hospital Psychiatry, 26*(2), 129–135.

Misra, M., Katzman, D., Miller, K. K., Mendes, N., Snelgrove, D., Russell, M., et al. (2011). Physiologic estrogen replacement increases bone density in adolescent girls with anorexia nervosa. *Journal of Bone and Mineral Research, 26*(10), 2430–2438.

Misra, M., & Klibanski, A. (2011). The neuroendocrine basis of anorexia nervosa and its impact on bone metabolism. *Neuroendocrinology, 93*(2), 65–73.

Misra, M., Miller, K. K., Tsai, P., Gallagher, K., Lin, A., Lee, N., et al. (2006). Elevated peptide YY levels in adolescent girls with anorexia nervosa. *The Journal of Clinical Endocrinology and Metabolism, 91*(3), 1027–1033.

Munoz, M., Morande, G., García-Centenera, J. A., Hervás, F., Pozo, J., & Argente, J. (2002). The effects of estrogen administration on bone mineral density in adolescents with anorexia nervosa. *European Journal of Endocrinology, 146*(1), 45–50.

Musatov, S., Chen, W., Pfaff, D. W., Kaplitt, M. G., & Ogawa, S. (2006). RNAi-mediated silencing of estrogen receptor alpha in the ventromedial nucleus of hypothalamus abolishes female sexual behaviors. *Proceedings of the National Academy of Sciences of the United States of America, 103*(27), 10456–10460.

Musatov, S., Chen, W., Pfaff, D. W., Mobbs, C. V., Yang, X. J., Clegg, D. J., et al. (2007). Silencing of estrogen receptor alpha in the ventromedial nucleus of hypothalamus leads to metabolic syndrome. *Proceedings of the National Academy of Sciences of the United States of America, 104*(7), 2501–2506.

Nance, D. M. (1983). The developmental and neural determinants of the effects of estrogen on feeding behavior in the rat: A theoretical perspective. *Neuroscience and Biobehavioral Reviews*, 7(2), 189–211.

Nilsson, M., Dahlman, I., Jiao, H., Gustafsson, J. A., Arner, P., & Dahlman-Wright, K. (2007). Impact of estrogen receptor gene polymorphisms and mRNA levels on obesity and lipolysis—A cohort study. *BMC Medical Genetics, 8*, 73.

Nilsson, M., Naessén, S., Dahlman, I., Lindén Hirschberg, A., Gustafsson, J. A., & Dahlman-Wright, K. (2004). Association of estrogen receptor beta gene polymorphisms with bulimic disease in women. *Molecular Psychiatry, 9*(1), 28–34.

Ohwada, R., Hotta, M., Sato, K., Shibasaki, T., & Takano, K. (2007). The relationship between serum levels of estradiol and osteoprotegerin in patients with anorexia nervosa. *Endocrine Journal, 54*(6), 953–959.

Olofsson, L. E., Pierce, A. A., & Xu, A. W. (2009). Functional requirement of AgRP and NPY neurons in ovarian cycle-dependent regulation of food intake. *Proceedings of the National Academy of Sciences of the United States of America, 106*(37), 15932–15937.

Olson, S. H., Bandera, E. V., & Orlow, I. (2007). Variants in estrogen biosynthesis genes, sex steroid hormone levels, and endometrial cancer: A HuGE review. *American Journal of Epidemiology, 165*(3), 235–245.

Ossenkopp, K. P., Rabi, Y. J., & Eckel, L. A. (1996). Oestradiol-induced taste avoidance is the result of a conditioned palatability shift. *Neuroreport*, 7(15–17), 2777–2780.

Osterlund, M. K., Gustafsson, J. A., Keller, E., & Hurd, Y. L. (2000). Estrogen receptor beta (ERbeta) messenger ribonucleic acid (mRNA) expression within the human forebrain: Distinct distribution pattern to ERalpha mRNA. *The Journal of Clinical Endocrinology and Metabolism, 85*(10), 3840–3846.

Osterlund, M. K., & Hurd, Y. L. (2001). Estrogen receptors in the human forebrain and the relation to neuropsychiatric disorders. *Progress in Neurobiology, 64*(3), 251–267.

Perry, A. N., Paramadilok, A., & Cushing, B. S. (2009). Neonatal oxytocin alters subsequent estrogen receptor alpha protein expression and estrogen sensitivity in the female rat. *Behavioural Brain Research, 205*(1), 154–161.

Pinheiro, A. P., Bulik, C. M., Thornton, L. M., Sullivan, P. F., Root, T. L., Bloss, C. S., et al. (2010). Association study of 182 candidate genes in anorexia nervosa. *American Journal of Medical Genetics. Part B, Neuropsychiatric Genetics, 153B*(5), 1070–1080.

Prossnitz, E. R., & Barton, M. (2011). The G-protein-coupled estrogen receptor GPER in health and disease. *Nature Reviews. Endocrinology*, 7(12), 715–726.

Qiu, J., Bosch, M. A., Tobias, S. C., Krust, A., Graham, S. M., Murphy, S. J., et al. (2006). A G-protein-coupled estrogen receptor is involved in hypothalamic control of energy homeostasis. *The Journal of Neuroscience, 26*(21), 5649–5655.

Raevuori, A., Kaprio, J., Hoek, H. W., Sihvola, E., Rissanen, A., & Keski-Rahkonen, A. (2008). Anorexia and bulimia nervosa in same-sex and opposite-sex twins: Lack of association with twin type in a nationwide study of Finnish twins. *The American Journal of Psychiatry, 165*(12), 1604–1610.

Ramoz, N., Versini, A., & Gorwood, P. (2007). Eating disorders: An overview of treatment responses and the potential impact of vulnerability genes and endophenotypes. *Expert Opinion on Pharmacotherapy, 8*(13), 2029–2044.

Rask-Andersen, M., Olszewski, P. K., Levine, A. S., & Schiöth, H. B. (2010). Molecular mechanisms underlying anorexia nervosa: Focus on human gene association studies and systems controlling food intake. *Brain Research Reviews, 62*(2), 147–164.

Reding, K. W., Chen, C., Lowe, K., Doody, D. R., Carlson, C. S., Chen, C. T., et al. (2012). Estrogen-related genes and their contribution to racial differences in breast cancer risk. *Cancer Causes & Control, 23*(5), 671–681.

Reed, S. C., Levin, F. R., & Evans, S. M. (2008). Changes in mood, cognitive performance and appetite in the late luteal and follicular phases of the menstrual cycle in women with and without PMDD (premenstrual dysphoric disorder). *Hormones and Behavior, 54*(1), 185–193.

Rivera, H. M., Santollo, J., Nikonova, L. V., & Eckel, L. A. (2012). Estradiol increases the anorexia associated with increased 5-HT(2C) receptor activation in ovariectomized rats. *Physiology & Behavior, 105*(2), 188–194.

Roepke, T. A., Bosch, M. A., Rick, E. A., Lee, B., Wagner, E. J., Seidlova-Wuttke, D., et al. (2010). Contribution of a membrane estrogen receptor to the estrogenic regulation of body temperature and energy homeostasis. *Endocrinology, 151*(10), 4926–4937.

Roepke, T. A., Qiu, J., Bosch, M. A., Rønnekleiv, O. K., & Kelly, M. J. (2009). Cross-talk between membrane-initiated and nuclear-initiated oestrogen signalling in the hypothalamus. *Journal of Neuroendocrinology, 21*(4), 263–270.

Roepke, T. A., Ronnekleiv, O. K., & Kelly, M. J. (2011). Physiological consequences of membrane-initiated estrogen signaling in the brain. *Frontiers in Bioscience, 16*, 1560–1573.

Roepke, T. A., Xue, C., Bosch, M. A., Scanlan, T. S., Kelly, M. J., & Rønnekleiv, O. K. (2008). Genes associated with membrane-initiated signaling of estrogen and energy homeostasis. *Endocrinology, 149*(12), 6113–6124.

Rosenkranz, K., Hinney, A., Ziegler, A., Hermann, H., Fichter, M., Mayer, H., et al. (1998). Systematic mutation screening of the estrogen receptor beta gene in probands of different weight extremes: Identification of several genetic variants. *The Journal of Clinical Endocrinology and Metabolism, 83*(12), 4524–4527.

Santollo, J., & Eckel, L. A. (2009). Effect of a putative ERalpha antagonist, MPP, on food intake in cycling and ovariectomized rats. *Physiology & Behavior, 97*(2), 193–198.

Santollo, J., Katzenellenbogen, B. S., Katzenellenbogen, J. A., & Eckel, L. A. (2010). Activation of ERα is necessary for estradiol's anorexigenic effect in female rats. *Hormones and Behavior, 58*(5), 872–877.

Santollo, J., Wiley, M. D., & Eckel, L. A. (2007). Acute activation of ER alpha decreases food intake, meal size, and body weight in ovariectomized rats. *American Journal of Physiology. Regulatory, Integrative and Comparative Physiology, 293*(6), R2194–R2201.

Scharfman, H. E., & MacLusky, N. J. (2006). Estrogen and brain-derived neurotrophic factor (BDNF) in hippocampus: Complexity of steroid hormone-growth factor interactions in the adult CNS. *Frontiers in Neuroendocrinology, 27*(4), 415–435.

Schioth, H. B., Kakizaki, Y., Kohsaka, A., Suda, T., & Watanobe, H. (2001). Agouti-related peptide prevents steroid-induced luteinizing hormone and prolactin surges in female rats. *Neuroreport, 12*(4), 687–690.

Schwartz, M. W., Woods, S. C., Porte, D. Jr., Seeley, R. J., & Baskin, D. G. (2000). Central nervous system control of food intake. *Nature, 404*(6778), 661–671.

Sieck, G. C., Nance, D. M., Ramaley, J. A., Taylor, A. N., & Gorski, R. A. (1977). Prepubertal cyclicity in feeding behavior and body weight regulation in the female rat. *Physiology & Behavior, 18*(2), 299–305.

Södersten, P., Nergårdh, R., Bergh, C., Zandian, M., & Scheurink, A. (2008). Behavioral neuroendocrinology and treatment of anorexia nervosa. *Frontiers in Neuroendocrinology, 29*(4), 445–462.

Suen, C. S., Berrodin, T. J., Mastroeni, R., Cheskis, B. J., Lyttle, C. R., & Frail, D. E. (1998). A transcriptional coactivator, steroid receptor coactivator-3, selectively augments steroid receptor transcriptional activity. *The Journal of Biological Chemistry, 273*(42), 27645–27653.

Taes, Y., Lapauw, B., Vandewalle, S., Zmierczak, H., Goemaere, S., Vanderschueren, D., et al. (2009). Estrogen-specific action on bone geometry and volumetric bone density: Longitudinal observations in an adult with complete androgen insensitivity. *Bone, 45*(2), 392–397.

Tetel, M. J. (2009). Modulation of steroid action in the central and peripheral nervous systems by nuclear receptor coactivators. *Psychoneuroendocrinology, 34*(Suppl. 1), S9–S19.

Tetel, M. J., & Pfaff, D. W. (2010). Contributions of estrogen receptor-α and estrogen receptor-ß to the regulation of behavior. *Biochimica et Biophysica Acta, 1800*(10), 1084–1089.

Thammacharoen, S., Geary, N., Lutz, T. A., Ogawa, S., & Asarian, L. (2009). Divergent effects of estradiol and the estrogen receptor-alpha agonist PPT on eating and activation of PVN CRH neurons in ovariectomized rats and mice. *Brain Research, 1268*, 88–96.

Thammacharoen, S., Lutz, T. A., Geary, N., & Asarian, L. (2008). Hindbrain administration of estradiol inhibits feeding and activates estrogen receptor-alpha-expressing cells in the nucleus tractus solitarius of ovariectomized rats. *Endocrinology, 149*(4), 1609–1617.

Toran-Allerand, C. D. (1996). Mechanisms of estrogen action during neural development: Mediation by interactions with the neurotrophins and their receptors? *The Journal of Steroid Biochemistry and Molecular Biology*, *56*(1–6 Spec. No.), 169–178.

Tucci, S. A., Murphy, L. E., Boyland, E. J., Dye, L., & Halford, J. C. (2010). Oral contraceptive effects on food choice during the follicular and luteal phases of the menstrual cycle. A laboratory based study. *Appetite*, *55*(3), 388–392.

Van de Stolpe, A., Slycke, A. J., Reinders, M. O., Zomer, A. W., Goodenough, S., Behl, C., et al. (2004). Estrogen receptor (ER)-mediated transcriptional regulation of the human corticotropin-releasing hormone-binding protein promoter: Differential effects of ERalpha and ERbeta. *Molecular Endocrinology*, *18*(12), 2908–2923.

Vandenput, L., & Ohlsson, C. (2009). Estrogens as regulators of bone health in men. *Nature Reviews. Endocrinology*, *5*(8), 437–443.

Versini, A., Ramoz, N., Le Strat, Y., Scherag, S., Ehrlich, S., Boni, C., et al. (2010). Estrogen receptor 1 gene (ESR1) is associated with restrictive anorexia nervosa. *Neuropsychopharmacology*, *35*(8), 1818–1825.

Vidal, O., Lindberg, M. K., Hollberg, K., Baylink, D. J., Andersson, G., Lubahn, D. B., et al. (2000). Estrogen receptor specificity in the regulation of skeletal growth and maturation in male mice. *Proceedings of the National Academy of Sciences of the United States of America*, *97* (10), 5474–5479.

Vidal, O., Lindberg, M., Sävendahl, L., Lubahn, D. B., Ritzen, E. M., Gustafsson, J. A., et al. (1999). Disproportional body growth in female estrogen receptor-alpha-inactivated mice. *Biochemical and Biophysical Research Communications*, *265*(2), 569–571.

Wade, G. N., & Gray, J. M. (1979). Gonadal effects on food intake and adiposity: A metabolic hypothesis. *Physiology & Behavior*, *22*, 583–593.

Wagner, A., Aizenstein, H., Venkatraman, V. K., Fudge, J., May, J. C., Mazurkewicz, L., et al. (2007). Altered reward processing in women recovered from anorexia nervosa. *The American Journal of Psychiatry*, *164*(12), 1842–1849.

Wang, S. S., Kamphuis, W., Huitinga, I., Zhou, J. N., & Swaab, D. F. (2008). Gene expression analysis in the human hypothalamus in depression by laser microdissection and real-time PCR: The presence of multiple receptor imbalances. *Molecular Psychiatry*, *13*(8), 786–799.

Wang, K., Zhang, H., Bloss, C. S., Duvvuri, V., Kaye, W., Schork, N. J., et al. (2011). A genome-wide association study on common SNPs and rare CNVs in anorexia nervosa. *Molecular Psychiatry*, *16*(9), 949–959.

Watanabe, H., Suzuki, A., Mizutani, T., Khono, S., Lubahn, D. B., Handa, H., et al. (2002). Genome-wide analysis of changes in early gene expression induced by oestrogen. *Genes to Cells*, 7(5), 497–507.

Westberg, L., & Eriksson, E. (2008). Sex steroid-related candidate genes in psychiatric disorders. *Journal of Psychiatry & Neuroscience*, *33*(4), 319–330.

Young, J. K. (1991). Estrogen and the etiology of anorexia nervosa. *Neuroscience and Biobehavioral Reviews*, *15*(3), 327–331.

Young, J. K. (2010). Anorexia nervosa and estrogen: Current status of the hypothesis. *Neuroscience and Biobehavioral Reviews*, *34*(8), 1195–1200.

Yu, Z., Geary, N., & Corwin, R. L. (2011). Individual effects of estradiol and progesterone on food intake and body weight in ovariectomized binge rats. *Physiology & Behavior*, *104* (5), 687–693.

CHAPTER SEVEN

Cannabinoid Receptors and Cholecystokinin in Feeding Inhibition

Francisco Alén[*], M. Teresa Ramírez-López[*], Raquel Gómez de Heras[*], Fernando Rodríguez de Fonseca[*,†,‡], Laura Orio[*,1]

[*]Departamento de Psicobiología, Facultad de Psicología, Universidad Complutense, Madrid, Spain
[†]Fundación IMABIS, Hospital Universitario Carlos Haya, Málaga, Spain
[‡]CIBEROBN, Instituto Salud Carlos III, Madrid, Spain
[1]Corresponding author: e-mail address: lorio@psi.ucm.es

Contents

1. Introduction: Peripheral Regulation of Food Intake: A Place for Endocannabinoids and Cholecystokinin 166
2. The Endocannabinoids and Feeding Regulation 168
   2.1 Endocannabinoids and its receptors 168
   2.2 Peripheral endocannabinoids and feeding 170
   2.3 Central endocannabinoids and feeding 172
3. CCK and Feeding Regulation 175
   3.1 CCK and its receptors 175
   3.2 Peripheral CCK and feeding 178
   3.3 Central CCK and feeding 180
4. Interactions Between CCK and Endocannabinoid Receptors in the Regulation of Feeding 181
5. Conclusions and Clinical Relevance 183
Acknowledgments 184
References 184

Abstract

The endocannabinoid system functions as a potent regulator of feeding behavior and energy balance through complex central and peripheral mechanisms. Recent findings have demonstrated the existence of cooperation between peripheral cannabinoid CB1 receptors and the satiety hormone cholecystokinin (CCK). The two systems have opposing actions in the modulation of feeding: while endocannabinoids such as anandamide promote feeding, CCK controls gastrointestinal motility and appetite suppression. In this review, we examine the individual contribution of endocannabinoids and CCK in the modulation of appetite and explore the interaction between the two systems. We also highlight the potential benefits of simultaneously targeting peripheral CB1 and CCK1 receptors to design new therapies to fight obesity.

Vitamins and Hormones, Volume 92
ISSN 0083-6729
http://dx.doi.org/10.1016/B978-0-12-410473-0.00007-6

1. INTRODUCTION: PERIPHERAL REGULATION OF FOOD INTAKE: A PLACE FOR ENDOCANNABINOIDS AND CHOLECYSTOKININ

Feeding is a complex behavior that emerges after the integration of central and peripheral signals that inform on nutritional status, energy expenditure, and food availability. Most of these signals arise either from the sensory organs or from peripheral systems involved in food processing and energy homeostasis. These peripheral signaling sources include the gastrointestinal tract, the liver, the adipose tissue, the muscle, and the peripheral endocrine glands. The signals generated are usually released into the blood stream and transported to the CNS structures involved in the regulation of feeding behavior and energy homeostasis. Specialized areas in the hypothalamus and the brainstem, including brain nuclei with open blood–brain barrier areas such as the median eminence and the area postrema, are responsible for detecting and integrating these signals. Other signals are directly transported through the blood–brain barrier and reach the hypothalamic and limbic centers regulating either hunger or motivational/rewarding aspects of feeding, respectively (Suzuki, Jayasena, & Bloom, 2011; Suzuki, Simpson, Minnion, Shillito, & Bloom, 2010). However, sensing of these signals involves not only hypothalamic and brainstem structures but also a direct stimulation of peripheral sensory terminals such as those included in the afferent projections of the vagus nerve (Rasoamanana, Darcel, Fromentin, & Tome, 2012). Vagal afferent pathways reach not only the dorsal vagal complex of the brain but also the lateral hypothalamic area controlling appetite. This anatomical disposition allows a rapid *on site* analysis of feeding/nutrition/energy expenditure processes in the different organs involved in the maintenance of body weight and energy stores (Owyang & Heldsinger, 2011). In fact, interference with vagal signals has been proposed as a potential therapy for complicated obesity (Das, 2011).

The main relevant signals arising from the peripheral nerve terminals are peptides. They are produced mainly by specialized endocrine cells located in the mucosa of the stomach or the intestine, the endocrine pancreas, or the adipose tissue. In the stomach, the main peptidic signal is ghrelin, the only orexigenic signal found to date. In the intestine, the main peptidic signals are cholecystokinin (CCK), peptide tyrosine tyrosine (PYY), glucagon-like peptides 1 & 2 (GLP-1 and GLP-2), and oxyntomodulin, all of which inhibit appetite and produce a feeling of satiety. In the pancreas, the main signals are the pancreatic polypeptide, amylin, insulin, and glucagon. In the adipose tissue, the main signal discovered to date is leptin, although the adipose tissue also produces many other signals (termed adipokines, and a heterogeneous family of new hormones such as adiponectin or cytokines such as interleukin-6 or tumor necrosis factor alpha), whose importance is currently being investigated (Suzuki et al., 2010, 2011).

Despite the CNS and the peripheral organs involved in feeding and nutrition, a much less studied third component contributes significantly to the regulation of feeding. It is the lumen of the gastrointestinal tract. Here, specific nutrients present in the diet and products produced by microbiota can act as potent independent signals regulating appetite, satiety, gastrointestinal motility, and enzymatic secretion. The signals generated in the lumen can act in receptors present in cells lining the gut mucosa, triggering the release of secondary signals that might activate peripheral sensory terminals or be released into the blood stream to reach the hypothalamus or the limbic system to control appetite (Schwartz, 2011; Serrano et al., 2011). In addition, they can be transported and incorporated into the organism to serve as either nutrients or regulatory signals for feeding and metabolism. Among the signals present in the nutrients or generated by processing diet components, lipid transmitters are gaining much relevance. Of them, the endocannabinoids *N*-arachidonoylethanolamine (anandamide, AEA) and 2-arachidonoylglycerol (2-AG), the peroxisome proliferator-activated alpha (PPAR-α) receptor agonist *N*-oleoylethanolamide (OEA), and the GPR119 receptor agonist 2-oleoylglycerol have been proposed to participate in both fat and glucose homeostasis. They act either as peripheral modulators of appetite or as signals activating what has been called a "fat sensor" (DiPatrizio, Astarita, Schwartz, Li, & Piomelli, 2011). While the endocannabinoids promote feeding, the OEA and GPR119 agonists inhibit it, making this new family of signals a very attractive target for pharmaceutical development (Gomez et al., 2002, Hansen, Rosenkilde, Holst, & Schwartz, 2012; Schwartz et al., 2008). The integration of fat sensing, appetite suppression, and the control of gastrointestinal motility had been traditionally attributed to intestinal CCK. However, the presence and physiological role of these lipid transmitters suggest the existence of a more complex network of regulatory signals for these functions. Recent findings have demonstrated the existence of cooperation between lipid transmitter signals and CCK. This review explores the role of the endocannabinoid system in feeding regulation, and its relationship with CCK. We first review the roles of the endocannabinoid system as a promoter of feeding and discuss the roles of CCK in the gastrointestinal tract, to finally examine the interaction between the two systems.

2. THE ENDOCANNABINOIDS AND FEEDING REGULATION

2.1. Endocannabinoids and its receptors

The Asiatic plant Cannabis Sativa/Indica has been known for more than 8000 years for its medical and psychotropic effects (Nagy, White, Paule, & Köfalvi, 2008), but it was not until 1964 that tetrahydrocannabinol (Δ9-THC), its major psychoactive compound, was isolated for the first time (Gaoni & Mechoulam, 1964). Its medical effects, which include anesthetic, antihypertensive, eye pressure reducing, as well as antiemetic effects, are mediated by the interaction of cannabinoid compounds with various types of receptors in the nervous system. To date, two main cannabinoid receptors have been identified, and various others are in different stages of characterization. Numbered in their order of discovery, the cannabinoid-type 1 (CB1) and cannabinoid-type 2 (CB2) receptors have been characterized (Gerard, Mollereau, Vassart, & Parmentier, 1990; Munro, Thomas, & Abu-Shaar, 1993). These two receptors exhibit only 48% amino acid sequence identity and are expressed in the brain and peripheral nervous system. Both CB1 and CB2 receptors are coupled through Gi/o-type G proteins, and their transduction pathways include inhibition of adenylyl cyclase and certain voltage-sensitive calcium channels, and activation of inwardly rectifying potassium channels, mitogen-activated protein kinase, and focal adhesion kinase (Howlett et al., 2002).

CB1 receptors are highly expressed in the brain; indeed, their densities are greater than those of most other G-protein-coupled receptors and comparable to that of the ionotropic GABA and glutamate receptors (Howlett et al., 2002). As the G-protein-coupled receptors are the targets of approximately 40% of all modern medicinal drugs, the cannabinoid system shows up as an important pharmacological target (Filmore, 2004). Within the CNS, the CB1 receptor is widely expressed in the cerebral cortex, hippocampus, basal ganglia, and cerebellum, with lower levels in the hypothalamus and spinal cord (Herkenham et al., 1990). Its expression, however, follows a complex pattern of distribution depending on cell type and brain region (Marsicano & Lutz, 1999). The majority of CB1 receptors are localized to the presynaptic terminals of neural axons, although they are also present in other neuronal areas to a lesser extent (Pamplona & Takahashi, 2012), and outside the brain in areas related with metabolic control such as adipocytes or muscle (Howlett et al., 2002). The CB2 receptor is also expressed in brain areas including the striatum, hypothalamus, cortex, substantia nigra, amygdala, and hippocampus (Onaivi et al., 2006), although it is primarily present in immune cells or peripheral organs such as thymus, tonsils, spleen, and pancreas (Galiègue et al., 1995; Howlett et al., 2002; Pettit, Anders, Harrison, & Cabral, 1996).

Several endogenous compounds have been shown to activate the CB receptors. The most studied endocannabinoids are AEA (Devane et al., 1992) and 2-AG (Mechoulam et al., 1995), although other analogues such as *N*-palmitoylethanolamine (PEA), noladin ether (2-arachidonylglycerol ether), or *N*-arachidonoyl dopamine have also shown cannabinomimetic activity (Calignano, La Rana, Giuffrida, & Piomelli, 1998; Conti, Costa, Colleoni, Parolaro, & Giagnoni, 2002; Hanuš et al., 2001; Huang et al., 2002). 2-AG is a natural ligand that binds weakly both CB1 and CB2 receptors (Mechoulam et al., 1995; Sigiura & Waku, 2000), whereas AEA shows higher affinity for CB1 receptors (Lin et al., 1998). Apart from CB1 and CB2 receptors, some endocannabinoids might activate other receptors such as the transient receptor potential vanilloid type-1 (TRPV1) receptor or the PPAR receptor, which would expand the mechanistic landscape of the endocannabinoid system (Huang et al., 2002; O'Sullivan, 2007; Zygmunt et al., 1999). Several articles have reported the ability of 2-AG, AEA, and other cannabinoids to interact with another G-protein-coupled receptor, the GPR55 (Ryberg et al., 2007), although its most potent ligand appears to be lysophosphatidylinositol (Oka, Nakajima, Yamashita, Kishimoto, & Sugiura, 2007). This receptor is highly expressed in brain areas such as the striatum and hypothalamus, frontal cortex, hippocampus, thalamus, and brainstem and peripheral regions such as the ileum, spleen, or adipocytes (Ryberg et al., 2007; Sharir & Abood, 2010). AEA, Δ9-THC, and the AEA metabolite *N*-arachidonylglycine also act as agonists of the GPR92 and the GPR18 receptors (McHugh, Page, Dunn, & Bradshaw, 2012; Oh et al., 2008). Another G-protein-coupled receptor, the GPR119, which is phylogenetically related to the endocannabinoids, is also activated by PEA and the non-cannabinomimetic analog OEA (Overton et al., 2006) predominantly in pancreatic and intestinal tissues, having important roles in feeding and energetic metabolism (Chu et al., 2007; Fu et al., 2003; Lauffer, Iakoubov, & Brubaker, 2009; Soga et al., 2005). OEA and, to a less extent, PEA activate the PPARα receptor, and this mechanism also appears to be involved in metabolic functions (Fu et al., 2003). This novel endocannabinoid machinery and its receptors need to be fully characterized together with their putative role in feeding and metabolic control.

The endocannabinoid system is a complex network of lipids comprising the endogenous ligands, their cannabinoid receptors, and the enzymes catalyzing the formation and degradation of endocannabinoids. As mentioned earlier, AEA and 2-AG are the most studied endocannabinoids, and their metabolic pathways are relatively well known. AEA is generated from enzymatic hydrolysis of *N*-arachidonoyl-phosphatidylethanolamine, a phospholipid precursor that is, in turn, produced from the *N*-acylation of phosphatidylethanolamine with arachidonic acid (Sun et al., 2004). Instead, 2-AG is generated through multiple routes of lipid metabolism, which explains its high concentration in brain tissue. For example, 2-AG is produced through the hydrolysis of the sn-2-arachidonate-containing diacylglycerols by a diacylglycerol lipase and is also generated through the hydrolyzation of a 2-arachidonoyl-lypophospholipid (Piomelli, 2003).

Because of their lipid nature, which allows them to diffuse throughout cellular membranes, endocannabinoids cannot be stored in vesicles; they are, therefore, synthesized on demand in response to elevations of intracellular calcium (Di Marzo, Bisogno, & Petrocellis, 2005). After their release in the extracellular space, they are rapidly removed by selective uptake into the cell and suffer intracellular enzymatic hydrolysis (Di Marzo, Bifulco, & De Petrocellis, 2004). Neural cells appear to internalize AEA and 2-AG by using energy-independent carriers. However, the protein or proteins responsible for this uptake have not yet been identified (Beltramo et al., 1997; Piomelli et al., 1999). Fatty acid amide hydrolase (FAAH), which breaks down AEA into arachidonic acid and ethanolamine, has been cloned, and its role in the hydrolysis of endocannabinoids and other bioactive fatty amides is well known (Piomelli, 2003). 2-AG, on the other hand, is hydrolyzed into arachidonic acid and glycerol by a monoacylglycerol lipase (MAGL), which appears to play a more important role than FAAH in 2-AG inactivation (Dinh et al., 2002). FAAH is expressed in postsynaptic structures, while MAGL is mostly present at nerve endings (Cravatt et al., 1996). Other metabolic pathways involve the cyclooxygenases, lipoxygenases, and P450 cytochromes (Kozak & Marnett, 2002; Van Der Stelt et al., 2002).

2.2. Peripheral endocannabinoids and feeding

The endocannabinoid system exerts a potent regulation of feeding behavior and energy balance by complex central, and recently highlighted, peripheral mechanisms. It was previously accepted that CB1 and CB2 receptors were preferentially expressed within the CNS and periphery, respectively (Gerard et al., 1990; Munro et al., 1993). However, investigations during the last two decades have described a functional presence of both CB1 and CB2 receptors within the CNS and peripheral organs. Hence, the discovery of CB1 receptors on nerve terminals innervating the gastrointestinal tract (Croci et al., 1998), in dorsal root ganglia (Hohmann & Herkenham, 1999), and in other peripheral organs related with the energetic metabolism, such as adipose tissue, pancreas, liver, or muscle (Bensaid et al., 2003; Bermudez-Silva et al., 2008; Cota et al., 2003; revisions in Hornby & Prouty, 2004; Kunos & Tam, 2011; Pagotto & Pasquali, 2006) allowed an extensive research into the contribution of the peripheral endocannabinoid system to the modulation of feeding and energy balance.

Up to 2002, the existence of a peripheral mechanism for CB1 receptors-dependent modulation of feeding was unknown. Gomez and colleagues described that food deprivation increases AEA levels in the small intestine but not in the brain or the stomach, which returned to normal levels after refeeding. AEA levels in the gut (and not in the brain) act as a hunger signal inducing hyperphagia. Such specific peripheral control of food intake appears to be mediated by CB1 receptors localized in sensory nerve terminals within the gut (Gomez et al., 2002). Interestingly, intestinal levels of AEA after food ingestion are inversely correlated with its non-cannabinomimetic analog OEA, acting in a coordinated manner to control feeding from the periphery (Gomez et al., 2002; Rodriguez de Fonseca et al., 2001).

There are other evidences for a diet-induced modulation of the endocannabinoid system. For example, refeeding induces a downregulation of CB1 receptor expression in vagal afferent neurons (Burdyga, Varro, Dimaline, Thompson, & Dockray, 2006b). It appears that the type and quantity of nutrients in the gastrointestinal tract influence the endocannabinoid production and regulation (Berger et al., 2001; Matias et al., 2008), which has important implications for high-fat-diet-induced obesity. In addition, endocannabinoids are capable of regulating gastrointestinal motility and secretion (reviewed in Storr & Sharkey, 2007) and influence the usage and storage of energy across different peripheral organs, playing a major role not only in feeding control but also in the regulation of energy balance (reviewed in Bermudez-Silva, Cardinal, & Cota, 2012). Nevertheless, studies with CB1 blockers reveal that CB1-mediated control of food intake and energy expenditure appears to follow independent mechanisms (Kunos & Tam, 2011).

In the periphery, the signals that regulate food intake may recruit both humeral and nervous pathways. The endocannabinoid system interacts with neuropeptides and hormones with an orexigenic (ghrelin) or satiety (leptin, CCK, GLP-1, PYY) action to regulate food intake, and there is a CB1-mediated neurochemical signal through the vagus nerve to central structures (mainly hypothalamic areas) involved in appetitive drive. The cross talk between different signals involved in energy homeostasis and the endocannabinoid system appears to be bidirectional: while endocannabinoids regulate the expression and action of mediators involved in nutrient intake such as ghrelin or leptin, endocannabinoid synthesis and activity are under the control of such neuropeptides (Matias, Bisogno, & Di Marzo, 2006). Such interplay involves complex interactions between metabolically relevant organs and the CNS. For example, the adiposity signal leptin reduces AEA and 2-AG levels in the hypothalamus (Di Marzo et al., 2001) and, interestingly, injection of leptin into the mediobasal hypothalamus inhibits AEA production in white adipose tissue (Buettner et al., 2008). Conversely, a lack of leptin increases endocannabinoid tone (Di Marzo et al., 2001), and endocannabinoids may feedback positively on leptin production from adipocytes, since less circulating levels of leptin were found in CB1 receptor knock-out mice (Ravinet Trillou, Delgorge, Menet, Arnone, & Soubrie, 2004). Similarly, the orexigenic gut hormone ghrelin increases endocannabinoid content in the hypothalamus (Kola et al., 2008) and, on the other hand, endocannabinoids might favor ghrelin synthesis since CB1 blockade reduces circulating levels of ghrelin (Cani, Montoya, Neyrinck, Delzenne, & Lambert, 2004). The endocannabinoid system might mediate the orexigenic effects of central ghrelin (Tucci, Rogers, Korbonits, & Kirkham, 2004) by a restricted action in the periphery (unpublished observations in our laboratory). The specific interplay between endocannabinoids and CCK is discussed in Section 4.

The endocannabinoid system appears to be altered in obesity and eating disorders. For example, the AEA content in plasma is increased in women affected by anorexia or binge-eating disorder, and there is also an overactivation of the endocannabinoid system in visceral obesity (Cervino, Vicennati, Pasquali, & Pagotto, 2009; Gaetani, Kaye, Cuomo, & Piomelli, 2008; Monteleone et al., 2005; but see Bennetzen et al., 2010). Investigations have focused their attention mainly on the role of CB1 receptors in the control of feeding and energy homeostasis, but little is known about the contribution of other cannabinoid receptors to these processes. CB2 receptors in the periphery seem to be associated with the inflammatory aspects of obesity. CB2 receptors are present in the endocrine pancreas and may contribute to maintain glucose homeostasis (Bermúdez-Silva, Suárez Pérez, Nadal, & Rodríguez de Fonseca, 2009; Li, Jones, & Persaud, 2011; Nogueiras et al., 2009). In addition, recent investigations describe a peripheral distribution of the putative cannabinoid receptor GPR55 and its possible role in obesity (Moreno-Navarrete et al., 2012).

2.3. Central endocannabinoids and feeding

The endocannabinoid system influences feeding and energy balance acting in a coordinated manner at several sites inside and outside the brain. In general, increased endocannabinoid activity enhances food intake and favors fat storage (Woods & Cota, 2007). Within the CNS, endocannabinoids may influence food intake acting mainly at two functional levels: in the hypothalamus, where they decrease satiety and enhance orexigenic signals, and in the limbic system, where they act enhancing food salience and/or palatability (Bermudez-Silva, Viveros, McPartland, & Rodriguez de Fonseca, 2010).

The hypothalamus is a major area for the integration of signals that regulate energy homeostasis (Sahu, 2004). CB1 receptors are expressed in the arcuate nuclei, the paraventricular nuclei (PVN), and the lateral hypothalamic area (Mackie, 2005; Sim, Selley, & Childers, 1995). Interestingly, hypothalamic areas containing CB1 receptors such as the arcuate nuclei are not completely protected by the blood–brain barrier because of its crucial role in the regulation of energy homeostasis (Merchenthaler, 1991). Though cannabinoid receptors are sparsely distributed in the hypothalamus (Moldrich & Wenger, 2000), their targeting shows a high-efficiency functional correlate (Breivogel & Childers, 1998). For example, THC administration facilitates feeding induced by electrical stimulation of the lateral hypothalamus (Trojniar & Wise, 1991), and AEA infusion into the ventromedial hypothalamus induces a CB1-mediated hyperphagia in presatiated rats (Jamshidi & Taylor, 2001). In addition, 2-AG levels in the hypothalamus are increased during fasting, and decline while animals eat (Kirkham, Williams, Fezza, & Di Marzo, 2002). Several mechanisms have been proposed to explain the orexigenic effects of hypothalamic endocannabinoids, such as disinhibition of the orexigenic neuropeptide melanin-concentrating hormone (MCH) release by the lateral hypothalamus, or inhibition of anorectic neurons in the PVN (Di Marzo, Ligresti, & Cristino, 2009). Other plausible mechanisms of action of endocannabinoids in the hypothalamus involve negative control of the corticotrophin-releasing hormone and the cocaine- and amphetamine-regulated transcript, and positive modulation of orexin-A signaling in the arcuate nucleus (Di Marzo et al., 2004).

Sensory pleasure or hedonic feelings constitute an important component in food reward. Long-known anecdotal reports refer to cravings for sweets after cannabinoid consumption (Tart, 1970), a phenomenon colloquially known as the "munchies." Basic research appears to support an important role for cannabinoids modulating food palatability (Yoshida et al., 2010). CB1 knock-out mice drink significantly more sucrose solution than their CB1 wild-type counterparts, and these differences are abolished if quinine, a bitter-flavored compound, is added to the sucrose solution, thus reducing its palatability (Sanchis-Segura, Cline, Marsicano, Lutz, & Spanagel, 2004). The intracerebroventricular administration of Δ9-THC potently increases intake of sweet food versus less palatable foods (Koch & Matthews, 2001), and administration of the CB1 antagonist/inverse agonist rimonabant specifically reduces the ingestion of more palatable food (Mathes, Ferrara, & Rowland, 2008). In a taste reactivity test, behavioral responses to various solutions infused into the animal's mouth are compared and can be used as an index of the perceived palatability of different solutions, other than merely the ingestion (Grill & Norgren, 1978). Using this technique, it has been shown that intra-accumbens shell administration of AEA doubles the number of positive ingestive responses to sweet solutions compared to intraoral infusions (Mahler, Smith, & Berridge, 2007). Indeed, among other brain sites, the accumbens shell is considered a key component mediating the perceived palatability of food (Berridge, 2000), and this structure is the only corticostriatal area that sends projections directly to the lateral hypothalamus, thus suggesting a unique interaction between both structures that may be mediated by endocannabinoids (Bermudez-Silva et al., 2012). CB1 receptor distribution in the nucleus accumbens shell closely colocalizes with opioid receptors, and both systems cooperate in the modulation of food palatability and ingestion (Cota, Tschöp, Horvath, & Levine, 2006). Dopaminergic activation in the accumbens shell is another important determinant of the hedonic value of stimuli and, interestingly, blockade of CB1 receptors in this area inhibits the dopamine release elicited by highly palatable food (Melis et al., 2007). Intra-accumbens injections of 2-AG induce a short-term feeding stimulation (Kirkham et al., 2002), and whereas food deprivation increases AEA and 2-AG levels, food consumption decreases both endocannabinoid levels in the limbic forebrain (Kirkham et al., 2002). However, it appears that the endocannabinoid system acts in multiple sites to control palatability-mediated food consumption. Besides the exposed role of the accumbal endocannabinoids in food palatability, the endocannabinoid system is also present in other brain areas receiving peripheral inputs, such as the brainstem. Specifically, it has been shown that an elevation of endocannabinoid tone via FAAH inhibition, or a 2-AG infusion in the pontine parabrachial nucleus, another structure involved in the processing of food gustatory properties, selectively stimulates the consumption of palatable food (DiPatrizio & Simansky, 2008a, 2008b).

It is noteworthy that high palatability is not a requirement to observe reductions in food consumption after the CB1 antagonist rimonabant administration, which suggests a wider role for endocannabinoids in food consumption (Freedland, Poston, & Porrino, 2000). Indeed, several data suggest a major role for endocannabinoids in general motivation for food. To test the motivational properties of a reward, variants of the self-administration paradigm, such as the progressive ratio schedules, are frequently used (Richardson & Roberts, 1996). Progressive ratio schedules generally assess the incentive value of rewards, and the number of responses that an animal is ready to complete in order to obtain the food (break-point) is considered an index of this incentive value (see Finger, Dinan, & Cryan, 2010). In this direction, endocannabinoid antagonists dose-dependently reduce the break-point of progressive responding for food, while CB1 agonists increase it (Higgs, Barber, Cooper, & Terry, 2005; Solinas & Goldberg, 2005; Wakley & Rasmussen, 2009; Ward & Dykstra, 2005). In addition, CB1 knock-out mice show reduced rates of responding for food and lower break-points than wild-type mice (Sanchis-Segura et al., 2004). The mesolimbic dopaminergic system is considered a key mediator of motivation and appetite, and a cross talk between the endocannabinoid and the dopaminergic systems in mesolimbic areas have been postulated. For example, dopamine inhibits endocannabinoid biosynthesis in the limbic forebrain and endocannabinoids are synthesized by dopaminergic neurons in the ventral tegmental area (VTA), which regulate mesolimbic areas (Melis et al., 2004). It is believed that endocannabinoid receptors modulate dopamine neurotransmission in a complex manner, probably by inhibiting glutamate release at the presynaptic level, which, in turn, inhibits GABAergic neurons that originate in the nucleus accumbens, resulting in an eventual disinhibition of VTA dopaminergic neurons (Maldonado, Valverde, & Berrendero, 2006). In addition, some endocannabinoids that target the excitatory TRPV1 receptors located in glutamatergic terminals may also increase the dopamine firing rate (Marinelli et al., 2007). In conclusion, any alteration in this motivational circuitry involving endocannabinoids may have important consequences for reward-related behaviors including food consumption.

3. CCK AND FEEDING REGULATION

3.1. CCK and its receptors

CCK is a peptide hormone belonging to a family of compounds acting at the gut–brain axis. It was discovered by Ivy and Olberg in 1943 as a hormone that contracts the gallbladder, soon after the discovery of other gastrointestinal hormones such as gastrin or secretin (revised in Konturek & Konturek, 2003). Since then, it is now well established the fundamental role of endogenously released or exogenously administered CCK in the regulation of the complex mechanisms underlying food intake.

CCK is composed of several peptides, being the 33-amino acid form (CCK-33) first isolated (Mutt & Jorpes, 1968). Each CCK peptide comes from the same mRNA molecule that is translated into an identical precursor or preprohormone (preproCCK) in the brain and the intestine. The existence of different CCK molecular forms might be explained by tissue-specific post-translational events (Deschenes et al., 1984; Gubler, Chua, Hoffman, Collier, & Eng, 1984). One of the most important posttranslational transformations of these peptides is the sulfatation of tyrosine or amidation of phenylalanyl residues located in the c-terminal (Eberlein et al., 1992; Rehfeld, 1998; Rehfeld & Hansen, 1986). Several bioactive forms of CCK have been described and named according to the number of amino acids: CCK-83, CCK-58, CCK-39, CCK-33, CCK-22, CCK-8, CCK-5 (Eng et al., 1984; Larsson & Rehfeld, 1979; Reeve, Eysselein, Walsh, Ben-Avram, & Shively, 1986; Rehfeld, 1978; Rehfeld, Sun, Christensen, & Hillingso, 2001). The bioactivity of different CCK forms depends on the polypeptidic length and the presence of sulfated forms, which are more potent (Bonetto et al., 1999; Dufresne, Seva, & Fourmy, 2006; Reeve, Eysselein, Walsh, Ben-Avram, & Shively, 1986; Rehfeld & Hansen, 1986). Further, CCK suffers a cell-specific processing: medium-size CCK forms have been found predominantly in endocrine cells, whereas CCK-33 and CCK-8 are located in plasma and neurons, respectively (Rehfeld, 1978; Rehfeld & Hansen, 1986; Rehfeld et al., 2001). In endocrine cells, the main stimulus to secrete CCK appears to be protein/fat-enriched food (Liddle, Goldfine, Rosen, Taplitz, & Williams, 1985; Rehfeld, 1998) and, within the brain, a calcium-dependent release of CCK-8 is effected by potassium-induced depolarization (Emson, Lee, & Rehfeld, 1980).

CCK is mainly synthesized in I-cells of small intestine, although it is produced in the CNS too (Miller, Jardine, Weissman, Go, & Speicher, 1984; Rehfeld, 1978). It has cholecystokinetic and pancreozymic actions, apart from being a growth factor and neurotransmitter. It has been found that it produces effects in smooth muscle as in the peripheral and central nervous system.

CCK exerts its actions by binding to CCK1 and CCK2 receptors, both members of the G-protein-coupled receptor superfamily (Wank, Harkins, et al., 1992; Wank, Pisegna, & de Weerth, 1992), which were first named type A (Alimentary) and type B (Brain), respectively (Dufresne et al., 2006; Noble et al., 1999). CCK1 is mainly localized in peripheral organs and discrete areas of the brain, whereas CCK2 is primarily expressed in the brain and in the stomach (Mutt & Jorpes, 1968; Wank, 1995).

The CCK1 receptor was first characterized in pancreatic acini cells (Sankaran, Goldfine, Deveney, Wong, & Williams, 1980), and it is distributed mainly in the gastric mucosa, where it inhibits acid secretion (Schmitz et al., 2001), the pancreas, and the gallbladder (Christophe, De Neef, Deschodt-Lanckman, & Robberecht, 1978; Jensen, Lemp, & Gardner, 1980; Tokunaga et al., 1993). The CCK1 receptor has been implicated in gallbladder contraction, relaxation of the sphincter of Oddi, pancreatic growth, inhibition of gastric acid secretion, stimulation of pancreatic secretion, and delay in gastric emptying, as well as the induction of satiety (revised in Cawston & Miller, 2010). Within the nervous system, there is a discrete presence of CCK1 receptors in several brain areas such as the area postrema, nucleus solitarius, hypothalamus, interpeduncular nucleus, and substantia nigra (revised in Cawston & Miller, 2010; van Megen, Westenberg, den Boer, & Kahn, 1996), and it has also been identified in vagal afferent neurons, where it might play a major role in the anorectic effects of CCK (Broberger, Holmberg, Shi, Dockray, & Hokfelt, 2001; Corp, McQuade, Moran, & Smith, 1993; Moran, Norgren, Crosby, & McHugh, 1990; Reidelberger, Castellanos, & Hulce, 2003; Reidelberger, Hernandez, Fritzsch, & Hulce, 2004; Ritter & Ladenheim, 1985; Smith, Jerome, Cushin, Eterno, & Simansky, 1981).

The CCK2 receptor is widely distributed in the brain (Innis & Snyder, 1980). Specifically, it is localized in the cortex, olfactory bulb, hypothalamus, nucleus accumbens, amygdala, hippocampus, caudate nucleus, and cerebellum (reviewed in van Megen et al., 1996), although it has been found in other organs such as the stomach (Reubi et al., 1997). The CCK2 receptor is involved in the regulation of food intake, pain, stress, neuroendocrine control, cardiovascular regulation, control of learning and memory, neuropsychiatric disorders including anxiety-related behaviors, modulation of dependence and withdrawal, and, in general, processes that are controlled by serotonergic, dopaminergic, and opiod systems (reviewed in Wang, Wong, Spiess, & Zhu, 2005).

While the CCK1 receptor shows high affinity to amidated and sulfated CCK forms, the CCK2 receptor appears to be less selective. For example, the CCK2 receptor binds with high affinity sulfated and nonsulfated CCK forms, short c-terminal fragments such as CCK-4 and CCK-5, and also gastrin (Rehfeld, 2004; Wang et al., 2005). The most abundant CCK form in the CNS is the CCK-8 sulfated peptide (CCK-8S), which is a natural ligand that activates CCK2 receptors. However, CCK-8S also binds CCK1 receptors with a 1000-fold higher affinity than unsulfated CCK-8,

CCK-4, or gastrin (Dufresne et al., 2006; Wang et al., 2005). It appears that the tetrapeptide form of CCK (CCK-4), which has high affinity for CCK2 receptors, might mediate CCK-induced anxiety, since it produces cardiovascular and stress hormone alterations as well as panic symptoms and other CNS alterations (Dauge & Lena, 1998; Eser et al., 2007). In addition, a polymorphism in the CCK2 receptor alleles has been associated with high risk of suffering panic disorders, although this hypothesis has not been confirmed in other studies (see Koszycki et al., 2012).

3.2. Peripheral CCK and feeding

Back in 1937, it was shown that administration of an extract of intestinal mucosa containing the active molecule for inhibition of gastric secretion and motility impaired appetite in rabbits (Maclagan, 1937). Some years later, in 1973 and 1975, the administration of the octapeptide CCK (CCK-8) was found to reduce food intake in rats (Gibbs, Young, & Smith, 1973; Antin, Gibbs, Holt, Young, & Smith, 1975). Subsequent studies extended the CCK-induced inhibition of feeding to numerous animal species and humans (Baldwin, Parrott, & Ebenezer, 1998; Kissileff, Pi-Sunyer, Thornton, & Smith, 1981), confirming its importance in postprandial satiety (Beglinger, Degen, Matzinger, D'Amato, & Drewe, 2001; Kissileff et al., 1981).

The induction of satiety by CCK might be explained by the existence of peripheral and central mechanisms. Peripheral CCK is involved in several actions related to feeding modulation, such as gallbladder contraction, bile release, pancreatic and intestine enzyme secretion, pancreatic endocrine secretion, pancreatic growth, gastrointestinal motility, intestinal blood flow, and inhibition of gastric acid secretion (reviewed in Rehfeld, 2004).

The discovery of CCK1 receptors in vagal afferent neurons has partially resolved the mechanistic aspects of CCK in satiety and its interaction with other systems in the modulation of feeding. Afferent neurons of the vagus nerve are an important target to gut hormones in the control of food intake. Vagal nerve afferents within the gastrointestinal tract and hepatoportal regions are stimulated by mechanical distension, chemical stimulation, and local production of gut hormones (Schwartz, 2000). The satiety action of CCK appears to be mediated by activation of peripheral CCK1 receptors located in the vagus nerve (Corp et al., 1993; Dourish, Ruckert, Tattersall, & Iversen, 1989). CCK is rapidly released from I-cells in the upper intestine (the duodenum and jejunum) in response to the intraluminal presence of the digestive products of fats and proteins (Cummings & Overduin,

2007), and its binding and axonal transport are evident in all abdominal vagal branches (Moran, Smith, Hostetler, & McHugh, 1987). Peripheral administration of CCK1 receptor antagonists increases food intake in several species (Hewson, Leighton, Hill, & Hughes, 1988) and, interestingly, abdominal vagotomy decreases the anorectic effects of peripheral CCK (Joyner, Smith, & Gibbs, 1993). Similar effects were found by selective vagal deafferentation using bilateral perineural application of the sensory neurotoxin capsaicin (Raybould & Tache, 1988). Apart from CCK1 receptors, CCK2 receptors have also been described in vagal afferent neurons. However, while there is a clear role for vagal CCK1 receptors in feeding, the specific role for CCK2 receptors in vagal afferent neurons requires further analysis. Some authors raise the hypothesis that activation of both CCK1 and CCK2 receptors, rather than specifically targeting CCK1 receptors, may a requirement to achieve a full satiety effect (Clerc et al., 2007).

In addition to CCK1 and CCK2 receptors, vagal afferent neurons also express ghrelin type 1 (GHS-1), orexin type 1 (OX-R1), MCH type 1 (MCH-1), cannabinoid CB1, and leptin receptors (***Burdyga et al., 2003, 2004, 2002; Burdyga, Varro, Dimaline, Thompson, & Dockray, 2006a; Burdyga et al., 2006b). An interaction between ghrelin and CCK has been described, since pretreatment with CCK inhibited the orexigenic effect of ghrelin and, conversely, the anorectic effect of CCK was blunted by preadministration of ghrelin. Interestingly, it is known that CCK1 and ghrelin receptors colocalize in the nodose ganglia, and, therefore, they might interfere with the signal transmission generated by each other (Date et al., 2005). For example, ghrelin and orexin are capable of inhibiting the discharge of vagal afferent neurons in response to CCK (Burdyga et al., 2003; Date et al., 2005).

CCK also appears to play a major role in body weight regulation by synergistic interaction with long-term adiposity signals, such as leptin (Morton, Cummings, Baskin, Barsh, & Schwartz, 2006). In response to chronic ingestion of a high-fat diet, the vagal afferent neurons develop resistance to leptin, and the onset of leptin resistance reduces the sensitivity of vagal afferent neurons to CCK, thus reducing the satiating effects of CCK. These results indicate that leptin signaling in vagal afferent neurons is required for appropriate CCK signaling and satiation (de Lartigue, Barbier de la Serre, Espero, Lee, & Raybould, 2012). CCK might also play a role in adaptive responses in pancreatic islets. It is upregulated by islet cells during obesity and functions as a paracrine or autocrine factor to increase β-cell survival and expand β-cell mass, thus compensating for the obesity-induced insulin resistance (Lavine et al., 2010).

3.3. Central CCK and feeding

The satiety effects of CCK might be mediated not only by peripheral but also by central mechanisms. Activation of the hypothalamic–pituitary–adrenal axis by fasting seems to involve CCK receptors. Indeed, an increase in plasma adrenocorticotropic hormone levels was observed after central and peripheral CCK treatment (Kamilaris et al., 1992). However, the central mechanisms whereby CCK may act as a modulator of food intake are still partly resolved (Baldwin et al., 1998; Blevins, Stanley, & Reidelberger, 2000). CCK is released in the hypothalamus after a meal (Schick, Reilly, Roddy, Yaksh, & Go, 1987), and, conversely, central administration of CCK into several hypothalamic nuclei appears to suppress food intake (Blevins et al., 2000; Inui et al., 1987). It is also known the presence of CCK receptors in brain areas related to food intake modulation (Carlberg, Gundlach, Mercer, & Beart, 1992; Hill, Campbell, Shaw, & Woodruff, 1987; Zajac, Gully, & Maffrand, 1996).

CCK is considered a satiety hormone since it inhibits food intake, meal size, and meal duration through activation of CCK1 receptors (Boguszewski, Paz-Filho, & Velloso, 2010; Hewson et al., 1988). Exogenous CCK also triggers a stereotyped sequence of behaviors normally displayed upon meal completion, suggesting that this peptide hormone evokes the perception of satiation without internal food stimuli (Antin et al., 1975). In addition, the consequences of CCK1 receptor suppression support a physiological role for this receptor in satiation. For example, CCK administration to mice lacking CCK1 receptors fails to decrease food intake (Kopin et al., 1999), and rats lacking CCK1 receptors showed an increase in meal size and gradually became obese (Moran, Katz, Plata-Salaman, & Schwartz, 1998).

As mentioned previously, CCK2 receptor is the predominant CCK receptor form found in the central nervous system, particularly in hypothalamic areas that control body energy balance (Barrachina, Martinez, Wang, Wei, & Tache, 1997). CCK2 receptors are also known to interact with opioids and the dopaminergic system, which regulates behavioral responses with a potent impact on food intake (Noble et al., 1999). Although generally considered a peripheral receptor type, CCK1 receptor is also found in the brain (Boden, Woodruff, & Pinnock, 1991). The contribution of each receptor to the central effects of CCK-induced satiety is still unclear. Central administration of proglumide, a mixed CCK1 and CCK2 receptor antagonist, blunted the satiating effect of peripheral CCK-8, and, similarly, the infusion of CCK1 receptor antagonists directly into the hypothalamus increased food consumption (Linden, Uvnas-Moberg, Forsberg, Bednar,

& Sodersten, 1989). Studies with functional magnetic resonance imaging showed that CCK1 receptor antagonists inhibit the activation of the brainstem, hypothalamus, and motor cortex observed in humans after ingestion of fatty acids (Lassman et al., 2010).

4. INTERACTIONS BETWEEN CCK AND ENDOCANNABINOID RECEPTORS IN THE REGULATION OF FEEDING

As reviewed earlier, both the endocannabinoids and CCK are positioned to interact not only in the regulation of appetite and satiety but also in the complex processes of nutrient sensing and the control of gastrointestinal motility. Interestingly, both systems are opposed in the promotion of feeding. CCK rises rapidly after a meal and induces satiety through the activation of the peripheral nerve terminals of the vagus and acting at peripheral nerve ganglia such as the nodose ganglia (Dockray, 2009; Owyang & Heldsinger, 2011). However, the effect of CCK on feeding is not permanent, and continuous infusion of CCK failed to decrease feeding and body weight gain because the animal compensate by increasing the meal frequency (Crawley & Beinfeld, 1983). Anandamide in the intestine, on the contrary, rises after food deprivation to promote feeding, and it rapidly decreases after refeeding (Gomez et al., 2002). Promotion of feeding by exogenous administered anandamide is greater when the animal is partially fed, that is, anandamide-induced overeating is greater in food deprived animals that has a short meal before the administration of the endocannabinoid (Williams & Kirkham, 1999). This effect is mediated by the vagus nerve, since abrogation of its peripheral nerve terminals with capsaicin abolished the feeding promotion effects of anandamide (Gomez et al., 2002). Thus, both, AEA and CCK converge in the vagus nerve to promote opposing actions on feeding behavior.

Because of this convergence between the CCK and AEA signaling systems, there is a growing interest in studying the existence of mutual interactions that may determine appetite/satiety status. From the anatomical point of view, cannabinoid CB1 receptors activated by AEA are located in vagal afferent neurons expressing CCK1 receptors. The coexistence of both signals goes beyond mere anatomical contiguity. The variations in the expression of cannabinoid CB1 receptors along with food deprivation are controlled by CCK (Burdyga et al., 2004). Food deprivation increased the expression of both cannabinoid CB1 receptors mRNA and protein in the rat nodose ganglia. This effect is prevented by refeeding and CCK-8, a CCK1 receptor agonist, treatment. Thus, CCK is capable of modulating the cannabinoid orexigenic machinery by limiting the number of active receptors in the vagal afferents that might be activated by AEA to promote feeding. This role of CCK is not new, since apparently CCK is capable of modulating the expression of other receptors for gastrointestinal peptides involved in appetite modulation (Burdyga et al., 2008; Dockray & Burdyga, 2011). In fact, this is the expression of a more generalized mechanism of plasticity of the vagus nerve, whose expression of receptors for gastrointestinal signals regulating appetite is widely modulated by nutritional status and hormonal/peptidic signals. This way, the vagus integrates peripherally the metabolic status with the nutritional information needed to establish a feeding pattern and the selection of macronutrients to be eaten (Burdyga, Varro, Dimaline, Thompson, & Dockray, 2010; Burdyga et al., 2006a, 2006b, Dockray & Burdyga, 2011).

The interaction between CCK and the endocannabinoid system in regulating appetite has been investigated recently (Orio et al., 2011). Since AEA promotes feeding, and the cannabinoid CB1 receptor antagonist rimonabant reduced appetite, it could be expected that a significant interaction between CCK-8 and the cannabinoid ligand may occur. The main results of this study are shown in Fig. 7.1. Pretreatment of animals with the cannabinoid CB1 receptor agonist WIN 55,212-2 antagonized the satiety induced by CCK-8 in rats. Conversely, pretreatment with the cannabinoid CB1 receptor antagonist/inverse agonist rimonabant produced additive effects on the satiety induced by CCK-8. This pharmacological demonstration sets in place the importance of a pharmacological design aiming to search for synergisms between regulatory systems.

The strategy of dual actions (i.e., activating CCK1 receptors and antagonizing CB1 receptors) might also avoid neuroadaptations that might result in loss of efficacy, as traditionally described for CCK. Moreover, in certain conditions, such as diet-induced obesity, the adaptations to high fat and the subsequent induction of leptin resistance leads to an inhibition of satiety signals such as those mediated by CCK. Both leptin-resistant Zucker rats and diet-induced obese rats are insensitive to CCK. The mechanisms of this inhibition involve intracellular pathways such as those of the early growth response 1. Any mechanism modulating leptin signaling (i.e., improving leptin resistance) might help to restore the efficacy of CCK (de Lartigue, Barbier de la Serre, Espero, Lee, & Raybould, 2011; de Lartigue et al., 2012). Up to date, cannabinoid CB1 receptor blockade has been proved to be an efficient

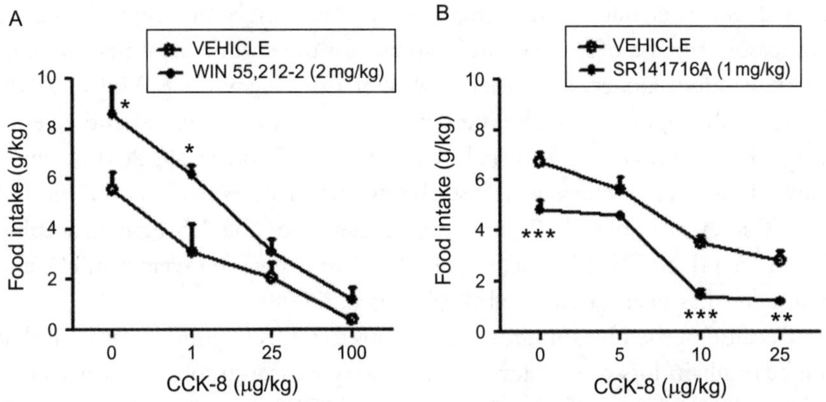

Figure 7.1 Interactions between CCK-8 and CB1 receptors in feeding behavior. (A) The inhibitory interaction between CCK-8, a CCK1 receptor agonist, and the CB1 receptor agonist WIN 55,212-2 in the modulation of food intake. Pretreatment of partially satiated rats with a single dose of WIN 55,212-2 (2 mg/kg) counteracts feeding suppression induced by different doses of CCK-8. On the contrary, (B) shows that the CB1 receptor antagonist SR141716A and CCK-8 have additive effects on feeding suppression. Pretreatments with WIN 55,212-2 (2 mg/kg, i.p.) and SR141716A (1 mg/kg, i.p.) were done 30 min before CCK-8 (1–100 μg/kg, i.p.). Food intake was measured 60 min posttreatment. Results shown as means ± SEM, $n = 9$–10. Different from vehicle-injected animals: $^{*}p < 0.05$, $^{**}p < 0.01$, $^{***}p < 0.001$ (two-way ANOVA followed by Bonferroni posttest). *Reproduced with permission from Orio et al. (2011).*

way of reducing appetite and body weight gain, and improving leptin resistance (Bermudez-Silva et al., 2010). From this perspective, a combinational therapy using a cannabinoid CB1 receptor antagonist and a CCK1 agonist might be a very useful combination therapy for reducing appetite. Considering the unwanted effects of central CB1 blockade (Bermudez-Silva et al., 2010), the use of a peripheral restricted / lower brain-penetrating CB1 antagonist might be a requisite to avoid the psychiatric effects that forced the withdrawal of cannabinoid CB1 antagonist from the market.

5. CONCLUSIONS AND CLINICAL RELEVANCE

In this review, we highlight the importance of combined therapies, such as CCK1 agonism and CB1 antagonism, to treat obesity in order to improve the efficacy of CCK1 agonism-based treatments. Several CCK1 agonists have been tested as a strategy to treat obesity but, unfortunately, clinical trials have been unsuccessful to date, due to physiological adaptations that resulted in loss of efficacy. It is to be noted that some CCK1 agonists could also bind

CCK2 receptors, due to the high homology between both receptors and, for this reason, the use of some CCK1 agonists for the chronic treatment of obesity may induce anxiety and other CNS alterations (Cawston & Miller, 2010). Some CCK1 agonists are in different phases of clinical trials as anti-obesity drugs. For example, the molecule CE-326597 (Elliott et al., 2010), which showed insufficient efficacy against obesity and diabetes in a phase II clinical trial (Cameron et al., 2012), and the efficiency of the 1,5-benzodiacepine derivative GI181771X (Castillo et al., 2004) in decreasing weight in chronic treatments has been questioned (Jordan et al., 2008).

Because of the physiological adaptations to CCK1 agonist treatment that might result in loss of efficacy, it is necessary to search for additional strategies. The additive effects of cannabinoid CB1 receptor blockade and CCK1 stimulation offer new alternatives not only because they are synergistic in feeding inhibition, but also because their effects in nutritional status and on mediators such as leptin, ghrelin, or PYY might determine the efficacy of CCK itself. Moreover, a therapeutics centered on peripheral signals offers the additional advantage of minimizing psychiatric side effects, which has been the leading cause of the failure of many new therapies designed to fight obesity.

ACKNOWLEDGMENTS

Research supported by [LO]: Spanish Ministry of Health PR28/11-18295 and Fundación Rodríguez Pascual; [FRF]: FIS 07/1226; VII European Framework Programme Grant "Reprobesity"; Proyectos de Excelencia Junta de Andalucía; Red de Trastornos Adictivos RD06/001 and CIBEROBN. MT.R.L. is the recipient of a fellowship (FPI) from the Spanish Ministry of Education and Science.

REFERENCES

Antin, J., Gibbs, J., Holt, J., Young, R. C., & Smith, G. P. (1975). Cholecystokinin elicits the complete behavioral sequence of satiety in rats. *Journal of Comparative and Physiological Psychology*, *89*, 784–790.

Baldwin, B. A., Parrott, R. F., & Ebenezer, I. S. (1998). Food for thought: A critique on the hypothesis that endogenous cholecystokinin acts as a physiological satiety factor. *Progress in Neurobiology*, *55*, 477–507.

Barrachina, M. D., Martinez, V., Wang, L., Wei, J. Y., & Tache, Y. (1997). Synergistic interaction between leptin and cholecystokinin to reduce short-term food intake in lean mice. *Proceedings of the National Academy of Sciences of the United States of America*, *94*, 10455–10460.

Beglinger, C., Degen, L., Matzinger, D., D'Amato, M., & Drewe, J. (2001). Loxiglumide, a CCK-A receptor antagonist, stimulates calorie intake and hunger feelings in humans. *American Journal of Physiology. Regulatory, Integrative and Comparative Physiology*, *280*, R1149–R1154.

Beltramo, M., Stella, N., Calignano, A., Lin, S. Y., Makriyannis, A., & Piomelli, D. (1997). Functional role of high-affinity anandamide transport, as revealed by selective inhibition. *Science, 277*, 1094–1097.

Bennetzen, M. F., Nielsen, T., Paulsen, S. K., Bendix, J., Fisker, S., Jessen, N., et al. (2010). Reduced cannabinoid receptor 1 protein in subcutaneous adipose tissue of obese. *European Journal of Clinical Investigation, 40*, 121–126 (Comprobar que en cita se refiera a esto, porque en realidad cita 2001).

Bensaid, M., Gary-Bobo, M., Esclangon, A., Maffrand, J. P., Le Fur, G., Oury-Donat, F., et al. (2003). The cannabinoid CB1 receptor antagonist SR141716 increases Acrp30 mRNA expression in adipose tissue of obese fa/fa rats and in cultured adipocyte cells. *Molecular Pharmacology, 63*, 908–914.

Berger, A., Crozier, G., Bisogno, T., Cavaliere, P., Innis, S., & Di Marzo, V. (2001). Anandamide and diet: Inclusion of dietary arachidonate and docosahexaenoate leads to increased brain levels of the corresponding N-acylethanolamines in piglets. *Proceedings of the National Academy of Sciences of the United States of America, 98*, 6402.

Bermudez-Silva, F. J., Cardinal, P., & Cota, D. (2012). The role of the endocannabinoid system in the neuroendocrine regulation of energy balance. *Journal of Psychopharmacology, 26*, 114–124.

Bermúdez-Silva, F. J., Suárez Pérez, J., Nadal, A., & Rodríguez de Fonseca, F. (2009). The role of the pancreatic endocannabinoid system in glucose metabolism. *Best Practice & Research. Clinical Endocrinology & Metabolism, 23*, 87–102.

Bermudez-Silva, F. J., Suarez, J., Baixeras, E., Cobo, N., Bautista, D., Cuesta-Munoz, A. L., et al. (2008). Presence of functional cannabinoid receptors in human endocrine pancreas. *Diabetologia, 51*, 476–487.

Bermudez-Silva, F. J., Viveros, M. P., McPartland, J. M., & Rodriguez de Fonseca, F. (2010). The endocannabinoid system, eating behavior and energy homeostasis: The end or a new beginning? *Pharmacology, Biochemistry, and Behavior, 95*, 375–382.

Berridge, K. C. (2000). Opioid site in nucleus accumbens shell mediates eating and hedonic 'liking'for food: Map based on microinjection Fos plumes. *Brain Research, 863*, 71–86.

Blevins, J. E., Stanley, B. G., & Reidelberger, R. D. (2000). Brain regions where cholecystokinin suppresses feeding in rats. *Brain Research, 860*, 1–10.

Boden, P. R., Woodruff, G. N., & Pinnock, R. D. (1991). Pharmacology of a cholecystokinin receptor on 5-hydroxytryptamine neurones in the dorsal raphe of the rat brain. *British Journal of Pharmacology, 102*, 635–638.

Boguszewski, C. L., Paz-Filho, G., & Velloso, L. A. (2010). Neuroendocrine body weight regulation: Integration between fat tissue, gastrointestinal tract, and the brain. *Endokrynologia Polska, 61*, 194–206.

Bonetto, V., Jornvall, H., Andersson, M., Renlund, S., Mutt, V., & Sillard, R. (1999). Isolation and characterization of sulphated and nonsulphated forms of cholecystokinin-58 and their action on gallbladder contraction. *European Journal of Biochemistry, 264*, 336–340.

Breivogel, C. S., & Childers, S. R. (1998). The functional neuroanatomy of brain cannabinoid receptors. *Neurobiology of Disease, 5*, 417–431.

Broberger, C., Holmberg, K., Shi, T. J., Dockray, G., & Hokfelt, T. (2001). Expression and regulation of cholecystokinin and cholecystokinin receptors in rat nodose and dorsal root ganglia. *Brain Research, 903*, 128–140.

Buettner, C., Muse, E. D., Cheng, A., Chen, L., Scherer, T., Pocai, A., et al. (2008). Leptin controls adipose tissue lipogenesis via central, STAT3–independent mechanisms. *Nature Medicine, 14*, 667–675.

Burdyga, G., de Lartigue, G., Raybould, H. E., Morris, R., Dimaline, R., Varro, A., et al. (2008). Cholecystokinin regulates expression of Y2 receptors in vagal afferent neurons serving the stomach. *Journal of Neuroscience, 28*, 11583–11592.

Burdyga, G., Lal, S., Spiller, D., Jiang, W., Thompson, D., Attwood, S., et al. (2003). Localization of orexin-1 receptors to vagal afferent neurons in the rat and humans. *Gastroenterology*, *124*, 129–139.

Burdyga, G., Lal, S., Varro, A., Dimaline, R., Thompson, D. G., & Dockray, G. J. (2004). Expression of cannabinoid CB1 receptors by vagal afferent neurons is inhibited by cholecystokinin. *Journal of Neuroscience*, *24*, 2708–2715.

Burdyga, G., Spiller, D., Morris, R., Lal, S., Thompson, D. G., Saeed, S., et al. (2002). Expression of the leptin receptor in rat and human nodose ganglion neurones. *Neuroscience*, *109*, 339–347.

Burdyga, G., Varro, A., Dimaline, R., Thompson, D. G., & Dockray, G. J. (2006a). Feeding-dependent depression of melanin-concentrating hormone and melanin-concentrating hormone receptor-1 expression in vagal afferent neurones. *Neuroscience*, *137*, 1405–1415.

Burdyga, G., Varro, A., Dimaline, R., Thompson, D. G., & Dockray, G. J. (2006b). Ghrelin receptors in rat and human nodose ganglia: Putative role in regulating CB-1 and MCH receptor abundance. *American Journal of Physiology. Gastrointestinal and Liver Physiology*, *290*, G1289–G1297.

Burdyga, G., Varro, A., Dimaline, R., Thompson, D. G., & Dockray, G. J. (2010). Expression of cannabinoid CB1 receptors by vagal afferent neurons: Kinetics and role in influencing neurochemical phenotype. *American Journal of Physiology. Gastrointestinal and Liver Physiology*, *299*, G63–G69.

Calignano, A., La Rana, G., Giuffrida, A., & Piomelli, D. (1998). Control of pain initiation by endogenous cannabinoids. *Nature*, *394*, 277–281.

Cameron, K. O., Beretta, E. E., Chen, Y., Chu-Moyer, M., Fernando, D., Gao, H., et al. (2012). Discovery of new piperidine amide triazolobenzodiazepinones as intestinal-selective CCK1 receptor agonists. *Bioorganic & Medicinal Chemistry Letters*, *22*, 2943–2947.

Cani, P., Montoya, M. L., Neyrinck, A. M., Delzenne, N. M., & Lambert, D. M. (2004). Short communication. Potential modulation of plasma ghrelin and glucagon-like peptide-1 by anorexigenic cannabinoid compounds, SR141716A (rimonabant) and oleoylethanolamide. *British Journal of Nutrition*, *92*, 757–761.

Carlberg, M., Gundlach, A. L., Mercer, L. D., & Beart, P. M. (1992). Autoradiographic localization of cholecystokinin A and B receptors in rat brain using [125I]d-Tyr25 (Nle28,31)-CCK 25–33S. *The European Journal of Neuroscience*, *4*, 563–573.

Castillo, E. J., Delgado-Aros, S., Camilleri, M., Burton, D., Stephens, D., O'Connor-Semmes, R., et al. (2004). Effect of oral CCK-1 agonist GI181771X on fasting and postprandial gastric functions in healthy volunteers. *American Journal of Physiology. Gastrointestinal and Liver Physiology*, *287*, G363–G369.

Cawston, E. E., & Miller, L. J. (2010). Therapeutic potential for novel drugs targeting the type 1 cholecystokinin receptor. *British Journal of Pharmacology*, *159*, 1009–1021.

Cervino, C., Vicennati, V., Pasquali, R., & Pagotto, U. (2009). Feeding disorders and obesity. *Current Topic in Behavioral Neurosciences*, *1*, 373–385.

Christophe, J., De Neef, P., Deschodt-Lanckman, M., & Robberecht, P. (1978). The interaction of caerulein with the rat pancreas. 2. Specific binding of [3H]caerulein on dispersed acinar cells. *European Journal of Biochemistry*, *91*, 31–38.

Chu, Z. L., Jones, R. M., He, H., Carroll, C., Gutierrez, V., Lucman, A., et al. (2007). A role for beta-cell-expressed G protein-coupled receptor 119 in glycemic control by enhancing glucose-dependent insulin release. *Endocrinology*, *148*, 2601–2609.

Clerc, P., Coll Constans, M. G., Lulka, H., Broussaud, S., Guigne, C., Leung-Theung-Long, S., et al. (2007). Involvement of cholecystokinin 2 receptor in food intake regulation: Hyperphagia and increased fat deposition in cholecystokinin 2 receptor-deficient mice. *Endocrinology*, *148*, 1039–1049.

Conti, S., Costa, B., Colleoni, M., Parolaro, D., & Giagnoni, G. (2002). Antiinflammatory action of endocannabinoid palmitoylethanolamide and the synthetic cannabinoid nabilone in a model of acute inflammation in the rat. *British Journal of Pharmacology, 135*, 181–187.

Corp, E. S., McQuade, J., Moran, T. H., & Smith, G. P. (1993). Characterization of type A and type B CCK receptor binding sites in rat vagus nerve. *Brain Research, 623*, 161–166.

Cota, D., Marsicano, G., Tschop, M., Grubler, Y., Flachskamm, C., Schubert, M., et al. (2003). The endogenous cannabinoid system affects energy balance via central orexigenic drive and peripheral lipogenesis. *The Journal of Clinical Investigation, 112*, 423–431.

Cota, D., Tschöp, M. H., Horvath, T. L., & Levine, A. S. (2006). Cannabinoids, opioids and eating behavior: The molecular face of hedonism? *Brain Research Reviews, 51*, 85–107.

Cravatt, B. F., Giang, D. K., Mayfield, S. P., Boger, D. L., Lerner, R. A., & Gilula, N. B. (1996). Molecular characterization of an enzyme that degrades neuromodulatory fatty-acid amides. *Nature, 384*, 83–87.

Crawley, J. N., & Beinfeld, M. C. (1983). Rapid development of tolerance to the behavioural actions of cholecystokinin. *Nature, 302*, 703–706.

Croci, T., Manara, L., Aureggi, G., Guagnini, F., Rinaldi-Carmona, M., Maffrand, J. P., et al. (1998). In vitro functional evidence of neuronal cannabinoid CB1 receptors in human ileum. *British Journal of Pharmacology, 125*, 1393–1395.

Cummings, D. E., & Overduin, J. (2007). Gastrointestinal regulation of food intake. *The Journal of Clinical Investigation, 117*, 13–23.

Das, U. N. (2011). Vagus nerve stimulation as a strategy to prevent and manage metabolic syndrome. *Medical Hypotheses, 76*, 429–433.

Date, Y., Toshinai, K., Koda, S., Miyazato, M., Shimbara, T., Tsuruta, T., et al. (2005). Peripheral interaction of ghrelin with cholecystokinin on feeding regulation. *Endocrinology, 146*, 3518–3525.

Dauge, V., & Lena, I. (1998). CCK in anxiety and cognitive processes. *Neuroscience and Biobehavioral Reviews, 22*, 815–825.

de Lartigue, G., Barbier de la Serre, C., Espero, E., Lee, J., & Raybould, H. E. (2011). Diet-induced obesity leads to the development of leptin resistance in vagal afferent neurons. *American Journal of Physiology, Endocrinology and Metabolism, 301*(1), 187–195.

de Lartigue, G., Barbier de la Serre, C., Espero, E., Lee, J., & Raybould, H. E. (2012). Leptin resistance in vagal afferent neurons inhibits cholecystokinin signaling and satiation in diet induced obese rats. *PLoS One*, 7, e32967.

Deschenes, R. J., Lorenz, L. J., Haun, R. S., Roos, B. A., Collier, K. J., & Dixon, J. E. (1984). Cloning and sequence analysis of a cDNA encoding rat preprocholecystokinin. *Proceedings of the National Academy of Sciences of the United States of America, 81*, 726–730.

Devane, W. A., Hanus, L., Breuer, A., Pertwee, R. G., Stevenson, L. A., Griffin, G., et al. (1992). Isolation and structure of a brain constituent that binds to the cannabinoid receptor. *Science, 258*, 1946–1949.

Di Marzo, V., Bifulco, M., & De Petrocellis, L. (2004). The endocannabinoid system and its therapeutic exploitation. *Nature Reviews. Drug Discovery, 3*, 771–784.

Di Marzo, V., Bisogno, T., & Petrocellis, L. (2005). The biosynthesis, fate and pharmacological properties of endocannabinoids. *Handbook of Experimental Pharmacology, 168*, 147–185.

Di Marzo, V., Goparaju, S. K., Wang, L., Liu, J., Batkal, S., Járai, Z., et al. (2001). Leptin-regulated endocannabinoids are involved in maintaining food intake. *Nature (London), 410*, 822–825.

Di Marzo, V., Ligresti, A., & Cristino, L. (2009). The endocannabinoid system as a link between homoeostatic and hedonic pathways involved in energy balance regulation. *International Journal of Obesity, 33*(Suppl. 2), S18–S24.

Dinh, T. P., Carpenter, D., Leslie, F. M., Freund, T. F., Katona, I., Sensi, S. L., et al. (2002). Brain monoglyceride lipase participating in endocannabinoid inactivation. *Proceedings of the National Academy of Sciences of the United States of America, 99*, 10819–10824.

DiPatrizio, N. V., Astarita, G., Schwartz, G., Li, X., & Piomelli, D. (2011). Endocannabinoid signal in the gut controls dietary fat intake. *Proceedings of the National Academy of Sciences of the United States of America, 108*, 12904–12908.

DiPatrizio, N. V., & Simansky, K. J. (2008a). Activating parabrachial cannabinoid CB1 receptors selectively stimulates feeding of palatable foods in rats. *Journal of Neuroscience, 28*, 9702–9709.

DiPatrizio, N. V., & Simansky, K. J. (2008b). Inhibiting parabrachial fatty acid amide hydrolase activity selectively increases the intake of palatable food via cannabinoid CB1 receptors. *American Journal of Physiology. Regulatory, Integrative and Comparative Physiology, 295*, R1409–R1414.

Dockray, G. J. (2009). Cholecystokinin and gut-brain signalling. *Regulatory Peptides, 155*, 6–10.

Dockray, G. J., & Burdyga, G. (2011). Plasticity in vagal afferent neurones during feeding and fasting: Mechanisms and significance. *Acta Physiologica, 201*, 313–321.

Dourish, C. T., Ruckert, A. C., Tattersall, F. D., & Iversen, S. D. (1989). Evidence that decreased feeding induced by systemic injection of cholecystokinin is mediated by CCK-A receptors. *European Journal of Pharmacology, 173*, 233–234.

Dufresne, M., Seva, C., & Fourmy, D. (2006). Cholecystokinin and gastrin receptors. *Physiological Reviews, 86*, 805–847.

Eberlein, G. A., Eysselein, V. E., Davis, M. T., Lee, T. D., Shively, J. E., Grandt, D., et al. (1992). Patterns of prohormone processing. Order revealed by a new procholecystokinin-derived peptide. *Journal of Biological Chemistry, 267*, 1517–1521.

Elliott, R. L., Cameron, K. O., Chin, J. E., Bartlett, J. A., Beretta, E. E., Chen, Y., et al. (2010). Discovery of N-benzyl-2-[(4S)-4-(1H-indol-3-ylmethyl)-5-oxo-1-phenyl-4,5-dihydro-6H-[1,2,4]triazolo[4,3-a][1,5]benzodiazepin-6-yl]-N-isopropylacetamide, an orally active, gut-selective CCK1 receptor agonist for the potential treatment of obesity. *Bioorganic & Medicinal Chemistry Letters, 20*, 6797–6801.

Emson, P. C., Lee, C. M., & Rehfeld, J. F. (1980). Cholecystokinin octapeptide: Vesicular localization and calcium dependent release from rat brain in vitro. *Life Sciences, 26*, 2157–2163.

Eng, J., Du, B., Pan, Y. E., Chang, M., Hulmes, J. D., & Yalow, R. S. (1984). Purification and sequencing of a rat intestinal 22 amino acid C-terminal CCK fragment. *Peptides, 5*, 1203–1206.

Eser, D., Schule, C., Baghai, T., Floesser, A., Krebs-Brown, A., Enunwa, M., et al. (2007). Evaluation of the CCK-4 model as a challenge paradigm in a population of healthy volunteers within a proof-of-concept study. *Psychopharmacology, 192*, 479–487.

Filmore, D. (2004). It's a GPCR world. *Modern Drug Discovery*, 7, 24–28.

Finger, B. C., Dinan, T. G., & Cryan, J. F. (2010). Progressive ratio responding in an obese mouse model: Effects of fenfluramine. *Neuropharmacology, 59*, 619–626.

Freedland, C. S., Poston, J. S., & Porrino, L. J. (2000). Effects of SR141716A, a central cannabinoid receptor antagonist, on food-maintained responding. *Pharmacology, Biochemistry, and Behavior, 67*, 265–270.

Fu, J., Gaetani, S., Oveisi, F., Lo Verme, J., Serrano, A., Rodriguez De Fonseca, F., et al. (2003). Oleylethanolamide regulates feeding and body weight through activation of the nuclear receptor PPAR-alpha. *Nature, 425*, 90–93.

Gaetani, S., Kaye, W., Cuomo, V., & Piomelli, D. (2008). Role of endocannabinoids and their analogues in obesity and eating disorders. *Eating and Weight Disorders, 13*, e42.

Galiègue, S., Mary, S., Marchand, J., Dussossoy, D., Carrière, D., Carayon, P., et al. (1995). Expression of central and peripheral cannabinoid receptors in human immune tissues and leukocyte subpopulations. *European Journal of Biochemistry, 232*, 54–61.

Gaoni, Y., & Mechoulam, R. (1964). Isolation, structure, and partial synthesis of an active constituent of hashish. *Journal of the American Chemical Society*, *86*, 1646–1647.
Gerard, C., Mollereau, C., Vassart, G., & Parmentier, M. (1990). Nucleotide sequence of a human cannabinoid receptor cDNA. *Nucleic Acids Research*, *18*, 7142.
Gibbs, J., Young, R. C., & Smith, G. P. (1973). Cholecystokinin decreases food intake in rats. *Journal of Comparative and Physiological Psychology*, *84*, 488–495.
Gomez, R., Navarro, M., Ferrer, B., Trigo, J. M., Bilbao, A., Del Arco, I., et al. (2002). A peripheral mechanism for CB1 cannabinoid receptor-dependent modulation of feeding. *Journal of Neuroscience*, *22*, 9612–9617.
Grill, H. J., & Norgren, R. (1978). The taste reactivity test. I. Mimetic responses to gustatory stimuli in neurologically normal rats. *Brain Research*, *143*, 263–279.
Gubler, U., Chua, A. O., Hoffman, B. J., Collier, K. J., & Eng, J. (1984). Cloned cDNA to cholecystokinin mRNA predicts an identical preprocholecystokinin in pig brain and gut. *Proceedings of the National Academy of Sciences of the United States of America*, *81*, 4307–4310.
Hansen, H. S., Rosenkilde, M. M., Holst, J. J., & Schwartz, T. W. (2012). GPR119 as a fat sensor. *Trends in Pharmacological Sciences*, *33*(7), 374–381.
Hanuš, L., Abu-Lafi, S., Fride, E., Breuer, A., Vogel, Z., Shalev, D. E., et al. (2001). 2-Arachidonyl glyceryl ether, an endogenous agonist of the cannabinoid CB1 receptor. *Proceedings of the National Academy of Sciences of the United States of America*, *98*, 3662.
Herkenham, M., Lynn, A. B., Little, M. D., Johnson, M. R., Melvin, L. S., De Costa, B. R., et al. (1990). Cannabinoid receptor localization in brain. *Proceedings of the National Academy of Sciences of the United States of America*, *87*, 1932.
Hewson, G., Leighton, G. E., Hill, R. G., & Hughes, J. (1988). The cholecystokinin receptor antagonist L364,718 increases food intake in the rat by attenuation of the action of endogenous cholecystokinin. *British Journal of Pharmacology*, *93*, 79–84.
Higgs, S., Barber, D. J., Cooper, A. J., & Terry, P. (2005). Differential effects of two cannabinoid receptor agonists on progressive ratio responding for food and free-feeding in rats. *Behavioural Pharmacology*, *16*, 389–393.
Hill, D. R., Campbell, N. J., Shaw, T. M., & Woodruff, G. N. (1987). Autoradiographic localization and biochemical characterization of peripheral type CCK receptors in rat CNS using highly selective nonpeptide CCK antagonists. *Journal of Neuroscience*, *7*, 2967–2976.
Hohmann, A. G., & Herkenham, M. (1999). Localization of central cannabinoid CB1 receptor messenger RNA in neuronal subpopulations of rat dorsal root ganglia: A double-label in situ hybridization study. *Neuroscience*, *90*, 923–931.
Hornby, P. J., & Prouty, S. M. (2004). Involvement of cannabinoid receptors in gut motility and visceral perception. *British Journal of Pharmacology*, *141*, 1335–1345.
Howlett, A. C., Barth, F., Bonner, T. I., Cabral, G., Casellas, P., Devane, W. A., et al. (2002). International Union of Pharmacology. XXVII. Classification of cannabinoid receptors. *Pharmacological Reviews*, *54*, 161–202.
Huang, S. M., Bisogno, T., Trevisani, M., Al-Hayani, A., De Petrocellis, L., Fezza, F., et al. (2002). An endogenous capsaicin-like substance with high potency at recombinant and native vanilloid VR1 receptors. *Proceedings of the National Academy of Sciences of the United States of America*, *99*, 8400.
Innis, R. B., & Snyder, S. H. (1980). Distinct cholecystokinin receptors in brain and pancreas. *Proceedings of the National Academy of Sciences of the United States of America*, 77, 6917–6921.
Inui, A., Inoue, T., Sakatani, N., Oya, M., Morioka, H., & Baba, S. (1987). Proglumide has access to brain and antagonizes the central satiety effect of cholecystokinin octapeptide in the dog. *Brain Research*, *417*, 355–359.
Jamshidi, N., & Taylor, D. A. (2001). Anandamide administration into the ventromedial hypothalamus stimulates appetite in rats. *British Journal of Pharmacology*, *134*, 1151–1154.

Jensen, R. T., Lemp, G. F., & Gardner, J. D. (1980). Interaction of cholecystokinin with specific membrane receptors on pancreatic acinar cells. *Proceedings of the National Academy of Sciences of the United States of America*, 77, 2079–2083.

Jordan, J., Greenway, F. L., Leiter, L. A., Li, Z., Jacobson, P., Murphy, K., et al. (2008). Stimulation of cholecystokinin-A receptors with GI181771X does not cause weight loss in overweight or obese patients. *Clinical Pharmacology and Therapeutics*, *83*, 281–287.

Joyner, K., Smith, G. P., & Gibbs, J. (1993). Abdominal vagotomy decreases the satiating potency of CCK-8 in sham and real feeding. *American Journal of Physiology. Regulatory, Integrative and Comparative Physiology*, *264*, R912–R916.

Kamilaris, T. C., Johnson, E. O., Calogero, A. E., Kalogeras, K. T., Bernardini, R., Chrousos, G. P., et al. (1992). Cholecystokinin-octapeptide stimulates hypothalamic-pituitary-adrenal function in rats: Role of corticotropin-releasing hormone. *Endocrinology*, *130*, 1764–1774.

Kirkham, T. C., Williams, C. M., Fezza, F., & Di Marzo, V. (2002). Endocannabinoid levels in rat limbic forebrain and hypothalamus in relation to fasting, feeding and satiation: Stimulation of eating by 2-arachidonoyl glycerol. *British Journal of Pharmacology*, *136*, 550–557.

Kissileff, H. R., Pi-Sunyer, F. X., Thornton, J., & Smith, G. P. (1981). C-terminal octapeptide of cholecystokinin decreases food intake in man. *American Journal of Clinical Nutrition*, *34*, 154–160.

Koch, J. E., & Matthews, S. M. (2001). Delta9-tetrahydrocannabinol stimulates palatable food intake in Lewis rats: Effects of peripheral and central administration. *Nutritional Neuroscience*, *4*, 179–187.

Kola, B., Farkas, I., Christ-Crain, M., Wittmann, G., Lolli, F., Amin, F., et al. (2008). The orexigenic effect of ghrelin is mediated through central activation of the endogenous cannabinoid system. *PLoS One*, *3*, e1797.

Konturek, P. C., & Konturek, S. J. (2003). The history of gastrointestinal hormones and the Polish contribution to elucidation of their biology and relation to nervous system. *Journal of Physiology and Pharmacology*, *54*(Suppl. 3), 83–98.

Kopin, A. S., Mathes, W. F., McBride, E. W., Nguyen, M., Al-Haider, W., Schmitz, F., et al. (1999). The cholecystokinin-A receptor mediates inhibition of food intake yet is not essential for the maintenance of body weight. *The Journal of Clinical Investigation*, *103*, 383–391.

Koszycki, D., Prichard, Z., Fiocco, A. J., Shlik, J., Kennedy, J. L., & Bradwejn, J. (2012). CCK-B receptor gene and response to cholecystokinin-tetrapeptide in healthy volunteers. *Peptides*, *35*, 9–13.

Kozak, K., & Marnett, L. (2002). Oxidative metabolism of endocannabinoids. *Prostaglandins, Leukotrienes, and Essential Fatty Acids*, *66*, 211–220.

Kunos, G., & Tam, J. (2011). The case for peripheral CB receptor blockade in the treatment of visceral obesity and its cardiometabolic complications. *British Journal of Pharmacology*, *163*, 1423–1431.

Larsson, L., & Rehfeld, J. F. (1979). Localization and molecular heterogeneity of cholecystokinin in the central and peripheral nervous system. *Brain Research*, *165*, 201–218.

Lassman, D. J., McKie, S., Gregory, L. J., Lal, S., D'Amato, M., Steele, I., et al. (2010). Defining the role of cholecystokinin in the lipid-induced human brain activation matrix. *Gastroenterology*, *138*, 1514–1524.

Lauffer, L. M., Iakoubov, R., & Brubaker, P. L. (2009). GPR119 is essential for oleoylethanolamide-induced glucagon-like peptide-1 secretion from the intestinal enteroendocrine L-cell. *Diabetes*, *58*, 1058–1066.

Lavine, J. A., Raess, P. W., Stapleton, D. S., Rabaglia, M. E., Suhonen, J. I., Schueler, K. L., et al. (2010). Cholecystokinin is up-regulated in obese mouse islets and expands beta-cell mass by increasing beta-cell survival. *Endocrinology*, *151*, 3577–3588.

Li, C., Jones, P. M., & Persaud, S. J. (2011). Role of the endocannabinoid system in food intake, energy homeostasis and regulation of the endocrine pancreas. *Pharmacology and Therapeutics*, *129*, 307–320.

Liddle, R. A., Goldfine, I. D., Rosen, M. S., Taplitz, R. A., & Williams, J. A. (1985). Cholecystokinin bioactivity in human plasma. Molecular forms, responses to feeding, and relationship to gallbladder contraction. *The Journal of Clinical Investigation*, *75*, 1144–1152.

Lin, S., Khanolkar, A. D., Fan, P., Goutopoulos, A., Qin, C., Papahadjis, D., et al. (1998). Novel analogues of arachidonylethanolamide (anandamide): Affinities for the CB1 and CB2 cannabinoid receptors and metabolic stability. *Journal of Medicinal Chemistry*, *41*, 5353–5361.

Linden, A., Uvnas-Moberg, K., Forsberg, G., Bednar, I., & Sodersten, P. (1989). Plasma concentrations of cholecystokinin octapeptide and food intake in male rats treated with cholecystokinin octapeptide. *Journal of Endocrinology*, *121*, 59–65.

Mackie, K. (2005). Distribution of cannabinoid receptors in the central and peripheral nervous system. *Handbook of Experimental Pharmacology*, *168*, 299–325.

Maclagan, N. F. (1937). The role of appetite in the control of body weight. *The Journal of Physiology (Oxford, UK)*, *90*, 385–394.

Mahler, S. V., Smith, K. S., & Berridge, K. C. (2007). Endocannabinoid hedonic hotspot for sensory pleasure: Anandamide in nucleus accumbens shell enhances 'liking' of a sweet reward. *Neuropsychopharmacology*, *32*, 2267–2278.

Maldonado, R., Valverde, O., & Berrendero, F. (2006). Involvement of the endocannabinoid system in drug addiction. *Trends in Neurosciences*, *29*, 225–232.

Marinelli, S., Di Marzo, V., Florenzano, F., Fezza, F., Viscomi, M. T., van der Stelt, M., et al. (2007). N-Arachidonoyl-dopamine tunes synaptic transmission onto dopaminergic neurons by activating both cannabinoid and vanilloid receptors. *Neuropsychopharmacology*, *32*, 298–308.

Marsicano, G., & Lutz, B. (1999). Expression of the cannabinoid receptor CB1 in distinct neuronal subpopulations in the adult mouse forebrain. *European Journal of Neuroscience*, *11*, 4213–4225.

Mathes, C. M., Ferrara, M., & Rowland, N. E. (2008). Cannabinoid-1 receptor antagonists reduce caloric intake by decreasing palatable diet selection in a novel dessert protocol in female rats. *American Journal of Physiology. Regulatory, Integrative and Comparative Physiology*, *295*, R67–R75.

Matias, I., Bisogno, T., & Di Marzo, V. (2006). Endogenous cannabinoids in the brain and peripheral tissues: Regulation of their levels and control of food intake. *International Journal of Obesity*, *30*, S7–S12.

Matias, I., Petrosino, S., Racioppi, A., Capasso, R., Izzo, A. A., & Di Marzo, V. (2008). Dysregulation of peripheral endocannabinoid levels in hyperglycemia and obesity: Effect of high fat diets. *Molecular and Cellular Endocrinology*, *286*, S66–S78.

McHugh, D., Page, J., Dunn, E., & Bradshaw, H. B. (2012). Delta(9)-tetrahydrocannabinol and N-arachidonyl glycine are full agonists at GPR18 receptors and induce migration in human endometrial HEC-1B cells. *British Journal of Pharmacology*, *165*, 2414–2424.

Mechoulam, R., Ben-Shabat, S., Hanus, L., Ligumsky, M., Kaminski, N. E., Schatz, A. R., et al. (1995). Identification of an endogenous 2-monoglyceride, present in canine gut, that binds to cannabinoid receptors. *Biochemical Pharmacology*, *50*, 83–90.

Melis, M., Pistis, M., Perra, S., Muntoni, A. L., Pillolla, G., & Gessa, G. L. (2004). Endocannabinoids mediate presynaptic inhibition of glutamatergic transmission in rat ventral tegmental area dopamine neurons through activation of CB1 receptors. *Journal of Neuroscience*, *24*, 53–62.

Melis, T., Succu, S., Sanna, F., Boi, A., Argiolas, A., & Melis, M. R. (2007). The cannabinoid antagonist SR 141716A (Rimonabant) reduces the increase of extra-cellular dopamine release in the rat nucleus accumbens induced by a novel high palatable food. *Neuroscience Letters*, *419*, 231–235.

Merchenthaler, I. (1991). Neurons with access to the general circulation in the central nervous system of the rat: A retrograde tracing study with fluoro-gold. *Neuroscience*, *44*, 655–662.

Miller, L. J., Jardine, I., Weissman, E., Go, V. L., & Speicher, D. (1984). Characterization of cholecystokinin from the human brain. *Journal of Neurochemistry*, *43*, 835–840.

Moldrich, G., & Wenger, T. (2000). Localization of the CB1 cannabinoid receptor in the rat brain. An immunohistochemical study. *Peptides*, *21*, 1735–1742.

Monteleone, P., Matias, I., Martiadis, V., De Petrocellis, L., Maj, M., & Di Marzo, V. (2005). Blood levels of the endocannabinoid anandamide are increased in anorexia nervosa and in binge-eating disorder, but not in bulimia nervosa. *Neuropsychopharmacology*, *30*, 1216–1221.

Moran, T. H., Katz, L. F., Plata-Salaman, C. R., & Schwartz, G. J. (1998). Disordered food intake and obesity in rats lacking cholecystokinin A receptors. *American Journal of Physiology*, *274*, R618–R625.

Moran, T. H., Norgren, R., Crosby, R. J., & McHugh, P. R. (1990). Central and peripheral vagal transport of cholecystokinin binding sites occurs in afferent fibers. *Brain Research*, *526*, 95–102.

Moran, T. H., Smith, G. P., Hostetler, A. M., & McHugh, P. R. (1987). Transport of cholecystokinin (CCK) binding sites in subdiaphragmatic vagal branches. *Brain Research*, *415*, 149–152.

Moreno-Navarrete, J. M., Catalan, V., Whyte, L., Diaz-Arteaga, A., Vazquez-Martinez, R., Rotellar, F., et al. (2012). The L-alpha-lysophosphatidylinositol/GPR55 system and its potential role in human obesity. *Diabetes*, *61*, 281–291.

Morton, G. J., Cummings, D. E., Baskin, D. G., Barsh, G. S., & Schwartz, M. W. (2006). Central nervous system control of food intake and body weight. *Nature*, *443*, 289–295.

Munro, S., Thomas, K. L., & Abu-Shaar, M. (1993). Molecular characterization of a peripheral receptor for cannabinoids. *Nature*, *365*, 61–65.

Mutt, V., & Jorpes, J. E. (1968). Structure of porcine cholecystokinin-pancreozymin. 1. Cleavage with thrombin and with trypsin. *European Journal of Biochemistry*, *6*, 156–162.

Nagy, I., White, J. P. M., Paule, C. C., & Köfalvi, A. (2008). An historical introduction to the endocannabinoid and endovanilloid systems. In A. Köfalvi (Ed.), *Cannabinoids and the brain* (pp. 3–13). New York: Springer Science.

Noble, F., Wank, S. A., Crawley, J. N., Bradwejn, J., Seroogy, K. B., Hamon, M., et al. (1999). International Union of Pharmacology. XXI. Structure, distribution, and functions of cholecystokinin receptors. *Pharmacological Reviews*, *51*, 745–781.

Nogueiras, R., Diaz-Arteaga, A., Lockie, S. H., Velasquez, D. A., Tschop, J., Lopez, M., et al. (2009). The endocannabinoid system: Role in glucose and energy metabolism. *Pharmacological Research*, *60*, 93–98.

O'Sullivan, S. E. (2007). Cannabinoids go nuclear: Evidence for activation of peroxisome proliferator-activated receptors. *British Journal of Pharmacology*, *152*, 576–582.

Oh, D. Y., Yoon, J. M., Moon, M. J., Hwang, J. I., Choe, H., Lee, J. Y., et al. (2008). Identification of farnesyl pyrophosphate and N-arachidonylglycine as endogenous ligands for GPR92. *Journal of Biological Chemistry*, *283*, 21054–21064.

Oka, S., Nakajima, K., Yamashita, A., Kishimoto, S., & Sugiura, T. (2007). Identification of GPR55 as a lysophosphatidylinositol receptor. *Biochemical and Biophysical Research Communications*, *362*, 928–934.

Onaivi, E. S., Ishiguro, H., Gong, J. P., Patel, S., Perchuk, A., Meozzi, P. A., et al. (2006). Discovery of the presence and functional expression of cannabinoid CB2 receptors in brain. *Annals of the New York Academy of Sciences*, *1074*, 514–536.

Orio, L., Crespo, I., Lopez-Moreno, J. A., Reyes-Cabello, C., Rodriguez de Fonseca, F., & Gomez de Heras, R. (2011). Additive effects of cannabinoid CB1 receptors blockade and cholecystokinin on feeding inhibition. *Pharmacology, Biochemistry, and Behavior, 98*, 220–226.

Overton, H. A., Babbs, A. J., Doel, S. M., Fyfe, M. C., Gardner, L. S., Griffin, G., et al. (2006). Deorphanization of a G protein-coupled receptor for oleoylethanolamide and its use in the discovery of small-molecule hypophagic agents. *Cell Metabolism, 3*, 167–175.

Owyang, C., & Heldsinger, A. (2011). Vagal control of satiety and hormonal regulation of appetite. *Journal of Neurogastroenterology and Motility, 17*, 338–348.

Pagotto, U., & Pasquali, R. (2006). Endocannabinoids and energy metabolism. *Journal of Endocrinological Investigation, 29*, 66–76.

Pamplona, F. A., & Takahashi, R. N. (2012). Psychopharmacology of the endocannabinoids: Far beyond anandamide. *Journal of Psychopharmacology, 26*, 7–22.

Pettit, D., Anders, D. L., Harrison, M. P., & Cabral, G. A. (1996). Cannabinoid receptor expression in immune cells. *Advances in Experimental Medicine and Biology, 402*, 119–129.

Piomelli, D. (2003). The molecular logic of endocannabinoid signalling. *Nature Reviews. Neuroscience, 4*, 873–884.

Piomelli, D., Beltramo, M., Glasnapp, S., Lin, S. Y., Goutopoulos, A., Xie, X. Q., et al. (1999). Structural determinants for recognition and translocation by the anandamide transporter. *Proceedings of the National Academy of Sciences of the United States of America, 96*, 5802–5807.

Rasoamanana, R., Darcel, N., Fromentin, G., & Tome, D. (2012). Nutrient sensing and signalling by the gut. *The Proceedings of the Nutrition Society, 27*, 1–10. http://dx.doi.org/10.1017/S0029665112000110.

Ravinet Trillou, C., Delgorge, C., Menet, C., Arnone, M., & Soubrie, P. (2004). CB1 cannabinoid receptor knockout in mice leads to leanness, resistance to diet-induced obesity and enhanced leptin sensitivity. *International Journal of Obesity and Related Metabolic Disorders: Journal of the International Association for the Study of Obesity, 28*, 640–648.

Raybould, H. E., & Tache, Y. (1988). Cholecystokinin inhibits gastric motility and emptying via a capsaicin-sensitive vagal pathway in rats. *American Journal of Physiology, 255*, G242–G246.

Reeve, J. R., Jr., Eysselein, V., Walsh, J. H., Ben-Avram, C. M., & Shively, J. E. (1986). New molecular forms of cholecystokinin. Microsequence analysis of forms previously characterized by chromatographic methods. *Journal of Biological Chemistry, 261*, 16392–16397.

Rehfeld, J. F. (1978). Immunochemical studies on cholecystokinin. II. Distribution and molecular heterogeneity in the central nervous system and small intestine of man and hog. *Journal of Biological Chemistry, 253*, 4022–4030.

Rehfeld, J. F. (1998). Accurate measurement of cholecystokinin in plasma. *Clinical Chemistry, 44*, 991–1001 (Whashington, DC, USA).

Rehfeld, J. F. (2004). Clinical endocrinology and metabolism. Cholecystokinin. *Best Practice & Research. Clinical Endocrinology & Metabolism, 18*, 569–586.

Rehfeld, J. F., & Hansen, H. F. (1986). Characterization of preprocholecystokinin products in the porcine cerebral cortex. Evidence of different processing pathways. *Journal of Biological Chemistry, 261*, 5832–5840.

Rehfeld, J. F., Sun, G., Christensen, T., & Hillingso, J. G. (2001). The predominant cholecystokinin in human plasma and intestine is cholecystokinin-33. *Journal of Clinical Endocrinology and Metabolism, 86*, 251–258.

Reidelberger, R. D., Castellanos, D. A., & Hulce, M. (2003). Effects of peripheral CCK receptor blockade on food intake in rats. *American Journal of Physiology. Regulatory, Integrative and Comparative Physiology, 285*, R429–R437.

Reidelberger, R. D., Hernandez, J., Fritzsch, B., & Hulce, M. (2004). Abdominal vagal mediation of the satiety effects of CCK in rats. *American Journal of Physiology. Regulatory, Integrative and Comparative Physiology, 286*, R1005–R1012.

Reubi, J., Waser, B., Laderach, U., Stettler, C., Friess, H., Halter, F., et al. (1997). Localization of cholecystokinin A and cholecystokinin B-gastrin receptors in the human stomach. *Gastroenterology, 112*, 1197–1205.

Richardson, N. R., & Roberts, D. C. (1996). Progressive ratio schedules in drug self-administration studies in rats: A method to evaluate reinforcing efficacy. *Journal of Neuroscience Methods, 66*, 1–11.

Ritter, R. C., & Ladenheim, E. E. (1985). Capsaicin pretreatment attenuates suppression of food intake by cholecystokinin. *American Journal of Physiology, 248*, R501–R504.

Rodriguez de Fonseca, F., Navarro, M., Gomez, R., Escuredo, L., Nava, F., Fu, J., et al. (2001). An anorexic lipid mediator regulated by feeding. *Nature, 414*, 209–212.

Ryberg, E., Larsson, N., Sjogren, S., Hjorth, S., Hermansson, N. O., Leonova, J., et al. (2007). The orphan receptor GPR55 is a novel cannabinoid receptor. *British Journal of Pharmacology, 152*, 1092–1101.

Sahu, A. (2004). Minireview: A hypothalamic role in energy balance with special emphasis on leptin. *Endocrinology, 145*, 2613–2620.

Sanchis-Segura, C., Cline, B. H., Marsicano, G., Lutz, B., & Spanagel, R. (2004). Reduced sensitivity to reward in CB1 knockout mice. *Psychopharmacology, 176*, 223–232.

Sankaran, H., Goldfine, I. D., Deveney, C. W., Wong, K. Y., & Williams, J. A. (1980). Binding of cholecystokinin to high affinity receptors on isolated rat pancreatic acini. *Journal of Biological Chemistry, 255*, 1849–1853.

Schick, R. R., Reilly, W. M., Roddy, D. R., Yaksh, T. L., & Go, V. L. (1987). Neuronal cholecystokinin-like immunoreactivity is postprandially released from primate hypothalamus. *Brain Research, 418*, 20–26.

Schmitz, F., Göke, M. N., Otte, J., Schrader, H., Reimann, B., Kruse, M., et al. (2001). Cellular expression of CCK-A and CCK-B/gastrin receptors in human gastric mucosa. *Regulatory Peptides, 102*, 101–110.

Schwartz, G. J. (2000). The role of gastrointestinal vagal afferents in the control of food intake: Current prospects. *Nutrition, 16*, 866–873.

Schwartz, G. J. (2011). Gut fat sensing in the negative feedback control of energy balance–recent advances. *Physiology and Behavior, 104*, 621–623.

Schwartz, G. J., Fu, J., Astarita, G., Li, X., Gaetani, S., Campolongo, P., et al. (2008). The lipid messenger OEA links dietary fat intake to satiety. *Cell Metabolism, 8*, 281–288.

Serrano, A., Pavon, F. J., Tovar, S., Casanueva, F., Senaris, R., Dieguez, C., et al. (2011). Oleoylethanolamide: Effects on hypothalamic transmitters and gut peptides regulating food intake. *Neuropharmacology, 60*, 593–601.

Sharir, H., & Abood, M. E. (2010). Pharmacological characterization of GPR55, a putative cannabinoid receptor. *Pharmacology and Therapeutics, 126*, 301–313.

Sigiura, T., & Waku, K. (2000). 2-Arachidonoylglycerol and the cannabinoid receptors. *Chemistry and Physics of Lipids, 108*(1–2), 89–106.

Sim, L. J., Selley, D. E., & Childers, S. R. (1995). In vitro autoradiography of receptor-activated G proteins in rat brain by agonist-stimulated guanylyl 5′-[gamma-[35S] thio]-triphosphate binding. *Proceedings of the National Academy of Sciences of the United States of America, 92*, 7242–7246.

Smith, G. P., Jerome, C., Cushin, B. J., Eterno, R., & Simansky, K. J. (1981). Abdominal vagotomy blocks the satiety effect of cholecystokinin in the rat. *Science, 213*, 1036–1037.

Soga, T., Ohishi, T., Matsui, T., Saito, T., Matsumoto, M., Takasaki, J., et al. (2005). Lysophosphatidylcholine enhances glucose-dependent insulin secretion via an orphan G-protein-coupled receptor. *Biochemical and Biophysical Research Communications, 326*, 744–751.

Solinas, M., & Goldberg, S. R. (2005). Motivational effects of cannabinoids and opioids on food reinforcement depend on simultaneous activation of cannabinoid and opioid systems. *Neuropsychopharmacology, 30*, 2035–2045.

Storr, M. A., & Sharkey, K. A. (2007). The endocannabinoid system and gut-brain signalling. *Current Opinion in Pharmacology*, *7*, 575–582.

Sun, Y. X., Tsuboi, K., Okamoto, Y., Tonai, T., Murakami, M., Kudo, I., et al. (2004). Biosynthesis of anandamide and N-palmitoylethanolamine by sequential actions of phospholipase A2 and lysophospholipase D. *The Biochemical Journal*, *380*, 749.

Suzuki, K., Jayasena, C. N., & Bloom, S. R. (2011). The gut hormones in appetite regulation. *Journal of Obesity*, *2011*, 528401. http://dx.doi.org/10.1155/2011/528401.

Suzuki, K., Simpson, K. A., Minnion, J. S., Shillito, J. C., & Bloom, S. R. (2010). The role of gut hormones and the hypothalamus in appetite regulation. *Endocrine Journal*, *57*, 359–372.

Tart, C. T. (1970). Marijuana intoxication common experiences. *Nature*, *226*, 701–704.

Tokunaga, Y., Cox, K. L., Coleman, R., Conception, W., Nakazato, P., & Esquivel, C. O. (1993). Characterization of cholecystokinin receptors on the human gallbladder. *Surgery*, *113*, 155–162.

Trojniar, W., & Wise, R. A. (1991). Facilitory effect of delta 9-tetrahydrocannabinol on hypothalamically induced feeding. *Psychopharmacology*, *103*, 172–176.

Tucci, S. A., Rogers, E. K., Korbonits, M., & Kirkham, T. C. (2004). The cannabinoid CB1 receptor antagonist SR141716 blocks the orexigenic effects of intrahypothalamic ghrelin. *British Journal of Pharmacology*, *143*, 520–523.

Van Der Stelt, M., Van Kuik, J. A., Bari, M., Van Zadelhoff, G., Leeflang, B. R., Veldink, G. A., et al. (2002). Oxygenated metabolites of anandamide and 2-arachidonoylglycerol: Conformational analysis and interaction with cannabinoid receptors, membrane transporter, and fatty acid amide hydrolase. *Journal of Medicinal Chemistry*, *45*, 3709–3720.

van Megen, H. J., Westenberg, H. G., den Boer, J. A., & Kahn, R. S. (1996). Cholecystokinin in anxiety. *European Neuropsychopharmacology: The Journal of the European College of Neuropsychopharmacology*, *6*, 263–280.

Wakley, A. A., & Rasmussen, E. B. (2009). Effects of cannabinoid drugs on the reinforcing properties of food in gestationally undernourished rats. *Pharmacology, Biochemistry, and Behavior*, *94*, 30–36.

Wang, H., Wong, P. T., Spiess, J., & Zhu, Y. Z. (2005). Cholecystokinin-2 (CCK2) receptor-mediated anxiety-like behaviors in rats. *Neuroscience and Biobehavioral Reviews*, *29*, 1361–1373.

Wank, S. A. (1995). Cholecystokinin receptors. *American Journal of Physiology*, *269*, G628–G646.

Wank, S. A., Harkins, R., Jensen, R. T., Shapira, H., de Weerth, A., & Slattery, T. (1992). Purification, molecular cloning, and functional expression of the cholecystokinin receptor from rat pancreas. *Proceedings of the National Academy of Sciences of the United States of America*, *89*, 3125–3129.

Wank, S. A., Pisegna, J. R., & de Weerth, A. (1992). Brain and gastrointestinal cholecystokinin receptor family: Structure and functional expression. *Proceedings of the National Academy of Sciences of the United States of America*, *89*, 8691–8695.

Ward, S. J., & Dykstra, L. A. (2005). The role of CB1 receptors in sweet versus fat reinforcement: Effect of CB1 receptor deletion, CB1 receptor antagonism (SR141716A) and CB1 receptor agonism (CP-55940). *Behavioural Pharmacology*, *16*, 381–388.

Williams, C. M., & Kirkham, T. C. (1999). Anandamide induces overeating: Mediation by central cannabinoid (CB1) receptors. *Psychopharmacology*, *143*, 315–317.

Woods, S. C., & Cota, D. (2007). Endocannabinoids and energy homeostasis. In R. F. Kushner & D. H. Bessesen (Eds.), *Treatment of the obese patient* (pp. 49–67). New Jersey: Humana Press.

Yoshida, R., Ohkuri, T., Jyotaki, M., Yasuo, T., Horio, N., Yasumatsu, K., et al. (2010). Endocannabinoids selectively enhance sweet taste. *Proceedings of the National Academy of Sciences of the United States of America*, *107*, 935–939.

Zajac, J. M., Gully, D., & Maffrand, J. P. (1996). [3H]-SR 27897B: A selective probe for autoradiographic labelling of CCK-A receptors in the brain. *Journal of Receptor and Signal Transduction Research*, *16*, 93–113.

Zygmunt, P. M., Petersson, J., Andersson, D. A., Chuang, H., Sorgard, M., Di Marzo, V., et al. (1999). Vanilloid receptors on sensory nerves mediate the vasodilator action of anandamide. *Nature*, *400*, 452–457.

CHAPTER EIGHT

Treatment of Cachexia: Melanocortin and Ghrelin Interventions

Jeremy Steinman, Mark Daniel DeBoer[1]

Division of Pediatric Endocrinology, Department of Pediatrics, P.O. Box 800386, University of Virginia, Charlottesville, Virginia, USA

[1]Corresponding author: e-mail address: deboer@virginia.edu

Contents

1. Introduction 198
2. Molecular Mediators of Cachexia 199
3. Peripheral and Central Appetite Regulation 201
   3.1 Basic anatomy 201
   3.2 Factors affecting POMC, AgRP, and NPY expression 206
4. Cancer Cachexia 209
   4.1 Basic science 209
   4.2 Clinical applications 210
5. Cardiac Cachexia 215
   5.1 Basic science 215
   5.2 Clinical applications 216
6. Renal Cachexia 219
   6.1 Basic science 219
   6.2 Clinical applications 219
7. Other Cachexia 220
   7.1 Burn/thermal injury 220
   7.2 Colitis 223
   7.3 HIV/AIDS 223
   7.4 Aging 224
   7.5 Cancer treatment-induced cachexia 225
8. Summary of Treatment Effects 225
9. Future Directions 226

References 227

Abstract

Cachexia is a condition typified by wasting of fat and LBM caused by anorexia and further endocrinological modulation of energy stores. Diseases known to cause cachectic symptoms include cancer, chronic kidney disease, and chronic heart failure; these conditions are associated with increased levels of proinflammatory cytokines and increased resting

Vitamins and Hormones, Volume 92
ISSN 0083-6729
http://dx.doi.org/10.1016/B978-0-12-410473-0.00008-8

energy expenditure. Early studies have suggested the central melanocortin system as one of the main mediators of the symptoms of cachexia. Pharmacological and genetic antagonism of these pathways attenuates cachectic symptoms in laboratory models; effects have yet to be studied in humans. In addition, ghrelin, an endogenous orexigenic hormone with receptors on melanocortinergic neurons, has been shown to ameliorate symptoms of cachexia, at least in part, by an increase in appetite via melanocortin modulation, in addition to its anticatabolic and anti-inflammatory effects. These effects of ghrelin have been confirmed in multiple types of cachexia in both laboratory and human studies, suggesting a positive future for cachexia treatments.

1. INTRODUCTION

Cachexia is a condition of anorexia and wasting that accompanies diseases such as cancer, chronic heart failure (CHF), and chronic kidney disease (CKD). This syndrome of wasting has emerged as an important condition related to the care of patients with chronic diseases (Anker, 2006; Deans & Wigmore, 2005; DeBoer & Marks, 2006a; Mak, Cheung, Cone, & Marks, 2006b) and is an important predictor of mortality (Lainscak, Podbregar, & Anker, 2007; Larkin, 1998; Tisdale, 1997).

Epidemiologic data over the last 10 years have affirmed that the symptoms associated with cachexia—namely, loss of appetite, loss of LBM, increased metabolism, and decreased quality of life—take a devastating toll on patients who are already suffering from serious underlying disease (Bossola, Tazza, Giungi, & Luciani, 2006; Fearon, Voss, Hustead, & Cancer Cachexia Study, 2006; Shinaberger et al., 2006; Tsai, Wu, Chiu, Hu, & Chen, 2006). Thus far, no treatment has been shown to be globally effective in the treatment of cachexia (DeBoer & Marks, 2006b; Springer, Filippatos, Akashi, & Anker, 2006; Tisdale, 2006). Perhaps the reason behind this observation is that the complete mechanism underlying cachexia has not been fully elicited, making it difficult to produce treatments to reverse cachexia in diverse settings. However, studies conducted in the last decade have provided a great deal of insight into the involved pathways by elucidating key processes involved in the mechanism and filling in details with further research. As will be seen, one of the more clinically relevant trends seen in these studies is that many proinflammatory molecules known to be associated with the onset of cachexia simultaneously play a role in both appetite regulation and progression of the underlying chronic diseases.

Significantly, another development in the field of cachexia has been the use of treatments that manipulate appetite-regulating centers. Two potentially useful treatments act on the melanocortin system of the hypothalamus. Antagonists of the melanocortin 4 receptor (MC4R) result in a decrease in anorexigenic signals from this system, thereby increasing food intake and weight gain. The orexigenic hormone ghrelin also acts, at least in part, at this center, increasing appetite-stimulating output from these centers. In this review, we consider what is known about appetite regulation in the setting of cachexia and how these two treatments, MC4R antagonists and ghrelin, have performed in cachexia for both humans and animal models. In these considerations, we pay particular attention to clinical issues related to this important disease process that need to be addressed.

2. MOLECULAR MEDIATORS OF CACHEXIA

Decreased food consumption is a phenotype of cachexia-associated diseases. Anorexia contributes to a lower overall mass due to decreases in caloric intake. This process is mediated, at least in part, through increases in levels of proinflammatory cytokines interleukin-1β (IL-1β) and tumor necrosis factor-α (TNF-α)—each of which is elevated in various forms of cachexia (DeBoer & Marks, 2006b; Kim et al., 2012; Mak et al., 2006b; Ramos et al., 2004; Torre-Amione, Kapadia, Lee, et al., 1996); one effect of these molecules is a suppression of food intake (Plata-Salamán, Oomura, & Kai, 1988; Sonti, Ilyin, & Plata-Salaman, 1996)—other effects are discussed in the following sections of this review. However, the loss of body mass associated with cachexia is not solely mediated by the decreased food intake. This is to say that compared to animals with experimental cachexia, pair-fed animals consuming identical amounts of food exhibit greater weight gain (Arruda et al., 2010). The additional weight loss is due to further related processes mediated by cytokines and other pathways altering an individual's metabolic state (Arruda et al., 2010).

In cachexia, lipid, protein, and carbohydrate stores decrease further than expected from decreased food intake alone, likely due to endocrinological modulation of energy utilization. TNF-α produces increasing levels of lipolysis and decreasing levels of lipogenesis (Arruda et al., 2010; Langhans, 2002), which leads to an overall decrease in fat stores. TNF-α acts, at least in part, by inhibiting the effects of peroxisome proliferator-activated receptor-gamma (PPAR-γ; Sethi & Hotamisligil, 1999); because PPAR-γ increases adipogenesis and lipid uptake (Braissant, Foufelle, Scotto, Dauça, & Wahli, 1996), the decreasing activity of PPAR-γ decreases fat stores. TNF-α also decreases carbohydrate stores through inhibition of insulin receptor activity; a downstream decrease in glut-4 transporter expression leads to a decrease in glucose uptake (Sethi & Hotamisligil, 1999). TNF-α can also decrease LBM by acting on the muscle to increase breakdown and decrease rebuilding of myofibers. This action proceeds via NF-κB (Lee, Lin, Lee, Lee, & Yang, 2010), a molecule that prevents the differentiation of muscle cells (Choy & Panayi, 2001; Dalla Libera et al., 2001; Gielen et al., 2003; Langhans, 2002; Li & Reid, 2001; Ling, Schwartz, & Bistrian, 1997; Reid & Li, 2001; Sethi & Hotamisligil, 1999). Despite LBM having been shown to be directly correlated with resting energy expenditure (REE) in healthy individuals (Cunningham, 1991), the mechanism of action of TNF-α may explain how REE can be increased in the setting of cachexia.

In addition to the effects described here, TNF-α has additional upstream and downstream effects in multiple tissue types. TNF-α acts in the central nervous system (CNS; Plata-Salamán et al., 1988) as a downstream and upstream upregulator of cytokine release (Choy & Panayi, 2001). These proinflammatory cytokines, such as Interleukin-6 (IL-6; Carson & Baltgalvis, 2010; Michalaki, 2004; Strassmann, 1993; Strassmann, Fong, Kenney, & Jacob, 1992; Yamashita & Ogawa, 2000), Interleukin-10 (Bober et al., 2000; Chen et al., 2005; Peruhype-Magalhaes et al., 2006), Interferon-gamma (Cannon et al., 2007; Eylar et al., 2001; Frost, Nystrom, & Lang, 2009; Le Goffic et al., 2002; Madihally, Toner, Yarmush, & Mitchell, 2002; Peruhype-Magalhaes et al., 2006), and IL-1β (Choy & Panayi, 2001) work in the CNS as mediators of inflammation and work to release further inflammation-related factors (Choy & Panayi, 2001), and are also comediators in the same appetite and metabolic regulatory pathways as TNF-α. In some scenarios, the presence of these inflammatory mediators reduces the rate of survival to as low as 22% (Falconer et al., 1995), thus suggesting that cachexia onset, presence of cytokines, and incidence of mortality are closely correlated.

Also found in the CNS are catecholamines, which act as neurotransmitters in the sympathetic nervous system (Kobayashi, 2001). These act further to increase energy expenditure, further depleting energy stores. Catecholamines lead to an increase in lipolytic enzymes (Theander-Carrillo et al., 2006) and REE (Müller et al., 1992) and a decrease in lipogenic enzymes (Theander-Carrillo et al., 2006). Catecholamines have also been associated with an increased immune response (Ashitani, Matsumoto, & Nakazato, 2009; Nagaya et al., 2005, 2001a), suggesting that the sympathetic nervous system is a prominent downstream mediator of cachexia.

Lower levels of albumin and prealbumin correlate with lower levels of survival in multiple forms of cachexia (Arques & Ambrosi, 2011; Asher, Lee, & Bali, 2011; Qureshi et al., 2002; Sreedhara, Avram, Blanco, Batish, & Mittman, 1996; Wang et al., 2004); this trend is most likely caused by lower rate of albumin synthesis (Kaysen, Rathore, Shearer, & Depner, 1995). Lower albumin levels are associated with greater REE, VO_2, LBM loss, and lower kidney function (in CKD; Wang et al., 2004). Other predictors of mortality include decreasing handgrip strength and plasma insulin-like growth factor-1 (IGF-1; Qureshi et al., 2002), potentially caused by hypoalbuminemia.

IGF-1 may also have an important role in these disease processes. Levels of IGF-1 are decreased in the setting of cachexia (Trobec, von Haehling, Anker, & Lainscak, 2011). IGF-1 has an effect on the regulation of body metabolic status (e.g., carbohydrate, lipid, and protein synthesis) and is also involved in the mechanism of activation of cytokines (Trobec et al., 2011). Cytokines reduce the efficacy of both IGF-1 and growth hormone (GH) and thus decrease muscle production (Bennani-Baiti & Davis, 2008), leading to a decrease in LBM. Modulation of IGF-1, indirectly or directly, has potential therapeutic implications in alleviating symptoms of cachexia.

Significant research has been performed to identify molecules which act peripherally and centrally to lead to the phenotype of cachexia. Further investigation has explored the central mechanisms involved in converting an incoming message (e.g., TNF-α) to a somatic response (e.g., sympathetic nervous system activation) in an effort to target cachexia treatment. In this sense, treatments may be able to reverse the phenotype of cachexia by antagonizing upstream action of mediators such as proinflammatory cytokines or by reversing downstream effects at the level of the tissue. As we will see, much of the research in this area has targeted upstream effects in appetite regulation centers.

3. PERIPHERAL AND CENTRAL APPETITE REGULATION

3.1. Basic anatomy

One of the neural centers involved in the propagation of many of these symptoms of cachexia is the melanocortin system in the hypothalamus and brainstem. Since the initial description of the role of the central melanocortin system in cachexia (Marks, Ling, & Cone, 2001), significant progress has been made understanding the pathophysiology involved with over- and underactivation of the melanocortin system regarding appetite regulation, including the mechanisms through which symptoms of cachexia are propagated, diseases which respond to melanocortin antagonism, and novel methods designed to inhibit the neuronal center.

The central melanocortin system is located principally in the arcuate nucleus of the hypothalamus, in an area adjacent to the third ventricle (see Fig. 8.1; Cone, 2005). This area is proximal to the semipermeable blood–brain barrier, which gives it exposure to circulating indicators of disease activity, including inflammatory cytokines (Cheunsuang & Morris, 2005). In the arcuate nucleus are two oppositely appetite-regulating neurons which comprise the melanocortin system: those that produce pro-opiomelanocortin (POMC) and those that produce both Agouti-related peptide (AgRP) and neuropeptide Y (NPY; Cone, 2005; DeBoer & Marks, 2006a). Each set of neurons has its cell bodies in the arcuate nucleus and sends axon and dendrite projections to second-order neurons in widespread nuclei throughout the hypothalamus including the paraventricular

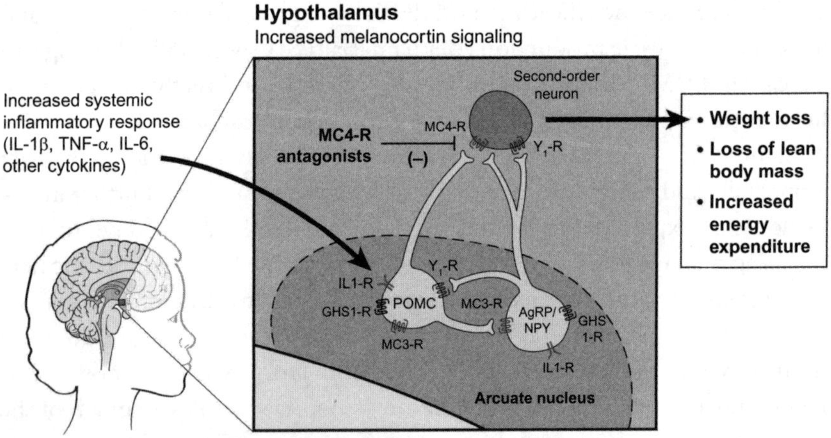

Figure 8.1 Model for activation of the central melanocortin system in the hypothalamus during cachexia. The melanocortin system comprises two sets of neurons, ones expressing either POMC or AgRP and NPY. Each set of these expresses receptors to IL-1β, Ghrelin, and α-MSH. During cachexia, inflammatory cytokines are released; IL-1β acts on the IL-1-RI to increase the release of α-MSH from POMC neurons and decrease the release of AgRP. This causes an increase in activity at the MC4-Rs at second-order neurons and downstream events characteristic of cachexia. Blockade of this signal by AgRP/NPY neurons attenuates these downstream events. Increased production of AgRP, as is caused by the effect of ghrelin at the GHS-1R, also blocks melanocortin output. AgRP, Agouti-related protein; GHS-1R, growth hormone secretagogue receptor 1; IL1-R, interleukin-1 receptor; IL-1β, interleukin-1b; IL-6, interleukin-6; MC3-R, melanocortin-3 receptor; MC4-R, melanocortin-4 receptor; NPY, neuropeptide Y; TNF-α, tumor necrosis factor-α; Y1-R, NPY receptor-1. *Figure adapted from DeBoer (2010); used with permission.* (See Color Insert.)

nucleus, which is an important center of multiple neuroendocrine responses such as appetite (DeBoer, 2010; Swanson & Sawchenko, 1980). Although these neurons send signals to similar hypothalamic centers, the functions of the POMC-expressing neurons and the AgRP/NPY-expressing neurons have opposing actions. Table 8.1 shows a summary of known receptor–ligand interactions and functionality associated with the central melanocortin system.

The neurons expressing POMC initiate an anorexic signal (Tritos et al., 1998). This starts by cleaving POMC—a large precursor peptide—into α-melanocyte-stimulating hormone (α-MSH). This hormone is then released into synapses with second-order neurons in multiple areas around the brain and brainstem, including the paraventricular nucleus of the hypothalamus (also involved in appetite regulation), the lateral hypothalamus, and the nucleus of the solitary tract in the brainstem (Cone, 2005). α-MSH acts on one of the two central melanocortin receptors, namely, the melanocortin 3 receptor (MC3R) or the MC4R, with stimulation of MC4R receptor

Table 8.1 Comparison of effects of ligand–receptor interaction on melanocortin signaling

		Effect on levels of neurons listed below		
Receptor type	**Ligand**	**POMC (a-MSH)**	**AgRP/NPY**	**Second order**
MC4-R	a-MSH	–	–	Up
MC3-R (AgRP neuron)	a-MSH	–	Down	Up[a]
Ob-R	Ob	Up	Down	Up[a]
IL1-R	IL-1	Up	Down	Up[a]
5-HT_{2C}-R	5-HT	Up	–	Up[a]
LIF-R	LIF	Up	–	Up[a]
MC4-R	AgRP	–	–	Down
MC3-R (POMC neuron)	a-MSH	Down	–	Down[a]
Y3-R (second-order neuron)	NPY	–	–	Down[a]
GHS1-R	Ghrelin	Down	Up	Down[a]
Y3-R (POMC neuron)	NPY	Down	–	Down[a]

The top shaded portion of the table describes anorexic interactions, whereas the bottom unshaded portion describes orexigenic interactions.

[a]Signifies receptor activity on upstream neurons, which have a downstream effect on second-order neurons. Ob, leptin; Ob-R, leptin receptor; 5-HT_{2C}-R, serotonin receptor; 5-HT, serotonin; LIF, leukemia inhibitory factor; LIF-R, LIF, leukemia inhibitory factor receptor.

being the main source of the anorexic output (Madison & Marks, 2006) and antagonism of MC3R being another, lesser source (Marks, Butler, Turner, Brookhart, & Cone, 2003). As such, activation of these POMC neurons appears to be a major source of symptoms seen consistently in cachexia. A separate group of neurons expressing POMC is also seen in the brainstem and are further involved in producing an anorexic signal (DeBoer, Scarlett, Levasseur, Grant, & Marks, 2009).

The class of neurons responsible for expression of NPY and AgRP is orexigenic in nature (Ollmann et al., 1997). The first output of these appetite-stimulating neurons is via a stimulatory action of NPY itself on second-order neurons. More pertinent to our discussion of cachexia, though (at least from the standpoint of treatment potential), is that the AgRP/NPY neurons release AgRP, which is natural inverse agonist of MC3R and MC4R (Nijenhuis, Oosterom, & Adan, 2001). Thus, administration of AgRP or a synthetic MC4R antagonist into the intraventricular space results in an increase in food-seeking behavior (Fan, Boston, Kesterson, Hruby, & Cone, 1997; Marks et al., 2001; Nicholson et al., 2006) by decreasing the signal of POMC neurons at the source and thus decreasing the efficacy of the signal that remains; it follows that NPY levels are increased in starved animals (Chance, Balasubramaniam, Dayal, Brown, & Fischer, 1994). Similarly, genetic mutation of the MC4R results in a decrease in melanocortin tone and is the most common monogenic cause of obesity (Farooqi et al., 2003, 2000). Together, then, POMC and AgRP neurons confer constant tone on the MC4R neurons, which influences them to promote feeding stimulation or feeding inhibition.

Experimentally, stimulation of MC4R via intracerebroventricular injection of α-MSH or another MC4R agonist results in a decrease in feeding behavior in rodent models (Li et al., 2007; Tritos et al., 1998), leading to widespread downstream effects, including a decrease in food-seeking behavior, an increase in basal metabolic rate, a decrease in LBM (Cowley et al., 1999; Krakoff et al., 2008; Markison et al., 2005; Whitaker & Reyes, 2008), and an increase in white adipocyte lipolysis (Wellhoner et al., 2011) suggesting that antagonism could increase lipogenesis. The converse of these results is also true: antagonizing the action of α-MSH at this receptor, either by introduction of an MC4R antagonist or by genetic mutation, results in an increase in feeding behavior (Chance et al., 1994; Fan et al., 1997; Farooqi et al., 2003; Huszar et al., 1997; Markison et al., 2005; Nicholson et al., 2006; Ollmann et al., 1997), total body mass (TBM; Dallmann et al., 2011), and fat mass (FM; Nicholson et al., 2006).

In addition, melanocortin antagonism results in a decrease in activity in brown adipocytes in MC4R KO and antagonized mice (Voss-Andreae et al., 2007). These brown adipocytes are responsible for lipolysis; thus, their antagonism decreases VO_2 and REE (Dallmann et al., 2011) as fat oxidation is decreased, leading to retention of fat stores. Opposite of the cachexia phenotype, it is likely that LBM is also increased in a similar manner, also allowing the REE to decrease. It should also be noted that heterozygous mice exhibit some of these phenotypes, but to a lesser extent than full MC4R KO mice (Srisai et al., 2011), reinforcing that dosage changes in tonic melanocortin activity exhibit physiologic effects that may be relevant to clinical care. As expected, in MC4R KO mice, treatment with a MC4R antagonist had no significant effects (Dallmann et al., 2011; Markison et al., 2005; Sutton, Josephine Babin, Gu, Hruby, & Butler, 2008).

The effects of MC3R modulation on cachexia signaling are less clear, at least in part due to the complexity of the system. MC3R is present on both POMC and AgRP/NPY neurons with downregulatory effects on both, leading to opposite effects on central melanocortin activity (Table 8.1). The presence of MC3R on POMC neurons (Fig. 8.1) confers a negative feedback (Cowley et al., 1999); data shown on MC3R KO mice demonstrate reduced lean mass gain, reduced linear growth, greater stress responses, and decreased exercise capacity (Butler & Cone, 2002). In the setting of anorexia through lipopolysaccharide (LPS) injection, mice lacking MC3R showed the opposite effects of knocking out MC4R in that it enhanced the cachexia-related effects. MC3R KO mice had decreased food intake and activity levels, but increased TBM loss and nonsignificantly increased VO_2. Similar effects were seen in IL-1β-treated mice as well (Marks et al., 2003), suggesting a significant increase in melanocortin activity in the absence of the negative feedback of α-MSH binding to MC3R.

In contrast, MC4R antagonism produced the opposite results to MC3R antagonism in the setting of LPS cachexia: improved food intake, increased activity levels, resisted weight loss, resisted body temperature changes, and decreased REE (Huang, Hruby, & Tatro, 1999; Marks et al., 2003, 2001; Sutton et al., 2008). These data suggest that signaling at the MC4R may be a central event in the propagation of the symptoms of cachexia, or at a minimum that inhibition of the melanocortin system can overcome some other system responsible for producing these symptoms. The potential to reverse the anorexia, loss of LBM, and increased REE that result from melanocortin activation has made antagonism of this system a major focus in the treatment of cachexia syndromes (DeBoer, 2007; Marks et al., 2001).

3.2. Factors affecting POMC, AgRP, and NPY expression

3.2.1 Ghrelin

Ghrelin is a 28 amino acid peptide produced mainly on the fundus of the stomach, which acts upon the growth hormone secretagogue receptor-1 (GHS-1; Kojima et al., 1999). Circulating ghrelin levels increase during the initial period of fasting and decrease after eating (Nakazato et al., 2001; Shiiya et al., 2002). Additionally, obese patients have lower levels of ghrelin and anorexia nervosa patients have higher levels (Shiiya et al., 2002; Soriano-Guillén, Barrios, Campos-Barros, & Argente, 2004), showing a direct correlation between ghrelin and appetite and an indirect correlation between ghrelin and BMI.

Treatment with synthetic ghrelin increases food intake (Adachi et al., 2010; Hanada et al., 2003; Nakazato et al., 2001; Neary et al., 2004; Theander-Carrillo et al., 2006; Wang, Andersson, Iresjo, Lonnroth, & Lundholm, 2006; Wren et al., 2000), plasma ghrelin and GH levels (Nass et al., 2008; Neary et al., 2004; Wang et al., 2006; Wren et al., 2000), and IGF-1 (Nass et al., 2008; Takeda et al., 2006). As summarized in Table 8.1, this orexigenic action is mediated by agonizing NPY (Nakazato et al., 2001; Seoane et al., 2003) and antagonizing POMC neurons (Nakazato et al., 2001) via direct action of ghrelin receptors (Cowley et al., 2003); this effect is seen regardless of route of administration of ghrelin (Asakawa et al., 2003). It should also be noted that ghrelin receptors are found on both types of melanocortin neurons; however, the number of receptors are less numerous on anorexic neurons than that of orexigenic neurons (Ashitani et al., 2009).

It follows that ghrelin administration results in an increase in TBM (Adachi et al., 2010; Hanada et al., 2003; Nakazato et al., 2001; Nass et al., 2008; Theander-Carrillo et al., 2006; Tschop, Smiley, & Heiman, 2000; Wang et al., 2006), LBM (Nass et al., 2008), and FM (Hanada et al., 2003; Theander-Carrillo et al., 2006; Tschop et al., 2000; Wang et al., 2006) in both humans and rodents in healthy controls. Ghrelin decreases the levels of catecholamines and catecholamine neuron activity (Cui, Li, & Appleyard, 2011; Soeki et al., 2008), leading to the downregulation of lipolytic enzymes and upregulation of lipogenic enzymes. Ghrelin's action in muscle mass is mediated, at least in part, through the decreasing activity of NF-κB (Wu et al., 2007), suggesting that ghrelin assists in preventing the upregulation of muscle breakdown, thus leading to increased LBM over time.

Ghrelin also possesses anti-inflammatory properties, which may contribute to its anti-cachectic effects. In multiple models, ghrelin has been shown to decrease the presence or effects of inflammatory markers (Ersahin et al., 2011; Li et al., 2004). Conversely, inflammatory response as stimulated by LPS showed a decrease in ghrelin levels (Stengel et al., 2010). If this occurs in the setting of cachexia, anti-inflammatory effects working upstream of the central melanocortin system would prevent downstream changes following ghrelin administration. Given its direct activity in the central melanocortin system, its ability to increase food intake and FM, and its anti-inflammatory effects, ghrelin could have potential therapeutic effects in the setting of cachexia caused by chronic underlying diseases (DeBoer et al., 2007).

3.2.2 Cytokines

Given their increased prevalence in the setting of cachexia and the integral role the melanocortin system plays in cachexia, TNF-α and other cytokines should have a central role in the modulation of the melanocortin system (Table 8.1) given their anorexigenic nature. Thus far, IL-1β receptors have been shown to be on both POMC (Scarlett et al., 2007) and AgRP (Scarlett et al., 2008) neurons in the arcuate nucleus, which are stimulatory and inhibitory in nature, respectively, leading to a net enhancement of the melanocortin system. A separate mouse model confirmed that IL-1β administration produced increases in metabolic rates similar to that seen in cachexia. Moreover, the site of action was shown to be in the melanocortin system as treatment with a MC4R antagonist attenuated the cachectic effects (Whitaker & Reyes, 2008), though it remains to be seen how varying doses of IL-1β and the antagonist would affect these outcomes. Administration of TNF-α instead of IL-1β in the same study revealed similar effects; however, these events occurred later than as seen in IL-1β administration. Additional cytokine receptors on melanocortinergic neurons include leukemia inhibitory factor (LIF), which also induces anorexic response (Grossberg et al., 2010). Finally, given the upstream modulation of IL-1β by other cytokines, proinflammatory cytokines could potentially be upstream mediators of melanocortin-related neuropeptides.

3.2.3 Leukemia inhibitory factor

LIF is another example of a proinflammatory cytokine. Levels of LIF have been shown to be elevated in chronic disease (Carroll, Bell, Wang, Chapman, & Mills, 1998; Cornish, Callon, King, Edgar, & Reid, 1993; Hamilton, Waring, & Filonzi, 1993; Metcalf, Nicola, & Gearing, 1990; Mori et al., 2011; Villiger, Geng, & Lotz, 1993) and have been associated with incidence of cachexia (Suzuki et al., 2011). LIF has also been shown to be active in the POMC-releasing neurons of the arcuate nucleus (Grossberg et al., 2010; Suzuki et al., 2011). It should be noted that animals do not desensitize to LIF, unlike in the setting of IL-1β, in which animals develop resistance to the effects of IL-1β (Grossberg et al., 2010; Metcalf & Gearing, 1989). LIF has also been shown to work via the same pathway as leptin (Febbraio, 2007; Suzuki et al., 2011) directly increasing levels of αMSH release in the hypothalamus (Grossberg et al., 2010; Table 8.1). While antagonism of LIF could be another potential therapeutic target in the setting of cachexia, this approach—as is true for many of the mediators affecting melanocortin activity—has thus far not been tested (ClinicalTrials.gov., 2012a).

3.2.4 Leptin

Leptin is a well-studied peptide with a structure similar to that of a cytokine (Zhang et al., 1997). Secreted by adipocytes in proportion to the amount of FM, leptin is correlated with BMI (Kim et al., 2012) and has been known to be a downregulator of food intake, TBM, and REE (Kim et al., 2012; Schwartz, 2000). Leptin receptors in the hypothalamus (Inui, 1999) interact with the central melanocortin neurons (Inui, 1999; Schwartz et al., 1997) to activate the melanocortin system (Table 8.1). The levels of orexigenic neuropeptides such as NPY and AgRP are suppressed by leptin, whereas the levels of anorexic neuropeptides such as α-MSH and POMC are increased by leptin (Inui, 1999; Schwartz et al., 1997). Specifically in the melanocortin system, leptin has direct effects on POMC (Cheung, Clifton, & Steiner, 1997) and AgRP (Wilson et al., 1999) neurons, causing stimulation of anorexic output (Cowley et al., 2001) and inhibition of orexigenic output (Hahn, Breininger, Baskin, & Schwartz, 1998), respectively.

Further studies have suggested other pathways for a leptin–hypophagia response. NPY KO mice are still sensitive to leptin, perhaps suggesting compensatory responses by POMC neurons or other pathways (Ramos et al., 2004). It was shown that the weights of NPY and leptin double-KO mice were halfway between wild-type and leptin KO phenotypes, suggesting a necessary role for NPY neurons in mediating hyperphagia in the absence of leptin (Inui, 1999). If leptin is involved in appetite suppression in the setting of cachexia, theoretically, antagonism of leptin could have therapeutic use in reversing its effects on the melanocortin system. Nevertheless, the levels of leptin are significantly decreased in the setting of cachexia (Kim et al., 2012) and further knockdown of leptin's anorectic effects may not exhibit additional effects.

3.2.5 Serotonin

Serotonin (5-HT) levels are directly correlated with satiety; as such, the drug fenfluramine was used as a powerful antiobesity drug (Pinder, Brogden, Sawyer, Speight, & Avery, 1975). Blocking uptake and stimulating the release of 5-HT has a direct effect on appetite suppression (Heisler et al., 2002; Table 8.1). Furthermore, 5-HT has been shown to have a receptor subtype, 2C, on POMC neurons, but not on AgRP neurons (Heisler et al., 2003), contributing to hypophagia (Vickers et al., 2003). Thus, 5-HT_{2C}-R-knockout mice are hyperphagic, whereas mice expressing 5-HT_{2C}-R only on POMC neurons experience eating habits similar to wild-type mice (Xu et al., 2008). While direct manipulation of serotonergic pathways seemed to be a promising clinical route, it was shown that drugs acting upon this pathway had the side effect of pulmonary hypertension and valvular heart disease, eliminating the opportunity of its clinical use (Connolly et al., 1997).

In spite of this, future potential for serotonin modulation exists through secondary pathways. A recent study has shown that fasting increased the level of an Abelson helper integration site 1 protein (Ahi1) in the arcuate nucleus (Doering et al., 2008; Wang et al., 2012). Investigators showed that Ahi1 decreased expression of 5-HT_{2C}-R (Vickers et al., 2003; Wang et al., 2012) and POMC and increased expression of NPY (Wang et al., 2012). Small inhibitory RNA overexpression of Ahi1 significantly decreased NPY levels by 40% and increased POMC levels by 40%; significant changes were also seen in knockdown of Ahi1, with NPY increased by 40% and POMC decreased by 40% (Wang et al., 2012). Thus, with the direct modulation of the serotonin receptor no longer a viable possibility, future direction could test for negative consequences of indirect modulation of this receptor subtype to manipulate the appetite regulation. This and other stimulators of the processes of cachexia underscore the complexity of inputs into the system as well as the potential to interrupt these processes in the setting of specific disease states, as we will see below.

4. CANCER CACHEXIA

4.1. Basic science

Various cancer types have long been known to cause cachexia (Donovan, 1954), largely because of reciprocal processes between the tumor and the host organism (Fearon & Carter, 1988). In the setting of cancer, patients without treatment significantly lost TBM (Kerem et al., 2008; Vos et al., 2004;

Weyermann et al., 2009), LBM (Fearon, 1992; Nicholson et al., 2006; Weyermann et al., 2009), and more significantly lost FM (Fearon, 1992; Fouladiun et al., 2005; Nicholson et al., 2006; Weyermann et al., 2009); a trend that holds true across most cancer types (Tisdale, 2009). Consistent with the loss of FM, levels of leptin are decreased (Fouladiun et al., 2005; Kerem et al., 2008) in cancer patients versus healthy humans over time; these data suggest that though leptin levels may increase due to inflammation, they are more strongly affected by loss of FM. In cancer patients, ghrelin levels were increased (Chopin et al., 2011; Hanada et al., 2003; Kerem et al., 2008; Shimizu et al., 2003) and even more so in cachectic patients compared to noncachectic patients (Kim et al., 2012). This suggests that cancer cachexia involves some degree of resistance to the orexigenic effects of increased ghrelin and decreased leptin (Garcia et al., 2005; Wang et al., 2006; Wisse, Frayo, Schwartz, & Cummings, 2001) as, overall, these levels are consistent with normal physiologic response to weight loss.

The resistance to physiologic signals of appetite regulation appears to be due, at least in part, to modulation of the melanocortin system. Levels of TNF-α, IL-6, IL-1β, LIF, and other proinflammatory cytokines are increased in human cancer (Hanada et al., 2003; Kim et al., 2012; Ramos et al., 2004; Tisdale, 2010) and serotonin is increased in tumor-bearing rats (Blaha et al., 1998). As these hormones are anorexigenic in nature, it follows that levels of POMC are relatively increased, and levels of AgRP and NPY are decreased in the setting of cancer (Chance et al., 1994; Davis, Dreicer, Walsh, Lagman, & LeGrand, 2004; Laviano et al., 2008) and are more potent in regulating appetite than the modulated levels of ghrelin and leptin. Tumor-bearing MC3R KO mice showed similar trends as previously described cachectic mice; TBM was significantly decreased, due mainly to the drop in LBM as FM change was nonsignificant (Marks et al., 2003), again suggesting melanocortin intervention to be a potential treatment.

4.2. Clinical applications

Overall, pharmacologic interventions for cancer cachexia have had limited success. An original Cochrane review and a follow-up deemed megestrol acetate (MA) to be effective in increasing weight gain and appetite in cancer patients; however, MA alone did not improve overall quality of life (Berenstein & Ortiz, 2005; Payne, Wiffen, & Martin, 2012), potentially due to persistent malabsorption; weight gain is thought to be due to increased water and FM (Simons et al., 1998), but not LBM. Treatment with ω-3 fatty acids increased TBM, LBM, and quality of life versus control

(Barber, Fearon, Tisdale, McMillan, & Ross, 2001; Barber et al., 2004; Fearon et al., 2003), but only at high enough doses; combination therapy of an ω-3 fatty acid and MA was not significantly different from MA therapy (Jatoi et al., 2004). Anti-inflammatory treatment increased chances of survival (Lundholm et al., 1994); this treatment supplemented with additional nutrition increased food intake as well as energy balance, but failed to ameliorate changes in REE, TBM, LBM, or FM (Lundholm, Daneryd, Bosaeus, Körner, & Lindholm, 2004). Administration of anti-inflammatory drugs, carnitine, and antioxidants in conjunction with MA in cachectic cancer patients was shown to be significantly better at increasing LBM, decreasing REE, and reducing proinflammatory cytokine levels than administration of MA alone (Madeddu et al., 2012).

In humans, heterozygosity for a single, neutral mutation decreased cachexia frequency in nonleukemic cancer patients (22% vs. 0%, $p < 0.05$; DeBoer, 2010; Knoll et al., 2008), suggesting that melanocortin antagonism may assist in reversing cancer cachexia. As seen in Table 8.2, MC4R antagonism significantly increases food intake (Chen et al., 2008; Jiang et al., 2007; Joppa, Gogas, Foster, & Markison, 2007; Markison et al., 2005; Marks et al., 2001; Tran et al., 2007; Weyermann et al., 2009), TBM (Chen et al., 2008; Joppa et al., 2007; Markison et al., 2005; Marks et al., 2001; Vos et al., 2004; Weyermann et al., 2009), LBM (Jiang et al., 2007; Joppa et al., 2007; Markison et al., 2005; Nicholson et al., 2006; Tran et al., 2007; Weyermann et al., 2009), and FM (Joppa et al., 2007; Markison et al., 2005; Weyermann et al., 2009) versus vehicle-treated controls. In one study, total food consumption did not change in tumor-bearing mice receiving a small molecule melanocortin antagonist versus vehicle controls, while LBM, FM, and light-phase food intake significantly increased (Nicholson et al., 2006). Other less studied outcomes include increased water consumption (Marks et al., 2001) in the presence of an antagonist, but more importantly, antagonism decreased the incidence of cachexia (Weyermann et al., 2009). In most studies, it is clear that the presence of an MC4R antagonist (or lack of MC4R) produces a significant improvement over tumor-bearing, vehicle-treated animals, even if treated mice are not rescued entirely to the level of food intake and weight gain of noncancer controls.

As seen in Table 8.2, ghrelin has similar effects to melanocortin antagonism; an overall effect of increasing food intake (Adachi et al., 2010; DeBoer et al., 2007; Neary et al., 2004; Strasser et al., 2008; Yamamoto et al., 2010), TBM (Adachi et al., 2010; DeBoer et al., 2007; Garcia & Polvino, 2007, 2009; Hanada et al., 2003; Wang et al., 2006; Yamamoto et al., 2010),

Table 8.2 MC4-R antagonism (top) and ghrelin administration (bottom) in cancer cachexia

References	Species/model of cachexia	Molecule × dose (route)	Duration of Tx	Effect	*p*
Marks et al. (2001)	Mice/sarcoma	MC4-R KO	16 days	FI: KO mice +5% versus WT −39.5% (vs. pretumor baseline); TBM change: KO +0.85 g versus WT −0.75 g	$p < 0.0001$, $p < 0.05$
Marks et al. (2001)	Mice/sarcoma	AgRP (3 injections) × 2.5 nmol (ICV)	5 days	TBM (over 19 days' experiment): AgRP 63% versus veh 30%; FI 76% versus ctrl (all % of AgRP sham)	$p < 0.01$, $p < 0.05$
Marks et al. (2003)	Mice/adenocarcinoma	MC4-R KO	15 days	LBM: KO +9% versus −0.5% WT versus +4% WT sham; FM: KO +20% versus WT −25% versus +4% WT sham	$p < 0.05$
Vos et al. (2004)	Mice/colorectal cancer	ML 00253764 × 32 mg/kg/day (SC)	11 days	TBM: ant +8% versus veh −3%	$p < 0.00001$
Nicholson et al. (2006)	Mice/LLC	ML 00253764 × 30 mg/kg/day (SC)	13 days	LBM: ant +0% versus veh −6.25%	$p < 0.01$
Markison et al. (2005)	Mice/LLC	NBI-12i × 6 mg/kg/day (IP)	3 days	FI: ant +100% from veh; TBM: ant +11.5% versus veh +2.9%; LBM: ant +13% versus +3.5%; FM: ant +19% versus +7.2% veh (%baseline)	$p < 0.001$, $p < 0.05$, $p < 0.01$, $p < 0.05$
Tran et al. (2007)	Mice/LLC	Phenyl piperazine (no name attributed) × 6.0 and 18.0 mg/kg/day (IP)	4 days	FI: low and high dose +2% over veh; LBM: high dose +15%, low dose +6.3%, veh +2.1% (%baseline)	$p < 0.05$
Chen et al. (2008)	Mice/LLC	Piperazine derivative (no name attributed) × 2.0 mg/kg/day (IP)	4 days	FI: ant 86% higher than veh; TBM: ant +2.8% versus veh −2.7% (% baseline); LBM: ant +4.1% versus veh −0.1% (% baseline)	$p < 0.05$, $p < 0.05$, NS

Jiang et al. (2007)	Mice/LLC	Pyrrolidinone (no name attributed) × 6.0 mg/kg/day (SC)	4 days	FI: ant +82% over veh; LBM: ant −0.5% versus −9.5% (%baseline)	$p < 0.05$
Weyermann et al. (2009)	Mice/colorectal cancer	SNT207707 × 30 mg/kg/day (oral)	15 days	TBM: ant +0.8% versus veh −9.5% versus (no tumor) +2.9%; LBM change ant 70% versus veh −10%; FM change ant 41.7% versus veh −41.7% (% of veh change)	$p < 0.001$, NS, $p < 0.05$
Weyermann et al. (2009)	Mice/colorectal cancer	SNT209858 × 30 mg/kg/day (oral)	15 days	TBM: ant +1.8% versus veh −13.4% versus (no tumor) +4.9%; LBM: ant 16% versus ant −150%; FM: ant 14.3% versus −171% veh (% of veh change)	$p < 0.001$, $p < 0.05$, $p < 0.01$, $p < 0.05$
Dallmann et al. (2011)	Rats/adenocarcinoma	BL-6020/979 (SNT207979) × 30 mg/kg/day (oral)	15 days	TBM: ant: −2.4% versus veh −9.6% versus (no tumor) +3.7%; LBM: ant 34% vs. −21% (% of sham change); FM: ant 39% versus −21% (% of sham change)	$p < 0.001$, $p < 0.01$, $p < 0.05$
Wisse et al. (2001)	Rats/prostate cancer	SHU 9119 × 0.35 nmol/day (ICV)	3 days	FI +39%; TBM gain +160% (vs. pretreatment anorectic baseline)	$p < 0.05$
Neary et al. (2004)	Humans/multiple cancers	Ghrelin × 0.450 nmol/kg (1.5 μg/kg) (IV)	1 dose	Single meal FI +31% over saline injection	$p < 0.01$
Strasser et al. (2008)	Humans/multiple cancers	Ghrelin × 8 μg/kg (2.4 nmol/kg) (IV)	17–18 days	Single-day nutritional intake ghrelin 250% greater than veh	$p < 0.10$
Lundholm et al. (2010)	Humans/gastrointestinal cancer	Ghrelin × 0.7 or 13 mg/kg/day (0.2 nmol/kg or 3.86 nmol/kg) (SQ)	8 weeks	LBM: high dose +6.7%, low dose +1.8% (NS); FM change: high dose 1%, low dose 2.3%	NS, $p < 0.05$

Continued

Table 8.2 MC4-R antagonism (top) and ghrelin administration (bottom) in cancer cachexia—cont'd

References	Species/model of cachexia	Molecule × dose (route)	Duration of Tx	Effect	*p*
Yamamoto et al. (2010)	Humans/ esophageal cancer	Ghrelin × 6 μg/kg/day (1.78 μmol/lkg/day) (IV)	10 days	Caloric intake +44.5% versus veh, total TBM loss: −1% ghrelin versus −3% in veh; LBM change: 0% versus −4% in veh	$p < 0.05$
Adachi et al. (2010)	Humans/gastric cancer	Ghrelin × 6 μg/kg/day (1.78 μmol/lkg/day) (IV)	10 days	FI: ghrelin +32.7% over veh; TBM loss: Ghrelin −1.4% versus placebo −3.7%	$p < 0.05$
Garcia and Polvino (2007)	Humans/ multiple cancers	RC-1291 × 50 mg/d (oral)	12 weeks	Total mass RC 1291 +1.54%, placebo −1.31%	$p < 0.05$
DeBoer et al. (2007)	Rats/sarcoma	Ghrelin, BIM −28131 × 500 nmol/kg each day (continuous IP)	5 days	FI: ghrelin +37% from veh, BIM +43% from veh; TBM: ghrelin +13%, BIM-28131 +19.5% veh −10.3%, untreated +10%	$p < 0.001$
Wang et al. (2006)	Mice/sarcoma	Ghrelin × 40 μg/day (2400 μg/kg/day, 700 nmol/ day) (IP)	5 days	TBM: +4%, FI: +13%, FM: +43% (increase over veh)	$p < 0.05$
Hanada et al. (2003)	Mice/human melanoma	Ghrelin 6 μg/kg/day (1.78 μmol/lkg) (IV)	6 days	TBM gain: ghrelin +0.01%, veh −0.4%, untreated +2.4%	$p < 0.05$

KO, knockout; WT, wild type; ICV, intracerebroventricular; SC, subcutaneous; IP, intraperitoneal; FI, food intake; TBM, total body mass; LBM, lean body mass; FM, fat mass; ant, MC4-R antagonist; veh, vehicle control; LLC, Lewis lung carcinoma.

LBM (Lundholm et al., 2010; Yamamoto et al., 2010), and FM (Lundholm et al., 2010; Wang et al., 2006) versus a vehicle control. While the mechanism for these effects is not certain, ghrelin's efficacy could be mediated by increases in plasma ghrelin and GH levels (Garcia & Polvino, 2009; Hanada et al., 2003; Lundholm et al., 2010; Neary et al., 2004; Strasser et al., 2008; Wang et al., 2006), IGF-1 (Garcia & Polvino, 2009), and serum albumin levels (Adachi et al., 2010). Treatment with ghrelin in the setting of cancer cachexia increased transcription of AgRP and NPY genes but had no significant effect on POMC expression in tumor-bearing rats (DeBoer et al., 2007). During ghrelin treatment, transcription levels of IL-1β were not significantly changed, but ghrelin decreased levels of IL-1β receptor transcription (DeBoer et al., 2007). These data suggest that ghrelin partially reverses the effects of anorexia and diminishes some of the harmful neuropeptide and inflammatory changes that are present in cachexia—effects that appear to be mediated in part through activation of orexigenic neurons of the central melanocortin system.

5. CARDIAC CACHEXIA

5.1. Basic science

Cardiac cachexia is a condition affecting 15% of CHF patients (Anker et al., 1997a), caused by cellular hypoxia, reduction in food intake, and hypermetabolism (Pittman & Cohen, 1964). Similar to other disease states associated with cachexia, TNF-α and IL-6 are significantly upregulated in these patients (Dutka, Elborn, Delamere, Shale, & Morris, 1993; Levine, Kalman, Mayer, Fillit, & Packer, 1990; McMurray, Abdullah, Dargie, & Shapiro, 1991; Torre-Amione, Kapadia, Benedict, et al., 1996). Cachexia carries a 50% mortality in CHF patients versus a 17% mortality in noncachectic patients (Anker et al., 1997c). Through action by different mediators, cardiac cachexia, similar to other cachexia, leads to LBM and FM decreases (Akashi et al., 2009; Anker & Sharma, 2002).

Much like in the setting of cancer, the damaged cardiac muscle can directly produce the proinflammatory cytokines. A stimulus of TNF-α can be released from the cardiac myocytes in response to a failing heart (Torre-Amione, Kapadia, Lee, et al., 1996). Another theory is that CHF-associated edema raises levels of TNF-α increasing absorption of endotoxin through an edematous bowel (Anker et al., 1997b; Anker & Sharma, 2002; Michie et al., 1988). Both these theories could contribute to the increase in TNF-α, which is associated with an increase in catecholamines (Anker &

Sharma, 2002) and leptin (Straburzynska-Migaj, Gwizdala, Siniawski, Ochotny, & Grajek, 2010); ghrelin levels overall are not different between all patients with CHF versus controls, but upon selection for cachectic individuals, ghrelin levels are increased (Nagaya et al., 2001b), again suggesting that pharmacologic orexigens could have a therapeutic impact.

5.2. Clinical applications

As is generally true in these settings, improving the underlying disease process also improves the degree of cachexia. As such, assisting cardiac function was shown to significantly reduce levels of TNF-α when compared to an unassisted heart (Torre-Amione et al., 1999). Infliximab, a monoclonal anti-TNF-α antibody, has been shown to be effective in a mouse model at reversing cachexia in CHF (Kadokami et al., 2001), while etanercept, a soluble TNF-α antagonist, has been shown to be ineffective at correcting the harmful effects of CHF in both rodents and humans (Anker & Coats, 2002; Chung et al., 2003; Haugen, Tang, Isic, Andersson, & Fu, 2008).

Table 8.3 shows that, similar to cancer cachexia, antagonism of the MC4R in cardiac cachexia produces the effect of increasing food intake, TBM, LBM, and FM in both pharmacological and genetic antagonism of the receptor (Scarlett et al., 2010). REE and O_2 consumption are decreased and survival is increased (Scarlett et al., 2010); however, comparatively few studies have been published on this subject.

Much like melanocortin antagonism, ghrelin and its analogues have been shown to increase food intake (Akashi et al., 2009; Kodama, Ashitani, Matsumoto, Kangawa, & Nakazato, 2008; Nagaya et al., 2005, 2004; Palus et al., 2011), attenuate loss of TBM (Akashi et al., 2009; Kodama et al., 2008; Nagaya et al., 2004; Nagaya, Uematsu, Kojima, Ikeda, et al., 2001; Palus et al., 2011; von Haehling, Stepney, & Anker, 2010), LBM (Akashi et al., 2009; Nagaya et al., 2005, 2004; Palus et al., 2011), and FM (Akashi et al., 2009; Nagaya et al., 2005; Palus et al., 2011) in both human and rat models of cardiac cachexia. Ghrelin treatment increased serum GH (Kodama et al., 2008; Nagaya et al., 2005, 2004) and IGF-1 (Kodama et al., 2008; Nagaya et al., 2004; Nagaya, Uematsu, Kojima, Ikeda, et al., 2001) by varying degrees of significance and decreased serum catecholamines along with sputum levels of MPO and TNF-α (Nagaya et al., 2005, 2004); cardiac function (Nagaya, Uematsu, Kojima, Ikeda, et al., 2001) and handgrip strength (Nagaya et al., 2005, 2004) also improved. Most importantly, it was shown that ghrelin increased survival rate in MI rats (Schwenke et al., 2008), suggesting an overall improvement due to ghrelin treatment.

Table 8.3 MC4-R antagonism (top) and ghrelin administration (bottom) in cardiac cachexia

References	Species/ model of cachexia	Molecule × dose (route)	Duration of Tx (days)	Effect	*p*
Scarlett et al. (2010)	Mouse/MI	MC4-R KO	56	FI: KO −2.1% versus WT −10.5%; TBM: KO +22.2% versus WT −2.2%; LBM: KO +13.9% versus WT −0.6%; FM: KO +10.3% versus WT +33.2% (% baseline)	$p < 0.05$
Scarlett et al. (2010)	Mouse/MI	AgRP × 1 nmol (8 injections ICV)	14	FI: AgRP +68% versus veh +18.1%; TBM: AgRP +27.7% versus veh +3.1%; LBM: AgRP +20.5% versus veh +3.3%; FM: AgRP +145.5% versus veh −1.3%	$p < 0.05$
Nagaya et al. (2004)	Humans/ CHF	Ghrelin × 4 μg/kg/day (1.2 nmol/kg/day) (IV)	21	TBM: ghrelin +1.6%; FI: +8%; LBM: +1.8% (% baseline, veh had all NS change from baseline)	$p < 0.10$, $p < 0.05$, $p < 0.05$
Nagaya et al. (2005)	Humans/ COPD	Ghrelin × 4 μg/kg/day (1.2 nmol/kg/day) (IV)	21	FI: +9.8%; TBM: +2%; LBM: 1.8% (% baseline, no ctrl)	$p < 0.05$
Kodama et al. (2008)	Humans/ recurrent lung infection	Ghrelin × 4 μg/kg/day (1.2 nmol/kg/day) (IV)	21	TBM: ghrelin +6% from baseline; FI: +25% from baseline (no ctrl)	$p < 0.05$
von Haehling et al. (2010)	Humans/ COPD	SUN11031 × 40 mg/kg/day (SC)	28	TBM: +4% versus veh +1%	$p < 0.05$

Continued

Table 8.3 MC4-R antagonism (top) and ghrelin administration (bottom) in cardiac cachexia—cont'd

References	Species/ model of cachexia	Molecule × dose (route)	Duration of Tx (days)	Effect	*p*
Nagaya, Uematsu, Kojima, Ikeda, et al. (2001)	Rats/ coronary artery ligation	Ghrelin × 200 μg/kg/day (60 nmol/kg/day)	21	TBM: ghrelin +10% versus saline +3%	$p < 0.05$
Palus et al. (2011)	Rats/CHF	Ghrelin, BIM 28125, BIM-28131 × 500 nmol/kg/day (1700 mg/kg/day) (IV)	21	FI: 125 +10%, 131 +14.5% ghrelin +8.6%; TBM: (125) +24.2% (131) +25.1%, ghrelin +22.5% versus +9% veh; LBM: 125 +14%, 131 +15.5%, ghrelin +14% versus veh +8%; FM: 125 +58%, 131 +85%, ghrelin +53% versus veh +15%	($p < 0.01$, $p < 0.001$, $p < 0.05$); all $p < 0.01$; $p < 0.001$; $p < 0.001$
Akashi et al. (2009)	Rats/MI	Ghrelin × 500 nmol/kg/day (1700 mg/kg/day) (SC)	28	FI: ghrelin +14.2% over veh, TBM: ghrelin +22% versus veh +8.5%; LBM: ghrelin +15.7% versus +7.7% veh; FM: +56.5% versus veh +1.9%	$p < 0.001$

MI, myocardial infarction; CHF, chronic heart failure; COPD, chronic obstructive pulmonary disorder; KO, knockout; WT, wild type; ICV, intracerebroventricular; SC, subcutaneous; IP, intraperitoneal; FI, food intake; TBM, total body mass; LBM, lean body mass; FM: fat mass; veh, vehicle control.

6. RENAL CACHEXIA

6.1. Basic science

CKD is characterized not only by malnutrition and anorexia (Mak, Cheung, Cone, & Marks, 2005) but also by the modified metabolic state associated with cachexia (Mak, Cheung, Zhan, Shen, & Foster, 2012; von Haehling & Anker, 2010). Unlike cancer cachexia in which the tumor secretes inflammatory cytokines, the cause of inflammation in CKD is not quite clear, though it is most likely caused by multiple factors (Mak et al., 2012), perhaps by uremia or acidosis. CKD models have increased levels of leptin (Bergstrom, 1995; Carrero et al., 2011; Cheung et al., 2005, 2007; Mak, Cheung, Cone, & Marks, 2006a; Mitch, 1998; Yoshimoto et al., 2002) which decrease over time (Beberashvili et al., 2011; Mak et al., 2012). Also of note regarding cachectic subjects is the decrease in the fraction of ghrelin expressed as active (acyl) ghrelin (Buscher, Buscher, Hauffa, & Hoyer, 2010; Naufel, Bordon, de Aquino, Ribeiro, & de Abreu Carvalhaes, 2010). Lower ghrelin levels were associated with higher leptin levels, even when corrected for BMI, and also correlated with survival (Carrero et al., 2011). These data, in conjunction with increased levels of proinflammatory cytokines (Cheung et al., 2007; Mak et al., 2006b), are consistent with the findings that food consumption, LBM, FM, IGF-1, and albumin decreased, and REE increased (Cheung et al., 2005; Cheung, Rosengren, Boyle, & Mak, 2008) with the progression of the underlying disease (Cheung et al., 2005, 2008; Mak et al., 2012; Naufel et al., 2010; Rodriguez et al., 2010). These changes are not seen in nephrectomized leptin KO mice (Cheung et al., 2005; Mak et al., 2006a), suggesting effects of CKD cachexia are at least partially mediated through leptin or leptin-associated pathways such as the central melanocortin system.

6.2. Clinical applications

Clinical trials and application in the setting of CKD cachexia are not as numerous as those of cancer cachexia. One trial of ω-3 fatty acids did not produce a decrease in inflammation for patients undergoing hemodialysis for kidney failure (Fiedler, Mall, Wand, & Osten, 2005; Vernaglione, Cristofano, & Chimienti, 2008). Other trials confirmed this result and also showed that it attenuated inflammation responses to hemodialysis (Szklarek-Kubicka et al., 2009). It was shown for a shorter time frame that twice the amount of ω-3 fatty acids could decrease inflammation (Rasic-Milutinovic et al., 2007), though this was not sustained. Additionally, MA was shown to be effective in increasing weight and leptin levels in patients with CKD (Rammohan, Kalantar-Zadeh, Liang, & Ghossein, 2005).

As shown in Table 8.4, antagonism by MC4R KO models (Cheung et al., 2005) or administration of an antagonist, either endogenous (Cheung et al., 2005, 2008) or synthetic (Cheung et al., 2007), shows consistent effects in rodent models of CKD. Treatment results in increases in food consumption, TBM, LBM, and FM versus vehicle-treated controls (Cheung et al., 2005, 2007, 2008), possibly modulated by decreasing IL-6 upon administration (Cheung et al., 2007). Antagonism decreased serum levels of leptin, increased feeding efficiency, and decreased REE significantly (Cheung et al., 2005, 2007, 2008). These two studies suggest a high degree of potential for melanocortin antagonism in CKD, though clinical trials are greatly needed for confirmation.

Regarding treatment with ghrelin and other GHR-1a agonists, administration of these compounds increased food consumption (Ashby et al., 2009; DeBoer et al., 2008; Wynne et al., 2005), TBM (DeBoer et al., 2008), LBM (DeBoer et al., 2008), and FM (DeBoer et al., 2008). While TBM, LBM, and FM have not been exhaustively studied, other outcomes of ghrelin treatment include an increase in GH levels, decreased levels of IL-1R transcriptions (DeBoer et al., 2008), and a decrease in kidney inflammatory markers and serum IL-6 (Rajan et al., 2012). Ghrelin also decreased blood pressure (Wynne et al., 2005), though this effect had disappeared 2 h after injection in human (Ashby et al., 2009). Ghrelin also significantly improved renal function using a variety of different measures, such as serum nitrogen levels and creatinine levels (Takeda et al., 2006), suggesting effects on the underlying disease process as a mediator of improvements in cachexia (DeBoer, 2011a).

7. OTHER CACHEXIA

7.1. Burn/thermal injury

Thermal injuries have been shown to lead to hypermetabolism, body catabolism, and an increase in inflammatory markers (Dasu et al., 2004; Yang, Berthiaume, & Androulakis, 2011), potentially leading to cachexia (Trop, Schintler, Spendel, & Stockenhuber, 2008). REE is increased due to metabolic changes in the body, including modulation of lipogenesis and lipolysis

Table 8.4 MC4-R antagonism (top) and ghrelin administration (bottom) in renal cachexia

References	Species/model of cachexia	Molecule × dose (route)	Duration of Tx	Effect	*p*
Cheung et al. (2005)	Mice/ nephrectomy	MC4-R KO	14 days	FI: KO +24.8% over WT; TBM: KO +4.4% versus WT +2%; LBM: KO +5.6% versus WT −6%; FM: KO +7.8% versus WT −15.8%	Significance not explicitly reported, but error bars suggest $p < 0.05$
Cheung et al. (2005)	Mice/ nephrectomy	AgRP × 2 nmol/dose, 5 injections (ICV)	14 days	FI: AgRP +1.29% over veh; TBM: AgRP +4.5% versus veh +2.3%; LBM: AgRP +1.3% versus veh −4.3%; FM: AgRP +5.6% versus veh −9.8%	$p < 0.001$
Cheung et al. (2007)	Mice/ nephrectomy	NBI-12i × 6 mg/kg/day (IP)	14 days	FI: ant +11.9% over veh; TBM: ant +6.2% versus veh +1.4%; LBM: ant +2.2% versus veh −2.5%; FM: ant +2.2% versus veh −4.5%	$p < 0.001$
Cheung et al. (2008)	Mice/ nephrectomy	AgRP × 2 nmol/dose, 5 injections (ICV)	14 days	TBM: AgRP +6.2% versus veh +2.6%; LBM: AgRP +2.2% versus veh −1.6%; FM: AgRP +3.2% versus veh −3.2%	$p < 0.001$
DeBoer et al. (2008)	Humans/end-stage kidney disease	Ghrelin × single 3.6 nmol/kg (12 μg/kg) (SC)	1 meal	FI: ghrelin +57% over placebo	$p < 0.01$

Continued

Table 8.4 MC4-R antagonism (top) and ghrelin administration (bottom) in renal cachexia—cont'd

References	Species/model of cachexia	Molecule × dose (route)	Duration of Tx	Effect	*p*
Wynne et al. (2005)	Humans/ malnourished dialysis patients	Acyl-ghrelin × 12 μg/kg/day (3.7 nmol/kg/day) (SC)	8 days	Total FI: ghrelin +24.6% over veh	$p<0.001$
Ashby et al. (2009)	Rats/ nephrectomy	Ghrelin, BIM 28125, BIM-28131 × 150 nmol/kg/day (478 μg/kg/day) (continuous SC pump)	14 days	For (ghrelin, BIM 28125, BIM28131, vehicle); cumulative FI: +19%, +19%, +20% (over vehicle); TBM: +22%, +27%, +21%, +1% (% baseline); LBM: +26%, +29%, +24%, +2.8% (% baseline)	$p<0.001$, $p<0.05$, $p<0.01$

KO, knockout; WT, wild type; ICV, intracerebroventricular; SC, subcutaneous; IP, intraperitoneal; FI, food intake; TBM, total body mass; LBM, lean body mass; FM, fat mass; ant, MC4-R antagonist; veh, vehicle control.

(Baumann & Gauldie, 1994). REE may be enhanced due to the heat loss through the injured tissue (Baumann & Gauldie, 1994). Endogenous ghrelin levels have been shown to be greatly decreased in rats with thermal injury (Balasubramaniam et al., 2006), suggesting ghrelin treatment could have therapeutic effects.

Treatment with ghrelin in thermally injured rats was shown to increase 2 h food intake in thermally injured rats (ghrelin +178% vs. −18% control) and increased GH (Balasubramaniam et al., 2006) and IGF-1 (Balasubramaniam et al., 2009) levels, while decreasing levels of TNF-α (Balasubramaniam et al., 2009; Sheriff et al., 2012) and IL-6 (Sheriff, Joshi, Friend, James, & Balasubramaniam, 2009). Muscle metabolism decreased in rat models (Balasubramaniam et al., 2009; Sheriff et al., 2009), mirroring *in vitro* results of increased levels of protein synthesis and decreased mediators of proteolysis (Sheriff et al., 2012). No known studies of melanocortin antagonism in the setting of thermal injury have been performed.

7.2. Colitis

In an experimental model of colitis, it was shown that weight decreased and macroscopic score increased; TNF-α, IL-6, and IL-1β also increased (Gonzalez-Rey, Chorny, & Delgado, 2006). In ulcerative colitis and Crohn's disease, levels of active ghrelin were decreased versus the disease in remission (Ates, Degertekin, Erdil, Yaman, & Dagalp, 2008) and healthy control subjects (Karmiris et al., 2006).

It was shown that treatment with ghrelin ameliorated the weight decrease and inflammation increase associated with colitis (Gonzalez-Rey et al., 2006; Konturek et al., 2009). Ghrelin treatment in the setting of colitis has not been studied in humans (DeBoer, 2011b). Antagonism of the melanocortin receptor in the setting of colitis has not been well studied in any model.

7.3. HIV/AIDS

Much like other forms of cachexia, weight loss, including LBM, is commonly associated with HIV and is a predictor of mortality (Palenicek et al., 1995; Thibault, Cano, & Pichard, 2011). In the setting of HIV, IL-6 levels, TNF-α levels, and REE are higher than in healthy individuals, leading to hypophagia (Kosmiski, 2011). Antiretroviral medications (Shevitz et al., 1999) and secondary infections (Melchior et al., 1993) have been shown to increase REE even further.

Ghrelin increases food consumption, LBM, and TBM versus untreated patients with HIV/AIDS (Esposito, Thomas, Kingdon, & Ezzat, 2004, 2005; Moyle et al., 2004; Schambelan et al., 1996). However, ghrelin treatment also decreases fat body mass more than as seen in vehicle-treated patients (Esposito et al., 2004, 2005; Moyle et al., 2004; Paton et al., 1999; Schambelan et al., 1996). This could potentially be due to some of the mitigating factors such as secondary infections and interactions with antiretroviral medications; this loss in FM is different than changes seen in other models of cachexia. This observation is further complicated by the initial abnormal distribution of fat in HIV (Stanley & Grinspoon, 2009); treatment with GH is known to decrease fat in visceral tissue (Stanley & Grinspoon, 2009). Other effects include a decrease in protein catabolism (Paton et al., 1999) and increases in grip strength (Paton et al., 1999), levels of IGF-1 (Esposito et al., 2004, 2005; Paton et al., 1999), maximal work output (Esposito et al., 2005; Moyle et al., 2004), and quality of life (Moyle et al., 2004). No known studies of melanocortin antagonism in the setting of AIDS have been performed.

7.4. Aging

In healthy individuals, older (>60 years) subjects had higher serum levels of cytokines than younger subjects (Alvarez-Rodriguez, Lopez-Hoyos, Munoz-Cacho, & Martinez-Taboada, 2012). In addition, it was shown in a mouse model that food intake was decreased, fasting ghrelin levels were decreased, feeding leptin levels were higher, and levels of NPY and AgRP were decreased in the older mice (Takeda et al., 2010); POMC levels were increased in the fasted condition, albeit nonsignificantly (Takeda et al., 2010). Activity of the hypothalamic receptors was decreased, potentially explaining these findings (Takeda et al., 2010).

In this model, treatment with ghrelin increased circulating levels of ghrelin but did not provide a significant increase in 1 and 24 h food consumption in older mice, though it did in younger control mice (Takeda et al., 2010). However, in other models, ghrelin stimulated food intake (Ariyasu et al., 2008; Toshinai et al., 2007), though at a lower observed in young rats–and the increase in food intake did not last long term (Toshinai et al., 2007). It was also shown that in older mice, ghrelin significantly increased LBM and decreased FM from controls (Ariyasu et al., 2008). A human trial of a ghrelin in older adults showed an increase in serum IGF-1 and GH, increased LBM and TBM, but not FM (Nass et al., 2008).

7.5. Cancer treatment-induced cachexia

While a tumor can be a main cause of cachexia, treatment of the cancer, such as chemotherapy drugs cisplatin and methotrexate (MTX) and radiation, has been shown to induce cachexia. Side effects associated with cisplatin administration include anorexia and loss of TBM, LBM (Garcia, Cata, Dougherty, & Smith, 2008; Maltoni et al., 1999; Sinno et al., 2010), and FM (Sinno et al., 2010); other effects include decreased water intake (Sinno et al., 2010) and IGF-1 protein (Garcia et al., 2008), and a decrease in NPY mRNA (Sinno et al., 2010). Interestingly, IL-1β protein and POMC mRNA were also decreased (Sinno et al., 2010); this is likely due to the effects of MTX on the cancer cell, decreasing IL-1β and thus decreasing release of POMC.

In animals, treatment with ghrelin after administration of cisplatin significantly increases weight gain and cumulative food intake versus animals receiving doses of saline; ghrelin attenuates the decrease in levels of IGF-1 in this setting as well (Garcia et al., 2008; Liu, Malik, Sanger, & Andrews, 2006). No significant changes were seen in LBM or FM (Liu et al., 2006).

Treatment with AgRP has also been shown to reverse the effects of radiation-induced cachexia by significantly increasing TBM (AgRP +0.2% vs. vehicle −2.3%) and food intake (AgRP 16.3% vs. vehicle 70.9% of nonirradiated mice; Joppa et al., 2007). No other experiments using antagonism of MC4R have been studied using a model of either cisplatin or radiation.

8. SUMMARY OF TREATMENT EFFECTS

Overall, ghrelin and ghrelin mimetics increase food consumption, TBM, and LBM, suggesting that not only are the anorectic effects of cachexia alleviated, but the hormonal changes are also corrected. Except for the aberration of AIDS cachexia, FM is also increased, thus leading to the reassertion that ghrelin has anticatabolic effects as it relates to both fat and protein levels, most likely through modulation of proinflammatory cytokines. Even though ghrelin levels are physiologically increased in cachectic patients, ghrelin treatment improves multiple outcomes related to cachectic.

A similar output is seen in melanocortin antagonists, though it is not as well studied; however, food consumption, TBM, LBM, and FM are generally increased. While MC4R antagonists have not been extensively evaluated for their effects on inflammation, one group reported a downstream anti-inflammatory response to MC4R agonists, raising this as a further desirable effect (Minutoli et al., 2011). Last, all MC4R studies have been performed in mouse and rat models; no human data exists.

9. FUTURE DIRECTIONS

Antagonism of the central melanocortin system may be a powerful therapy in the alleviation of cachectic symptoms. This appears to be particularly true in using ghrelin and other GHS-1a agonists, though it may also be true using MC4R agonists should clinical studies confirm basic science models of cachexia (DeBoer, 2007). In the case of ghrelin agonists, early work has been instructive in characterizing the effects of ghrelin in disease and further publications have shown the effect and safety of potential routes of treatment in both animal and human models. One side effect noted at a higher rate in treated individuals versus controls was gastrointestinal complaints, which warrants further study (DeBoer, 2008). Other studies have suggested potential reproductive effects of ghrelin treatment, including decreased testosterone levels (Barreiro & Tena-Sempere, 2004) and testes weight (Sirotkin et al., 2008) in the setting of ghrelin treatment in rats, a consequence which was exacerbated in the setting of food restriction (Sirotkin et al., 2008). Further research regarding these effects is still needed in the setting of treatment in cachexia in humans. Continuing this work to provide a more comprehensive picture on effects of ghrelin agonism would prove to be fruitful as a treatment for cachexia.

The future is much less clear regarding treatment using other direct antagonists of the central melanocortin system. Despite seemingly promising short-term results, studies of longer duration in rodent models are limited by ethical concerns surrounding the morbidity of cachectic animals. Thus, questions persist regarding tolerance- and potential-diminished efficacy of continued antagonism. At this point, the longest treatment in a study using melanocortin antagonism is 2 weeks.

The lack of published clinical trials regarding the efficacy of melanocortin antagonism in the setting of cachexia is also noteworthy (ClinicalTrials.gov., 2012b). If at some point safety were able to be assessed, these questions surrounding the safety of treated patients could not be immediately applied to a human model; for example, antagonism of MC4R could lead to drops in blood pressure (Greenfield et al., 2009).

As main components of cachexia include significant decreases in food intake, TBM, FM, and LBM, wasting can severely inhibit the body's capacity to survive. Thus far, MC4R antagonism has shown cautiously optimistic results regarding the reversal of the cachectic phenotype. A note of caution needs to be sounded because of the lack of studies in human disease models, even healthy subjects (ClinicalTrials.gov., 2012c), and the lack of long-term studies in laboratory models; the longest any pharmacological blockade was studied in mice was 16 days. On the brighter side, ghrelin is further along in its human efficacy and safety studies in cachectic patients and provides more short-term optimism regarding potential therapy. Both appetite regulation drugs seem to have a positive outlook on mitigating some of the harmful characteristics of cachexia. Further research in humans remains an important need.

REFERENCES

Adachi, S., Takiguchi, S., Okada, K., Yamamoto, K., Yamasaki, M., Miyata, H., et al. (2010). Effects of ghrelin administration after total gastrectomy: A prospective, randomized, placebo-controlled phase II study. *Gastroenterology*, *138*, 1312–1320.

Akashi, Y. J., Palus, S., Datta, R., Halem, H., Taylor, J. E., Thoene-Reineke, C., et al. (2009). No effects of human ghrelin on cardiac function despite profound effects on body composition in a rat model of heart failure. *International Journal of Cardiology*, *137*, 267–275.

Alvarez-Rodriguez, L., Lopez-Hoyos, M., Munoz-Cacho, P., & Martinez-Taboada, V. M. (2012). Aging is associated with circulating cytokine dysregulation. *Cellular Immunology*, *273*, 124–132.

Anker, S. (2006). European perspectives. *Circulation*, *113*, f53–f56.

Anker, S. D., Chua, T. P., Ponikowski, P., Harrington, D., Swan, J. W., Kox, W. J., et al. (1997). Hormonal changes and catabolic/anabolic imbalance in chronic heart failure and their importance for cardiac cachexia. *Circulation*, *96*, 526–534.

Anker, S. D., & Coats, A. J. (2002). How to RECOVER from RENAISSANCE? The significance of the results of RECOVER, RENAISSANCE, RENEWAL and ATTACH. *International Journal of Cardiology*, *86*, 123–130.

Anker, S. D., Egerer, K. R., Volk, H.-D., Kox, W. J., Poole-Wilson, P. A., & Coats, A. J. S. (1997). Elevated soluble CD14 receptors and altered cytokines in chronic heart failure. *The American Journal of Cardiology*, *79*, 1426–1430.

Anker, S. D., Ponikowski, P., Varney, S., Chua, T. P., Clark, A. L., Webb-Peploe, K. M., et al. (1997). Wasting as independent risk factor for mortality in chronic heart failure. *Lancet*, *349*, 1050–1053.

Anker, S. D., & Sharma, R. (2002). The syndrome of cardiac cachexia. *International Journal of Cardiology*, *85*, 51–66.

Ariyasu, H., Iwakura, H., Yamada, G., Nakao, K., Kangawa, K., & Akamizu, T. (2008). Efficacy of ghrelin as a therapeutic approach for age-related physiological changes. *Endocrinology*, *149*, 3722–3728.

Arques, S., & Ambrosi, P. (2011). Human serum albumin in the clinical syndrome of heart failure. *Journal of Cardiac Failure*, *17*, 451–458.

Arruda, A. P., Milanski, M., Romanatto, T., Solon, C., Coope, A., Alberici, L. C., et al. (2010). Hypothalamic actions of tumor necrosis factor α provide the thermogenic core for the wastage syndrome in cachexia. *Endocrinology*, *151*, 683–694.

Asakawa, A., Inui, A., Kaga, T., Katsuura, G., Fujimiya, M., Fujino, M. A., et al. (2003). Antagonism of ghrelin receptor reduces food intake and body weight gain in mice. *Gut*, *52*, 947–952.

Ashby, D. R., Ford, H. E., Wynne, K. J., Wren, A. M., Murphy, K. G., Busbridge, M., et al. (2009). Sustained appetite improvement in malnourished dialysis patients by daily ghrelin treatment. *Kidney International, 76*, 199–206.

Asher, V., Lee, J., & Bali, A. (2011). Preoperative serum albumin is an independent prognostic predictor of survival in ovarian cancer. *Medical Oncology (Northwood, London, England), 29*, 2005–2009.

Ashitani, J.-i, Matsumoto, N., & Nakazato, M. (2009). Ghrelin and its therapeutic potential for cachectic patients. *Peptides, 30*, 1951–1956.

Ates, Y., Degertekin, B., Erdil, A., Yaman, H., & Dagalp, K. (2008). Serum ghrelin levels in inflammatory bowel disease with relation to disease activity and nutritional status. *Digestive Diseases and Sciences, 53*, 2215–2221.

Balasubramaniam, A., Joshi, R., Su, C., Friend, L. A., Sheriff, S., Kagan, R. J., et al. (2009). Ghrelin inhibits skeletal muscle protein breakdown in rats with thermal injury through normalizing elevated expression of E3 ubiquitin ligases MuRF1 and MAFbx. *American Journal of Physiology—Regulatory, Integrative and Comparative Physiology, 296*, R893–R901.

Balasubramaniam, A., Wood, S., Joshi, R., Su, C., Friend, L. A., Sheriff, S., et al. (2006). Ghrelin stimulates food intake and growth hormone release in rats with thermal injury: Synthesis of ghrelin. *Peptides, 27*, 1624–1631.

Barber, M. D., Fearon, K. C., Tisdale, M. J., McMillan, D. C., & Ross, J. A. (2001). Effect of a fish oil-enriched nutritional supplement on metabolic mediators in patients with pancreatic cancer cachexia. *Nutrition and Cancer, 40*, 118–124.

Barber, M. D., Preston, T., McMillan, D. C., Slater, C., Ross, J. A., & Fearon, K. C. (2004). Modulation of the liver export protein synthetic response to feeding by an n-3 fatty-acid-enriched nutritional supplement is associated with anabolism in cachectic cancer patients. *Clinical Science (London, England), 106*, 359–364.

Barreiro, M. L., & Tena-Sempere, M. (2004). Ghrelin and reproduction: A novel signal linking energy status and fertility? *Molecular and Cellular Endocrinology, 226*, 1–9.

Baumann, H., & Gauldie, J. (1994). The acute phase response. *Immunology Today, 15*, 74–80.

Beberashvili, I., Sinuani, I., Azar, A., Yasur, H., Feldman, L., Averbukh, Z., et al. (2011). Longitudinal study of leptin levels in chronic hemodialysis patients. *Nutrition Journal, 10*, 68.

Bennani-Baiti, N., & Davis, M. P. (2008). Cytokines and cancer anorexia cachexia syndrome. *The American Journal of Hospice & Palliative Care, 25*, 407–411.

Berenstein, E. G., & Ortiz, Z. (2005). Megestrol acetate for the treatment of anorexia-cachexia syndrome. *Cochrane Database Systematic Reviews, 18*(2), CD004310.

Bergstrom, J. (1995). Why are dialysis patients malnourished? *American Journal of Kidney Diseases: The Official Journal of the National Kidney Foundation, 26*, 229–241.

Blaha, V., Yang, Z. J., Meguid, M. M., Chai, J. K., Oler, A., & Zadak, Z. (1998). Ventromedial nucleus of hypothalamus is related to the development of cancer-induced anorexia: in vivo microdialysis study. *Acta Medica (Hradec Kralove)/Universitas Carolina, Facultas Medica Hradec Kralove, 41*, 3–11.

Bober, L. A., Rojas-Triana, A., Jackson, J. V., Leach, M. W., Manfra, D., Narula, S. K., et al. (2000). Regulatory effects of interleukin-4 and interleukin-10 on human neutrophil function ex vivo and on neutrophil influx in a rat model of arthritis. *Arthritis and Rheumatism, 43*, 2660–2667.

Bossola, M., Tazza, L., Giungi, S., & Luciani, G. (2006). Anorexia in hemodialysis patients: An update. *Kidney International, 70*, 417–422.

Braissant, O., Foufelle, F., Scotto, C., Dauça, M., & Wahli, W. (1996). Differential expression of peroxisome proliferator-activated receptors (PPARs): Tissue distribution of PPAR-alpha, -beta, and -gamma in the adult rat. *Endocrinology, 137*, 354–366.

Buscher, A. K., Buscher, R., Hauffa, B. P., & Hoyer, P. F. (2010). Alterations in appetite-regulating hormones influence protein-energy wasting in pediatric patients with chronic kidney disease. *Pediatric Nephrology (Berlin, Germany)*, *25*, 2295–2301.

Butler, A. A., & Cone, R. D. (2002). The melanocortin receptors: Lessons from knockout models. *Neuropeptides*, *36*, 77–84.

Cannon, T., Couch, M., Yin, X., Guttridge, D., Lai, V., & Shores, C. (2007). Comparison of animal models for head and neck cancer cachexia. *The Laryngoscope*, *117*, 2152–2158.

Carrero, J. J., Nakashima, A., Qureshi, A. R., Lindholm, B., Heimburger, O., Barany, P., et al. (2011). Protein-energy wasting modifies the association of ghrelin with inflammation, leptin, and mortality in hemodialysis patients. *Kidney International*, *79*, 749–756.

Carroll, G., Bell, M., Wang, H., Chapman, H., & Mills, J. (1998). Antagonism of the IL-6 cytokine subfamily—A potential strategy for more effective therapy in rheumatoid arthritis. *Inflammation Research: Official Journal of the European Histamine Research Society ... [et al.]*, *47*, 1–7.

Carson, J. A., & Baltgalvis, K. A. (2010). Interleukin 6 as a Key regulator of muscle mass during cachexia. *Exercise and Sport Sciences Reviews*, *38*, 168–176.

Chance, W. T., Balasubramaniam, A., Dayal, R., Brown, J., & Fischer, J. E. (1994). Hypothalamic concentration and release of neuropeptide Y into microdialysates is reduced in anorectic tumor-bearing rats. *Life Sciences*, *54*, 1869–1874.

Chen, M.-C., Chang, H.-W., Wu, C.-J., Yang, C.-H., Yu, T.-H., Chen, C.-J., et al. (2005). Balance between plasma levels of tumor necrosis factor-[alpha] and interleukin-10 in rheumatic mitral stenosis. *Cardiology*, *104*, 171–175.

Chen, C., Tucci, F. C., Jiang, W., Tran, J. A., Fleck, B. A., Hoare, S. R., et al. (2008). Pharmacological and pharmacokinetic characterization of 2-piperazine-α-isopropyl benzylamine derivatives as melanocortin-4 receptor antagonists. *Bioorganic & Medicinal Chemistry*, *16*, 5606–5618.

Cheung, C. C., Clifton, D. K., & Steiner, R. A. (1997). Proopiomelanocortin neurons are direct targets for leptin in the hypothalamus. *Endocrinology*, *138*, 4489–4492.

Cheung, W. W., Kuo, H.-J., Markison, S., Chen, C., Foster, A. C., Marks, D. L., et al. (2007). Peripheral administration of the melanocortin-4 receptor antagonist NBI-12i ameliorates uremia-associated cachexia in mice. *Journal of the American Society of Nephrology*, *18*, 2517–2524.

Cheung, W. W., Rosengren, S., Boyle, D. L., & Mak, R. H. (2008). Modulation of melanocortin signaling ameliorates uremic cachexia. *Kidney International*, *74*, 180–186.

Cheung, W., Yu, P. X., Little, B. M., Cone, R. D., Marks, D. L., & Mak, R. H. (2005). Role of leptin and melanocortin signaling in uremia-associated cachexia. *The Journal of Clinical Investigation*, *115*, 1659–1665.

Cheunsuang, O., & Morris, R. (2005). Astrocytes in the arcuate nucleus and median eminence that take up a fluorescent dye from the circulation express leptin receptors and neuropeptide Y Y1 receptors. *Glia*, *52*, 228–233.

Chopin, L., Walpole, C., Seim, I., Cunningham, P., Murray, R., Whiteside, E., et al. (2011). Ghrelin and cancer. *Molecular and Cellular Endocrinology*, *340*, 65–69.

Choy, E. H. S., & Panayi, G. S. (2001). Cytokine pathways and joint inflammation in rheumatoid arthritis. *The New England Journal of Medicine*, *344*, 907–916.

Chung, E. S., Packer, M., Lo, K. H., Fasanmade, A. A., Willerson, J. T., & Anti, T. N. F. T. A. C. H. F. I. (2003). Randomized, double-blind, placebo-controlled, pilot trial of infliximab, a chimeric monoclonal antibody to tumor necrosis factor-alpha, in patients with moderate-to-severe heart failure: Results of the anti-TNF therapy against congestive heart failure (ATTACH) trial. *Circulation*, *107*, 3133–3140.

ClinicalTrials.gov. (2012a). Search of: Cachexia LIF—Search Details—ClinicalTrials.gov.

ClinicalTrials.gov. (2012b). Search of: Cachexia melanocortin—Search Details—ClinicalTrials.gov.

ClinicalTrials.gov. (2012c). Search of: Melanocortin 4 receptor antagonist—Search Details—ClinicalTrials.gov.

Cone, R. D. (2005). Anatomy and regulation of the central melanocortin system. *Nature Neuroscience*, *8*, 571–578.

Connolly, H. M., Crary, J. L., McGoon, M. D., Hensrud, D. D., Edwards, B. S., Edwards, W. D., et al. (1997). Valvular heart disease associated with fenfluramine–Phentermine. *The New England Journal of Medicine*, *337*, 581–588.

Cornish, J., Callon, K., King, A., Edgar, S., & Reid, I. R. (1993). The effect of leukemia inhibitory factor on bone in vivo. *Endocrinology*, *132*, 1359–1366.

Cowley, M. A., Pronchuk, N., Fan, W., Dinulescu, D. M., Colmers, W. F., & Cone, R. D. (1999). Integration of NPY, AGRP, and melanocortin signals in the hypothalamic paraventricular nucleus: Evidence of a cellular basis for the adipostat. *Neuron*, *24*, 155–163.

Cowley, M. A., Smart, J. L., Rubinstein, M., Cerdan, M. G., Diano, S., Horvath, T. L., et al. (2001). Leptin activates anorexigenic POMC neurons through a neural network in the arcuate nucleus. *Nature*, *411*, 480–484.

Cowley, M. A., Smith, R. G., Diano, S., Tschop, M., Pronchuk, N., Grove, K. L., et al. (2003). The distribution and mechanism of action of ghrelin in the CNS demonstrates a novel hypothalamic circuit regulating energy homeostasis. *Neuron*, *37*, 649–661.

Cui, R. J., Li, X., & Appleyard, S. M. (2011). Ghrelin inhibits visceral afferent activation of catecholamine neurons in the solitary tract nucleus. *The Journal of Neuroscience: The Official Journal of the Society for Neuroscience*, *31*, 3484–3492.

Cunningham, J. (1991). Body composition as a determinant of energy expenditure: A synthetic review and a proposed general prediction equation. *The American Journal of Clinical Nutrition*, *54*, 963–969.

Dalla Libera, L., Sabbadini, R., Renken, C., Ravara, B., Sandri, M., Betto, R., et al. (2001). Apoptosis in the skeletal muscle of rats with heart failure is associated with increased serum levels of TNF-α and sphingosine. *Journal of Molecular and Cellular Cardiology*, *33*, 1871–1878.

Dallmann, R., Weyermann, P., Anklin, C., Boroff, M., Bray-French, K., Cardel, B., et al. (2011). The orally active melanocortin-4 receptor antagonist BL-6020/979: A promising candidate for the treatment of cancer cachexia. *Journal of Cachexia Sarcopenia Muscle*, *2*, 163–174.

Dasu, M. R. K., Cobb, J. P., Laramie, J. M., Chung, T. P., Spies, M., & Barrow, R. E. (2004). Gene expression profiles of livers from thermally injured rats. *Gene*, *327*, 51–60.

Davis, M. P., Dreicer, R., Walsh, D., Lagman, R., & LeGrand, S. B. (2004). Appetite and cancer-associated anorexia: A review. *Journal of Clinical Oncology*, *22*, 1510–1517.

Deans, C., & Wigmore, S. J. (2005). Systemic inflammation, cachexia and prognosis in patients with cancer. *Current Opinion in Clinical Nutrition and Metabolic Care*, *8*, 265–269.

DeBoer, M. D. (2007). Melanocortin interventions in cachexia: How soon from bench to bedside? *Current Opinion in Clinical Nutrition and Metabolic Care*, *10*, 457–462. http://dx.doi.org/10.1097/MCO.1090b1013e328108f328441.

DeBoer, M. D. (2008). Emergence of ghrelin as a treatment for cachexia syndromes. *Nutrition*, *24*, 806–814.

DeBoer, M. D. (2010). Update on melanocortin interventions for cachexia: Progress toward clinical application (burbank, Los angeles county, calif.). *Nutrition*, *26*, 146–151.

DeBoer, M. D. (2011a). Ghrelin and cachexia: Will treatment with GHSR-1a agonists make a difference for patients suffering from chronic wasting syndromes? *Molecular and Cellular Endocrinology*, *340*, 97–105.

DeBoer, M. D. (2011b). Use of ghrelin as a treatment for inflammatory bowel disease: Mechanistic considerations. *International Journal of Peptides*, *2011*, 189242.

DeBoer, M. D., & Marks, D. L. (2006a). Cachexia: Lessons from melanocortin antagonism. *Trends in Endocrinology and Metabolism*, *17*, 199–204.

DeBoer, M. D., & Marks, D. L. (2006b). Therapy insight: Use of melanocortin antagonists in the treatment of cachexia in chronic disease. *Nature Clinical Practice, Endocrinology & Metabolism*, *2*, 459–466.

DeBoer, M. D., Scarlett, J. M., Levasseur, P. R., Grant, W. F., & Marks, D. L. (2009). Administration of IL-1beta to the 4th ventricle causes anorexia that is blocked by agouti-related peptide and that coincides with activation of tyrosine-hydroxylase neurons in the nucleus of the solitary tract. *Peptides*, *30*, 210–218.

DeBoer, M. D., Zhu, X., Levasseur, P. R., Inui, A., Hu, Z., Han, G., et al. (2008). Ghrelin treatment of chronic kidney disease: Improvements in lean body mass and cytokine profile. *Endocrinology*, *149*, 827–835.

DeBoer, M. D., Zhu, X. X., Levasseur, P., Meguid, M. M., Suzuki, S., Inui, A., et al. (2007). Ghrelin treatment causes increased food intake and retention of lean body mass in a Rat model of cancer cachexia. *Endocrinology*, *148*, 3004–3012.

Doering, J. E., Kane, K., Hsiao, Y.-C., Yao, C., Shi, B., Slowik, A. D., et al. (2008). Species differences in the expression of Ahi1, a protein implicated in the neurodevelopmental disorder joubert syndrome, with preferential accumulation to stigmoid bodies. *The Journal of Comparative Neurology*, *511*, 238–256.

Donovan, H. (1954). Malignant cachexia. *Proceedings of the Royal Society of Medicine*, *47*, 27–31.

Dutka, D. P., Elborn, J. S., Delamere, F., Shale, D. J., & Morris, G. K. (1993). Tumour necrosis factor alpha in severe congestive cardiac failure. *British Heart Journal*, *70*, 141–143.

Ersahin, M., Toklu, H. Z., Erzik, C., Akakin, D., Tetik, S., Sener, G., et al. (2011). Ghrelin alleviates spinal cord injury in rats via its anti-inflammatory effects. *Turkish Neurosurgery*, *21*, 599–605.

Esposito, J. G., Thomas, S. G., Kingdon, L., & Ezzat, S. (2004). Growth hormone treatment improves peripheral muscle oxygen extraction-utilization during exercise in patients with human immunodeficiency virus-associated wasting: A randomized controlled trial. *Journal of Clinical Endocrinology and Metabolism*, *89*, 5124–5131.

Esposito, J. G., Thomas, S. G., Kingdon, L., & Ezzat, S. (2005). Anabolic growth hormone action improves submaximal measures of physical performance in patients with HIV-associated wasting. *American Journal of Physiology—Endocrinology and Metabolism*, *289*, E494–E503.

Eylar, E. H., Lefranc, C., Baez, I., Colon-Martinez, S. L., Yamamura, Y., Rodriguez, N., et al. (2001). Enhanced interferon-[gamma] by CD8+ CD28- lymphocytes from HIV+patients. *Journal of Clinical Immunology*, *21*, 135–144.

Falconer, J. S., Fearon, K. C., Ross, J. A., Elton, R., Wigmore, S. J., Garden, O. J., et al. (1995). Acute-phase protein response and survival duration of patients with pancreatic cancer. *Cancer*, *75*, 2077–2082.

Fan, W., Boston, B. A., Kesterson, R. A., Hruby, V. J., & Cone, R. D. (1997). Role of melanocortinergic neurons in feeding and the agouti obesity syndrome. *Nature*, *385*, 165–168.

Farooqi, I. S., Keogh, J. M., Yeo, G. S. H., Lank, E. J., Cheetham, T., & O'Rahilly, S. (2003). Clinical spectrum of obesity and mutations in the melanocortin 4 receptor gene. *The New England Journal of Medicine*, *348*, 1085–1095.

Farooqi, I. S., Yeo, G. S., Keogh, J. M., Aminian, S., Jebb, S. A., Butler, G., et al. (2000). Dominant and recessive inheritance of morbid obesity associated with melanocortin 4 receptor deficiency. *The Journal of Clinical Investigation*, *106*, 271–279.

Fearon, K. C. H. (1992). The mechanisms and treatment of weight loss in cancer. *The Proceedings of the Nutrition Society*, *51*, 251–265.

Fearon, K. C., & Carter, D. C. (1988). Cancer cachexia. *Annals of Surgery*, *208*, 1–5.

Fearon, K. C., Von Meyenfeldt, M. F., Moses, A. G., Van Geenen, R., Roy, A., Gouma, D. J., et al. (2003). Effect of a protein and energy dense N-3 fatty acid enriched oral supplement on loss of weight and lean tissue in cancer cachexia: A randomised double blind trial. *Gut*, *52*, 1479–1486.

Fearon, K. C., Voss, A. C., Hustead, D. S., & Cancer Cachexia Study Group, (2006). Definition of cancer cachexia: Effect of weight loss, reduced food intake, and systemic inflammation on functional status and prognosis. *The American Journal of Clinical Nutrition*, *83*, 1345–1350.

Febbraio, M. A. (2007). gp130 Receptor ligands as potential therapeutic targets for obesity. *The Journal of Clinical Investigation*, *117*, 841–849.

Fiedler, R., Mall, M., Wand, C., & Osten, B. (2005). Short-term administration of omega-3 fatty acids in hemodialysis patients with balanced lipid metabolism. *Journal of Renal Nutrition*, *15*, 253–256.

Fouladiun, M., Korner, U., Bosaeus, I., Daneryd, P., Hyltander, A., & Lundholm, K. G. (2005). Body composition and time course changes in regional distribution of fat and lean tissue in unselected cancer patients on palliative care—Correlations with food intake, metabolism, exercise capacity, and hormones. *Cancer*, *103*, 2189–2198.

Frost, R. A., Nystrom, G. J., & Lang, C. H. (2009). Endotoxin and interferon-gamma inhibit translation in skeletal muscle cells by stimulating nitric oxide synthase activity. *Shock*, *32*, 416–426.

Garcia, J. M., Cata, J. P., Dougherty, P. M., & Smith, R. G. (2008). Ghrelin prevents cisplatin-induced mechanical hyperalgesia and cachexia. *Endocrinology*, *149*, 455–460.

Garcia, J. M., Garcia-Touza, M., Hijazi, R. A., Taffet, G., Epner, D., Mann, D., et al. (2005). Active ghrelin levels and active to total ghrelin ratio in cancer-induced cachexia. *The Journal of Clinical Endocrinology and Metabolism*, *90*, 2920–2926.

Garcia, J. M., & Polvino, W. J. (2007). Effect on body weight and safety of RC-1291, a novel, orally available ghrelin mimetic and growth hormone secretagogue: Results of a phase I, randomized, placebo-controlled, multiple-dose study in healthy volunteers. *The Oncologist*, *12*, 594–600.

Garcia, J. M., & Polvino, W. J. (2009). Pharmacodynamic hormonal effects of anamorelin, a novel oral ghrelin mimetic and growth hormone secretagogue in healthy volunteers. *Growth Hormone & IGF Research*, *19*, 267–273.

Gielen, S., Adams, V., Möbius-Winkler, S., Linke, A., Erbs, S., Yu, J., et al. (2003). Anti-inflammatory effects of exercise training in the skeletal muscle of patients with chronic heart failure. *Journal of the American College of Cardiology*, *42*, 861–868.

Gonzalez-Rey, E., Chorny, A., & Delgado, M. (2006). Therapeutic action of ghrelin in a mouse model of colitis. *Gastroenterology*, *130*, 1707–1720.

Greenfield, J. R., Miller, J. W., Keogh, J. M., Henning, E., Satterwhite, J. H., Cameron, G. S., et al. (2009). Modulation of blood pressure by central melanocortinergic pathways. *The New England Journal of Medicine*, *360*, 44–52.

Grossberg, A. J., Scarlett, J. M., Zhu, X., Bowe, D. D., Batra, A. K., Braun, T. P., et al. (2010). Arcuate nucleus proopiomelanocortin neurons mediate the acute anorectic actions of leukemia inhibitory factor via gp130. *Endocrinology*, *151*, 606–616.

Hahn, T. M., Breininger, J. F., Baskin, D. G., & Schwartz, M. W. (1998). Coexpression of agrp and NPY in fasting-activated hypothalamic neurons. *Nature Neuroscience*, *1*, 271–272.

Hamilton, J. A., Waring, P. M., & Filonzi, E. L. (1993). Induction of leukemia inhibitory factor in human synovial fibroblasts by IL-1 and tumor necrosis factor-alpha. *Journal of Immunology (Baltimore, Md.: 1950)*, *150*, 1496–1502.

Hanada, T., Toshinai, K., Kajimura, N., Nara-Ashizawa, N., Tsukada, T., Hayashi, Y., et al. (2003). Anti-cachectic effect of ghrelin in nude mice bearing human melanoma cells. *Biochemical and Biophysical Research Communications*, *301*, 275–279.

Haugen, E., Tang, M. S., Isic, A., Andersson, B., & Fu, M. (2008). TNF alpha antagonist upregulates interleukin-6 in rats with hypertensive heart failure. *International Journal of Cardiology*, *130*, 64–68.

Heisler, L. K., Cowley, M. A., Kishi, T., Tecott, L. H., Fan, W. E. I., Low, M. J., et al. (2003). Central serotonin and melanocortin pathways regulating energy homeostasis. *Annals of the New York Academy of Sciences*, *994*, 169–174.

Heisler, L. K., Cowley, M. A., Tecott, L. H., Fan, W., Low, M. J., Smart, J. L., et al. (2002). Activation of central melanocortin pathways by fenfluramine. *Science*, *297*, 609–611.

Huang, Q. H., Hruby, V. J., & Tatro, J. B. (1999). Role of central melanocortins in endotoxin-induced anorexia. *The American Journal of Physiology*, *276*, R864–R871.

Huszar, D., Lynch, C. A., Fairchild-Huntress, V., Dunmore, J. H., Fang, Q., Berkemeier, L. R., et al. (1997). Targeted disruption of the melanocortin-4 receptor results in obesity in mice. *Cell*, *88*, 131–141.

Inui, A. (1999). Feeding and body-weight regulation by hypothalamic neuropeptides—Mediation of the actions of leptin. *Trends in Neurosciences*, *22*, 62–67.

Jatoi, A., Rowland, K., Loprinzi, C. L., Sloan, J. A., Dakhil, S. R., MacDonald, N., et al. (2004). An eicosapentaenoic acid supplement versus megestrol acetate versus both for patients with cancer-associated wasting: A north central cancer treatment group and national cancer institute of Canada collaborative effort. *Journal of Clinical Oncology: Official Journal of the American Society of Clinical Oncology*, *22*, 2469–2476.

Jiang, W., Tucci, F. C., Tran, J. A., Fleck, B. A., Wen, J., Markison, S., et al. (2007). Pyrrolidinones as potent functional antagonists of the human melanocortin-4 receptor. *Bioorganic & Medicinal Chemistry Letters*, *17*, 5610–5613.

Joppa, M. A., Gogas, K. R., Foster, A. C., & Markison, S. (2007). Central infusion of the melanocortin receptor antagonist agouti-related peptide (AgRP(83-132)) prevents cachexia-related symptoms induced by radiation and colon-26 tumors in mice. *Peptides*, *28*, 636–642.

Kadokami, T., Frye, C., Lemster, B., Wagner, C. L., Feldman, A. M., & McTiernan, C. F. (2001). Anti-tumor necrosis factor-α antibody limits heart failure in a transgenic model. *Circulation*, *104*, 1094–1097.

Karmiris, K., Koutroubakis, I. E., Xidakis, C., Polychronaki, M., Voudouri, T., & Kouroumalis, E. A. (2006). Circulating levels of leptin, adiponectin, resistin, and ghrelin in inflammatory bowel disease. *Inflammatory Bowel Diseases*, *12*, 100–105.

Kaysen, G. A., Rathore, V., Shearer, G. C., & Depner, T. A. (1995). Mechanisms of hypoalbuminemia in hemodialysis patients. *Kidney International*, *48*, 510–516.

Kerem, M., Ferahkose, Z., Yilmaz, U. T., Pasaoglu, H., Ofluoglu, E., Bedirli, A., et al. (2008). Adipokines and ghrelin in gastric cancer cachexia. *World Journal of Gastroenterology: WJG*, *14*, 3633–3641.

Kim, H. J., Kim, H. J., Yun, J., Kim, K. H., Kim, S. H., Lee, S.-C., et al. (2012). Pathophysiological role of hormones and cytokines in cancer cachexia. *Journal of Korean Medical Science*, *27*, 128–134.

Knoll, S., Zimmer, S., Hinney, A., Scherag, A., Neubauer, A., & Hebebrand, J. (2008). Val103Ile Polymorphism of the melanocortin-4 receptor gene (MC4R) in cancer cachexia. *BMC Cancer*, *8*, 85.

Kobayashi, K. (2001). Role of catecholamine signaling in brain and nervous system functions: New insights from mouse molecular genetic study. *The Journal of Investigative Dermatology. Symposium Proceedings*, *6*, 115–121.

Kodama, T., Ashitani, J.-I., Matsumoto, N., Kangawa, K., & Nakazato, M. (2008). Ghrelin treatment suppresses neutrophil-dominant inflammation in airways of patients with chronic respiratory infection. *Pulmonary Pharmacology & Therapeutics*, *21*, 774–779.

Kojima, M., Hosoda, H., Date, Y., Nakazato, M., Matsuo, H., & Kangawa, K. (1999). Ghrelin is a growth-hormone-releasing acylated peptide from stomach. *Nature, 402*, 656–660.

Konturek, P. C., Brzozowski, T., Engel, M., Burnat, G., Gaca, P., Kwiecien, S., et al. (2009). Ghrelin ameliorates colonic inflammation. Role of nitric oxide and sensory nerves. *Journal of Physiology and Pharmacology, 60*, 41–47.

Kosmiski, L. (2011). Energy expenditure in HIV infection. *The American Journal of Clinical Nutrition, 94*, 1677S–1682S.

Krakoff, J., Ma, L., Kobes, S., Knowler, W. C., Hanson, R. L., Bogardus, C., et al. (2008). Lower metabolic rate in individuals heterozygous for either a frameshift or a functional missense MC4R variant. *Diabetes, 57*, 3267–3272.

Lainscak, M., Podbregar, M., & Anker, S. D. (2007). How does cachexia influence survival in cancer, heart failure and other chronic diseases? *Current Opinion in Supportive and Palliative Care, 1*, 299–305.

Langhans, W. (2002). Peripheral mechanisms involved with catabolism. *Current Opinion in Clinical Nutrition and Metabolic Care, 5*, 419–426.

Larkin, M. (1998). Thwarting the dwindling progression of cachexia. *Lancet, 351*, 1336.

Laviano, A., Inui, A., Meguid, M. M., Molfino, A., Conte, C., & Rossi Fanelli, F. (2008). NPY and brain monoamines in the pathogenesis of cancer anorexia. *Nutrition, 24*, 802–805.

Le Goffic, R., Mouchel, T., Aubry, F., Patard, J.-J., Ruffault, A., Jegou, B., et al. (2002). Production of the chemokines monocyte chemotactic protein-1, regulated on activation normal T cell expressed and secreted protein, growth-related oncogene, and interferon-[gamma]-inducible protein-10 is induced by the Sendai virus in human and rat testicular cells. *Endocrinology, 143*, 1434–1440.

Lee, C. W., Lin, C. C., Lee, I. T., Lee, H. C., & Yang, C. M. (2010). Activation and induction of cytosolic phospholipase A(2) by TNF-alpha mediated through Nox2, MAPKs, NF-kappa B, and p300 in human tracheal smooth muscle cells. *Journal of Cellular Physiology, 226*, 2103–2114.

Levine, B., Kalman, J., Mayer, L., Fillit, H. M., & Packer, M. (1990). Elevated circulating levels of tumor necrosis factor in severe chronic heart failure. *The New England Journal of Medicine, 323*, 236–241.

Li, W. G., Gavrila, D., Liu, X., Wang, L., Gunnlaugsson, S., Stoll, L. L., et al. (2004). Ghrelin inhibits proinflammatory responses and nuclear factor-κB activation in human endothelial cells. *Circulation, 109*, 2221–2226.

Li, Y.-P., & Reid, M. B. (2001). Effect of tumor necrosis factor-[alpha] on skeletal muscle metabolism. *Current Opinion in Rheumatology, 13*, 483–487.

Li, G., Zhang, Y., Rodrigues, E., Zheng, D., Matheny, M., Cheng, K. Y., et al. (2007). Melanocortin activation of nucleus of the solitary tract avoids anorectic tachyphylaxis and induces prolonged weight loss. *American Journal of Physiology. Endocrinology and Metabolism, 293*, E252–E258.

Ling, P. R., Schwartz, J. H., & Bistrian, B. R. (1997). Mechanisms of host wasting induced by administration of cytokines in rats. *American Journal of Physiology—Endocrinology and Metabolism, 272*, E333–E339.

Liu, Y. L., Malik, N., Sanger, G., & Andrews, P. (2006). Ghrelin alleviates cancer chemotherapy-associated dyspepsia in rodents. *Cancer Chemotherapy and Pharmacology, 58*, 326–333.

Lundholm, K., Daneryd, P., Bosaeus, I., Körner, U., & Lindholm, E. (2004). Palliative nutritional intervention in addition to cyclooxygenase and erythropoietin treatment for patients with malignant disease: Effects on survival, metabolism, and function. *Cancer, 100*, 1967–1977.

Lundholm, K., Gelin, J., Hyltander, A., Lönnroth, C., Sandström, R., Svaninger, G., et al. (1994). Anti-inflammatory treatment May prolong survival in undernourished patients with metastatic solid tumors. *Cancer Research, 54*, 5602–5606.

Lundholm, K., Gunnebo, L., Körner, U., Iresjö, B.-M., Engström, C., Hyltander, A., et al. (2010). Effects by daily long term provision of ghrelin to unselected weight-losing cancer patients. *Cancer, 116*, 2044–2052.

Madeddu, C., Dessì, M., Panzone, F., Serpe, R., Antoni, G., Cau, M. C., et al. (2012). Randomized phase III clinical trial of a combined treatment with carnitine + celecoxib ± megestrol acetate for patients with cancer-related anorexia/cachexia syndrome. *Clinical Nutrition, 31*, 176–182.

Madihally, S. V. P., Toner, M. P., Yarmush, M. L. M. D. P., & Mitchell, R. N. M. D. P. (2002). Interferon gamma modulates trauma-induced muscle wasting and immune dysfunction. *Annals of Surgery, 236*, 649–657.

Madison, L. D., & Marks, D. L. (2006). Anticatabolic properties of melanocortin-4 receptor antagonists. *Current Opinion in Clinical Nutrition and Metabolic Care, 9*, 196–200. http://dx.doi.org/10.1097/1001.mco.0000222099.0000236632.0000222081.

Mak, R. H., Cheung, W., Cone, R. D., & Marks, D. L. (2005). Orexigenic and anorexigenic mechanisms in the control of nutrition in chronic kidney disease. *Pediatric Nephrology (Berlin, Germany), 20*, 427–431.

Mak, R. H., Cheung, W., Cone, R. D., & Marks, D. L. (2006a). Leptin and inflammation-associated cachexia in chronic kidney disease. *Kidney International, 69*, 794–797.

Mak, R. H., Cheung, W., Cone, R. D., & Marks, D. L. (2006b). Mechanisms of disease: Cytokine and adipokine signaling in uremic cachexia. *Nature Clinical Practice. Nephrology, 2*, 527–534.

Mak, R. H., Cheung, W. W., Zhan, J. Y., Shen, Q., & Foster, B. J. (2012). Cachexia and protein-energy wasting in children with chronic kidney disease. *Pediatric Nephrology (Berlin, Germany), 27*, 173–181.

Maltoni, M., Nanni, O., Pirovano, M., Scarpi, E., Indelli, M., Martini, C., et al. (1999). Successful validation of the palliative prognostic score in terminally Ill cancer patients. *Journal of Pain and Symptom Management, 17*, 240–247.

Markison, S., Foster, A. C., Chen, C., Brookhart, G. B., Hesse, A., Hoare, S. R. J., et al. (2005). The regulation of feeding and metabolic rate and the prevention of murine cancer cachexia with a small-molecule melanocortin-4 receptor antagonist. *Endocrinology, 146*, 2766–2773.

Marks, D. L., Butler, A. A., Turner, R., Brookhart, G., & Cone, R. D. (2003). Differential role of melanocortin receptor subtypes in cachexia. *Endocrinology, 144*, 1513–1523.

Marks, D. L., Ling, N., & Cone, R. D. (2001). Role of the central melanocortin system in cachexia. *Cancer Research, 61*, 1432–1438.

McMurray, J., Abdullah, I., Dargie, H. J., & Shapiro, D. (1991). Increased concentrations of tumour necrosis factor in "cachectic" patients with severe chronic heart failure. *British Heart Journal, 66*, 356–358.

Melchior, J. C., Raguin, G., Boulier, A., Bouvet, E., Rigaud, D., Matheron, S., et al. (1993). Resting energy expenditure in human immunodeficiency virus-infected patients: Comparison between patients with and without secondary infections. *The American Journal of Clinical Nutrition, 57*, 614–619.

Metcalf, D., & Gearing, D. P. (1989). A myelosclerotic syndrome in mice engrafted with cells producing high levels of leukemia inhibitory factor (LIF). *Leukemia: Official Journal of the Leukemia Society of America, Leukemia Research Fund, UK, 3*, 847–852.

Metcalf, D., Nicola, N. A., & Gearing, D. P. (1990). Effects of injected leukemia inhibitory factor on hematopoietic and other tissues in mice. *Blood, 76*, 50–56.

Michalaki, V. (2004). The prognostic significance of serum levels of tumour necrosis factor-alpha and interleukin-6 and their association with cachexia in patients with prostate cancer. *Journal of Clinical Oncology, 22*, 4743.

Michie, H. R., Manogue, K. R., Spriggs, D. R., Revhaug, A., O'Dwyer, S., Dinarello, C. A., et al. (1988). Detection of circulating tumor necrosis factor after endotoxin administration. *The New England Journal of Medicine, 318*, 1481–1486.

Minutoli, L., Squadrito, F., Nicotina, P. A., Giuliani, D., Ottani, A., Polito, F., et al. (2011). Melanocortin 4 receptor stimulation decreases pancreatitis severity in rats by activation of the cholinergic anti-inflammatory pathway. *Critical Care Medicine, 39*, 1089–1096.

Mitch, W. (1998). Mechanisms causing loss of lean body mass in kidney disease. *The American Journal of Clinical Nutrition, 67*, 359–366.

Mori, T., Miyamoto, T., Yoshida, H., Asakawa, M., Kawasumi, M., Kobayashi, T., et al. (2011). IL-1beta and TNFalpha-initiated IL-6-STAT3 pathway is critical in mediating inflammatory cytokines and RANKL expression in inflammatory arthritis. *International Immunology, 23*, 701–712.

Moyle, G. J., Daar, E. S., Gertner, J. M., Kotler, D. P., Melchior, J.-C., O'Brien, F., et al. (2004). Growth hormone improves lean body mass, physical performance, and quality of life in subjects with HIV-associated weight loss or wasting on highly active antiretroviral therapy. *JAIDS Journal of Acquired Immune Deficiency Syndromes, 35*, 367–375.

Müller, M. J., Lautz, H. U., Plogmann, B., Bürger, M., Körber, J., & Schmidt, F. W. (1992). Energy expenditure and substrate oxidation in patients with cirrhosis: The impact of cause, clinical staging and nutritional state. *Hepatology, 15*, 782–794.

Nagaya, N., Itoh, T., Murakami, S., Oya, H., Uematsu, M., Miyatake, K., et al. (2005). Treatment of cachexia with ghrelin in patients with COPD. *Chest, 128*, 1187–1193.

Nagaya, N., Moriya, J., Yasumura, Y., Uematsu, M., Ono, F., Shimizu, W., et al. (2004). Effects of ghrelin administration on left ventricular function, exercise capacity, and muscle wasting in patients with chronic heart failure. *Circulation, 110*, 3674–3679.

Nagaya, N., Uematsu, M., Kojima, M., Date, Y., Nakazato, M., Okumura, H., et al. (2001a). Elevated circulating level of ghrelin in cachexia associated with chronic heart failure. *Circulation, 104*, 2034–2038.

Nagaya, N., Uematsu, M., Kojima, M., Date, Y., Nakazato, M., Okumura, H., et al. (2001b). Elevated circulating level of ghrelin in cachexia associated with chronic heart failure: Relationships between ghrelin and anabolic/catabolic factors. *Circulation, 104*, 2034–2038.

Nagaya, N., Uematsu, M., Kojima, M., Ikeda, Y., Yoshihara, F., Shimizu, W., et al. (2001). Chronic administration of ghrelin improves left ventricular dysfunction and attenuates development of cardiac cachexia in rats with heart failure. *Circulation, 104*, 1430–1435.

Nakazato, M., Murakami, N., Date, Y., Kojima, M., Matsuo, H., Kangawa, K., et al. (2001). A role for ghrelin in the central regulation of feeding. *Nature, 409*, 194–198.

Nass, R., Pezzoli, S. S., Oliveri, M. C., Patrie, J. T., Harrell, F. E., Jr., Clasey, J. L., et al. (2008). Effects of an oral ghrelin mimetic on body composition and clinical outcomes in healthy older adults: A randomized trial. *Annals of Internal Medicine, 149*, 601–611.

Naufel, M. F., Bordon, M., de Aquino, T. M., Ribeiro, E. B., & de Abreu Carvalhaes, J. T. (2010). Plasma levels of acylated and total ghrelin in pediatric patients with chronic kidney disease. *Pediatric Nephrology (Berlin, Germany), 25*, 2477–2482.

Neary, N. M., Small, C. J., Wren, A. M., Lee, J. L., Druce, M. R., Palmieri, C., et al. (2004). Ghrelin increases energy intake in cancer patients with impaired appetite: Acute, randomized, placebo-controlled trial. *Journal of Clinical Endocrinology and Metabolism, 89*, 2832–2836.

Nicholson, J. R., Kohler, G., Schaerer, F., Senn, C., Weyermann, P., & Hofbauer, K. G. (2006). Peripheral administration of a melanocortin 4-receptor inverse agonist prevents loss of lean body mass in tumor-bearing mice. *Journal of Pharmacology and Experimental Therapeutics, 317*, 771–777.

Nijenhuis, W. A. J., Oosterom, J., & Adan, R. A. H. (2001). AgRP(83–132) acts as an inverse agonist on the human-melanocortin-4 receptor. *Molecular Endocrinology, 15*, 164–171.

Ollmann, M. M., Wilson, B. D., Yang, Y.-K., Kerns, J. A., Chen, Y., Gantz, I., et al. (1997). Antagonism of central melanocortin receptors in vitro and in vivo by agouti-related protein. *Science, 278*, 135–138.

Palenicek, J. P., Graham, N. M., He, Y. D., Hoover, D. A., Oishi, J. S., Kingsley, L., et al. (1995). Weight loss prior to clinical AIDS as a predictor of survival. Multicenter AIDS Cohort Study Investigators. *Journal of Acquired Immune Deficiency Syndromes and Human Retrovirology: Official Publication of the International Retrovirology Association*, *10*, 366–373.

Palus, S., Schur, R., Akashi, Y. J., Bockmeyer, B., Datta, R., Halem, H., et al. (2011). Ghrelin and its analogues, BIM-28131 and BIM-28125, improve body weight and regulate the expression of MuRF-1 and MAFbx in a Rat heart failure model. *PLoS One*, *6*, e26865.

Paton, N. I., Newton, P. J., Sharpstone, D. R., Ross, H. M., Cotton, J., Calder, A. G., et al. (1999). Short-term growth hormone administration at the time of opportunistic infections in HIV-positive patients. *AIDS (London, England)*, *13*, 1195–1202.

Payne, C., Wiffen, P. J., & Martin, S. (2012). Interventions for fatigue and weight loss in adults with advanced progressive illness. *Cochrane Database of Systematic Reviews (Online)*, *1*, CD008427.

Peruhype-Magalhaes, V., Martins-Filho, O. A., Prata, A., Silva, L. De. A., Rabello, A., Teixeira-Carvalho, A., et al. (2006). Mixed inflammatory/regulatory cytokine profile marked by simultaneous raise of interferon-[gamma] and interleukin-10 and low frequency of tumour necrosis factor-[alpha] + monocytes are hallmarks of active human visceral leishmaniasis due to leishmania chagasi infection. *Clinical and Experimental Immunology*, *146*(1), 124–132.

Pinder, R. M., Brogden, R. N., Sawyer, P. R., Speight, T. M., & Avery, G. S. (1975). Fenfluramine: A review of its pharmacological properties and therapeutic efficacy in obesity. *Drugs*, *10*, 241–323.

Pittman, J. G., & Cohen, P. (1964). The pathogenesis of cardiac cachexia. *The New England Journal of Medicine*, *271*, 453–460.

Plata-Salamán, C. R., Oomura, Y., & Kai, Y. (1988). Tumor necrosis factor and interleukin-1β: Suppression of food intake by direct action in the central nervous system. *Brain Research*, *448*, 106–114.

Qureshi, A. R., Alvestrand, A., Divino-Filho, J. C., Gutierrez, A., Heimburger, O., Lindholm, B., et al. (2002). Inflammation, malnutrition, and cardiac disease as predictors of mortality in hemodialysis patients. *Journal of the American Society of Nephrology: JASN*, *13*(Suppl. 1), S28–S36.

Rajan, D., Wu, R., Shah, K. G., Jacob, A., Coppa, G. F., & Wang, P. (2012). Human ghrelin protects animals from renal ischemia-reperfusion injury through the vagus nerve. *Surgery*, *151*, 37–47.

Rammohan, M., Kalantar-Zadeh, K., Liang, A., & Ghossein, C. (2005). Megestrol acetate in a moderate dose for the treatment of malnutrition-inflammation complex in maintenance dialysis patients. *Journal of Renal Nutrition: The Official Journal of the Council on Renal Nutrition of the National Kidney Foundation*, *15*, 345–355.

Ramos, E. J., Suzuki, S., Marks, D., Inui, A., Asakawa, A., & Meguid, M. M. (2004). Cancer anorexia-cachexia syndrome: Cytokines and neuropeptides. *Current Opinion in Clinical Nutrition and Metabolic Care*, *7*, 427–434.

Rasic-Milutinovic, Z., Perunicic, G., Pljesa, S., Gluvic, Z., Sobajic, S., Djuric, I., et al. (2007). Effects of N-3 PUFAs supplementation on insulin resistance and inflammatory biomarkers in hemodialysis patients. *Renal Failure*, *29*, 321–329.

Reid, M. B., & Li, Y. P. (2001). Cytokines and oxidative signalling in skeletal muscle. *Acta Physiologica Scandinavica*, *171*, 225–232.

Rodriguez, A., Gomez-Ambrosi, J., Catalan, V., Becerril, S., Sainz, N., Gil, M. J., et al. (2010). Association of plasma acylated ghrelin with blood pressure and left ventricular mass in patients with metabolic syndrome. *Journal of Hypertension*, *28*, 560–567.

Scarlett, J. M., Bowe, D. D., Zhu, X., Batra, A. K., Grant, W. F., & Marks, D. L. (2010). Genetic and pharmacologic blockade of central melanocortin signaling attenuates cardiac cachexia in rodent models of heart failure. *Journal of Endocrinology*, *206*, 121–130.

Scarlett, J. M., Jobst, E. E., Enriori, P. J., Bowe, D. D., Batra, A. K., Grant, W. F., et al. (2007). Regulation of central melanocortin signaling by interleukin-1 beta. *Endocrinology, 148*, 4217–4225.

Scarlett, J. M., Zhu, X., Enriori, P. J., Bowe, D. D., Batra, A. K., Levasseur, P. R., et al. (2008). Regulation of agouti-related protein messenger ribonucleic acid transcription and peptide secretion by acute and chronic inflammation. *Endocrinology, 149*, 4837–4845.

Schambelan, M., Mulligan, K., Grunfeld, C., Daar, E. S., LaMarca, A., Kotler, D. P., et al. (1996). Recombinant human growth hormone in patients with HIV-associated wasting. *Annals of Internal Medicine, 125*, 873–882.

Schwartz, M. W. (2000). Central nervous system control of food intake. *Nature (London), 404*, 661.

Schwartz, M. W., Seeley, R. J., Woods, S. C., Weigle, D. S., Campfield, L. A., Burn, P., et al. (1997). Leptin increases hypothalamic pro-opiomelanocortin mRNA expression in the rostral arcuate nucleus. *Diabetes, 46*, 2119–2123.

Schwenke, D. O., Tokudome, T., Kishimoto, I., Horio, T., Shirai, M., Cragg, P. A., et al. (2008). Early ghrelin treatment after myocardial infarction prevents an increase in cardiac sympathetic tone and reduces mortality. *Endocrinology, 149*, 5172–5176.

Seoane, L. M., Lopez, M., Tovar, S., Casanueva, F. F., Senaris, R., & Dieguez, C. (2003). Agouti-related peptide, neuropeptide Y, and somatostatin-producing neurons are targets for ghrelin actions in the rat hypothalamus. *Endocrinology, 144*, 544–551.

Sethi, J. K., & Hotamisligil, G. S. (1999). The role of TNFα in adipocyte metabolism. *Seminars in Cell & Developmental Biology, 10*, 19–29.

Sheriff, S., Joshi, R., Friend, L. A., James, J. H., & Balasubramaniam, A. (2009). Ghrelin receptor agonist, GHRP-2, attenuates burn injury-induced MuRF-1 and MAFbx expression and muscle proteolysis in rats. *Peptides, 30*, 1909–1913.

Sheriff, S., Kadeer, N., Joshi, R., Friend, L. A., Howard James, J., & Balasubramaniam, A. (2012). Des-acyl ghrelin exhibits pro-anabolic and anti-catabolic effects on C2C12 myotubes exposed to cytokines and reduces burn-induced muscle proteolysis in rats. *Molecular and Cellular Endocrinology, 351*, 286–295.

Shevitz, A. H., Knox, T. A., Spiegelman, D., Roubenoff, R., Gorbach, S. L., & Skolnik, P. R. (1999). Elevated resting energy expenditure among HIV-seropositive persons receiving highly active antiretroviral therapy. *AIDS (London, England), 13*, 1351–1357.

Shiiya, T., Nakazato, M., Mizuta, M., Date, Y., Mondal, M. S., Tanaka, M., et al. (2002). Plasma ghrelin levels in lean and obese humans and the effect of glucose on ghrelin secretion. *Journal of Clinical Endocrinology and Metabolism, 87*, 240–244.

Shimizu, Y., Nagaya, N., Isobe, T., Imazu, M., Okumura, H., Hosoda, H., et al. (2003). Increased plasma ghrelin level in lung cancer cachexia. *Clinical Cancer Research: An Official Journal of the American Association for Cancer Research, 9*, 774–778.

Shinaberger, C. S., Kilpatrick, R. D., Regidor, D. L., McAllister, C. J., Greenland, S., Kopple, J. D., et al. (2006). Longitudinal associations between dietary protein intake and survival in hemodialysis patients. *American Journal of Kidney Diseases, 48*, 37–49.

Simons, J. P., Schols, A. M., Hoefnagels, J. M., Westerterp, K. R., ten Velde, G. P., & Wouters, E. F. (1998). Effects of medroxyprogesterone acetate on food intake, body composition, and resting energy expenditure in patients with advanced, nonhormone-sensitive cancer: A randomized, placebo-controlled trial. *Cancer, 82*, 553–560.

Sinno, M. H., Coquerel, Q., Boukhettala, N., Coëffier, M., Gallas, S., Terashi, M., et al. (2010). Chemotherapy-induced anorexia is accompanied by activation of brain pathways signaling dehydration. *Physiology & Behavior, 101*, 639–648.

Sirotkin, A. V., Chrenkova, M., Nitrayova, S., Patras, P., Darlak, K., Valenzuela, F., et al. (2008). Effects of chronic food restriction and treatments with leptin or ghrelin on different reproductive parameters of male rats. *Peptides, 29*, 1362–1368.

Soeki, T., Kishimoto, I., Schwenke, D. O., Tokudome, T., Horio, T., Yoshida, M., et al. (2008). Ghrelin suppresses cardiac sympathetic activity and prevents early left ventricular remodeling in rats with myocardial infarction. *American Journal of Physiology—Heart and Circulatory Physiology, 294*, H426–H432.

Sonti, G., Ilyin, S. E., & Plata-Salaman, C. R. (1996). Anorexia induced by cytokine interactions at pathophysiological concentrations. *The American Journal of Physiology, 270*, R1394–R1402.

Soriano-Guillén, L., Barrios, V., Campos-Barros, Á., & Argente, J. (2004). Ghrelin levels in obesity and anorexia nervosa: Effect of weight reduction or recuperation. *The Journal of Pediatrics, 144*, 36–42.

Springer, J., Filippatos, G., Akashi, Y. J., & Anker, S. D. (2006). Prognosis and therapy approaches of cardiac cachexia. *Current Opinion in Cardiology, 21*, 229–233. http://dx.doi.org/10.1097/1001.hco.0000221585.0000294490.0000221509.

Sreedhara, R., Avram, M. M., Blanco, M., Batish, R., & Mittman, N. (1996). Prealbumin is the best nutritional predictor of survival in hemodialysis and peritoneal dialysis. *American Journal of Kidney Diseases: The Official Journal of the National Kidney Foundation, 28*, 937–942.

Srisai, D., Gillum, M. P., Panaro, B. L., Zhang, X. M., Kotchabhakdi, N., Shulman, G. I., et al. (2011). Characterization of the hyperphagic response to dietary fat in the MC4R knockout mouse. *Endocrinology, 152*, 890–902.

Stanley, T., & Grinspoon, S. (2009). GH/GHRH axis in HIV lipodystrophy. *Pituitary, 12*, 143–152.

Stengel, A., Goebel, M., Wang, L., Reeve, J. R., Jr., Tache, Y., & Lambrecht, N. W. (2010). Lipopolysaccharide differentially decreases plasma acyl and desacyl ghrelin levels in rats: Potential role of the circulating ghrelin-acylating enzyme GOAT. *Peptides, 31*, 1689–1696.

Straburzynska-Migaj, E., Gwizdala, A., Siniawski, A., Ochotny, R., & Grajek, S. (2010). Leptin and inflammation in patients with chronic heart failure. *Kardiologia Polska, 68*, 1243–1247.

Strasser, F., Lutz, T. A., Maeder, M. T., Thuerlimann, B., Bueche, D., Tschop, M., et al. (2008). Safety, tolerability and pharmacokinetics of intravenous ghrelin for cancer-related anorexia/cachexia: A randomised, placebo-controlled, double-blind, double-crossover study. *British Journal of Cancer, 98*, 300–308.

Strassmann, G. (1993). Role of interleukin-6 in experimental cancer cachexia. *Journal of Immunotherapy, 13*, 73.

Strassmann, G., Fong, M., Kenney, J. S., & Jacob, C. O. (1992). Evidence for the involvement of interleukin 6 in experimental cancer cachexia. *The Journal of Clinical Investigation, 89*, 1681–1684.

Sutton, G. M., Josephine Babin, M., Gu, X., Hruby, V. J., & Butler, A. A. (2008). A derivative of the melanocortin receptor antagonist SHU9119 (PG932) increases food intake when administered peripherally. *Peptides, 29*, 104–111.

Suzuki, H., Hashimoto, H., Kawasaki, M., Watanabe, M., Otsubo, H., Ishikura, T., et al. (2011). Similar changes of hypothalamic feeding-regulating peptides mRNAs and plasma leptin levels in PTHrP-, LIF-secreting tumors-induced cachectic rats and adjuvant arthritic rats. *International Journal of Cancer, 128*, 2215–2223.

Swanson, L. W., & Sawchenko, P. E. (1980). Paraventricular nucleus: A site for the integration of neuroendocrine and autonomic mechanisms. *Neuroendocrinology, 31*, 410–417.

Szklarek-Kubicka, M., Fijalkowska-Morawska, J., Zaremba-Drobnik, D., Ucinski, A., Czekalski, S., & Nowicki, M. (2009). Effect of intradialytic intravenous administration of omega-3 fatty acids on nutritional status and inflammatory response in hemodialysis patients: A pilot study. *Journal of Renal Nutrition: The Official Journal of the Council on Renal Nutrition of the National Kidney Foundation, 19*, 487–493.

Takeda, H., Muto, S., Hattori, T., Sadakane, C., Tsuchiya, K., Katsurada, T., et al. (2010). Rikkunshito ameliorates the aging-associated decrease in ghrelin receptor reactivity via phosphodiesterase III inhibition. *Endocrinology, 151*, 244–252.

Takeda, R., Nishimatsu, H., Suzuki, E., Satonaka, H., Nagata, D., Oba, S., et al. (2006). Ghrelin improves renal function in mice with ischemic acute renal failure. *Journal of the American Society of Nephrology: JASN, 17*, 113–121.

Theander-Carrillo, C., Wiedmer, P., Cettour-Rose, P., Nogueiras, R., Perez-Tilve, D., Pfluger, P., et al. (2006). Ghrelin action in the brain controls adipocyte metabolism. *The Journal of Clinical Investigation, 116*, 1983–1993.

Thibault, R., Cano, N., & Pichard, C. (2011). Quantification of lean tissue losses during cancer and HIV infection/AIDS. *Current Opinion in Clinical Nutrition and Metabolic Care, 14*, 261–267.

Tisdale, M. J. (1997). Biology of cachexia. *Journal of the National Cancer Institute, 89*, 1763–1773.

Tisdale, M. J. (2006). Clinical anticachexia treatments. *Nutrition in Clinical Practice, 21*, 168–174.

Tisdale, M. J. (2009). Mechanisms of cancer cachexia. *Physiological Reviews, 89*, 381–410.

Tisdale, M. J. (2010). Cancer cachexia. *Current Opinion in Gastroenterology, 26*, 146–151.

Torre-Amione, G., Kapadia, S., Benedict, C., Oral, H., Young, J. B., & Mann, D. L. (1996). Proinflammatory cytokine levels in patients with depressed left ventricular ejection fraction: A report from the studies of left ventricular dysfunction (SOLVD). *Journal of the American College of Cardiology, 27*, 1201–1206.

Torre-Amione, G., Kapadia, S., Lee, J., Durand, J.-B., Bies, R. D., Young, J. B., et al. (1996). Tumor necrosis factor-α and tumor necrosis factor receptors in the failing human heart. *Circulation, 93*, 704–711.

Torre-Amione, G., Stetson, S. J., Youker, K. A., Durand, J.-B., Radovancevic, B., Delgado, R. M., et al. (1999). Decreased expression of tumor necrosis factor-α in failing human myocardium after mechanical circulatory support: A potential mechanism for cardiac recovery. *Circulation, 100*, 1189–1193.

Toshinai, K., Mondal, M. S., Shimbara, T., Yamaguchi, H., Date, Y., Kangawa, K., et al. (2007). Ghrelin stimulates growth hormone secretion and food intake in aged rats. *Mechanisms of Ageing and Development, 128*, 182–186.

Tran, J. A., Jiang, W., Tucci, F. C., Fleck, B. A., Wen, J., Sai, Y., et al. (2007). Design, synthesis, in vitro, and in vivo characterization of phenylpiperazines and pyridinylpiperazines as potent and selective antagonists of the melanocortin-4 receptor. *Journal of Medicinal Chemistry, 50*, 6356–6366.

Tritos, N. A., Vicent, D., Gillette, J., Ludwig, D. S., Flier, E. S., & Maratos-Flier, E. (1998). Functional interactions between melanin-concentrating hormone, neuropeptide Y, and anorectic neuropeptides in the rat hypothalamus. *Diabetes, 47*, 1687–1692.

Trobec, K., von Haehling, S., Anker, S. D., & Lainscak, M. (2011). Growth hormone, insulin-like growth factor 1, and insulin signaling-a pharmacological target in body wasting and cachexia. *Journal of Cachexia Sarcopenia Muscle, 2*, 191–200.

Trop, M., Schintler, M., Spendel, S., & Stockenhuber, A. (2008). Unhealed wounds, hypoalbuminemia and cachexia in a burned child—Where is the limit? *Annals of Burns and Fire Disasters, 21*, 59–62.

Tsai, J.-S., Wu, C.-H., Chiu, T.-Y., Hu, W.-Y., & Chen, C.-Y. (2006). Symptom patterns of advanced cancer patients in a palliative care unit. *Palliative Medicine, 20*, 617–622.

Tschop, M., Smiley, D. L., & Heiman, M. L. (2000). Ghrelin induces adiposity in rodents. *Nature, 407*, 908–913.

Vernaglione, L., Cristofano, C., & Chimienti, S. (2008). Omega-3 polyunsaturated fatty acids and proxies of cardiovascular disease in hemodialysis: A prospective cohort study. *Journal of Nephrology, 21*, 99–105.

Vickers, S. P., Easton, N., Webster, L. J., Wyatt, A., Bickerdike, M. J., Dourish, C. T., et al. (2003). Oral administration of the 5-HT_{2C} receptor agonist, mCPP, reduces body weight gain in rats over 28 days as a result of maintained hypophagia. *Psychopharmacology*, *167*, 274–280.

Villiger, P. M., Geng, Y., & Lotz, M. (1993). Induction of cytokine expression by leukemia inhibitory factor. *The Journal of Clinical Investigation*, *91*, 1575–1581.

von Haehling, S., & Anker, S. D. (2010). Cachexia as a major underestimated and unmet medical need: Facts and numbers. *Journal of Cachexia Sarcopenia Muscle*, *1*, 1–5.

von Haehling, S., Stepney, R., & Anker, S. D. (2010). Advances in understanding and treating cardiac cachexia: Highlights from the 5th cachexia conference. *International Journal of Cardiology*, *144*, 347–349 2010 Elsevier Ireland Ltd, Netherlands.

Vos, T. J., Caracoti, A., Che, J. L., Dai, M., Farrer, C. A., Forsyth, N. E., et al. (2004). Identification of 2-{2-[2-(5-bromo-2- methoxyphenyl)-ethyl]-3-fluorophenyl}-4,5-dihydro-1H-imidazole (ML00253764), a small molecule melanocortin 4 receptor antagonist that effectively reduces tumor-induced weight loss in a mouse model. *Journal of Medicinal Chemistry*, *47*, 1602–1604.

Voss-Andreae, A., Murphy, J. G., Ellacott, K. L., Stuart, R. C., Nillni, E. A., Cone, R. D., et al. (2007). Role of the central melanocortin circuitry in adaptive thermogenesis of brown adipose tissue. *Endocrinology*, *148*, 1550–1560.

Wang, W., Andersson, M., Iresjo, B. M., Lonnroth, C., & Lundholm, K. (2006). Effects of ghrelin on anorexia in tumor-bearing mice with eicosanoid-related cachexia. *International Journal of Oncology*, *28*, 1393–1400.

Wang, H., Huang, Z., Huang, L., Niu, S., Rao, X., Xu, J., et al. (2012). Hypothalamic Ahi1 mediates feeding behavior through interaction with 5-HT2C receptor. *Journal of Biological Chemistry*, *287*, 2237–2246.

Wang, A. Y., Sea, M. M., Tang, N., Sanderson, J. E., Lui, S. F., Li, P. K., et al. (2004). Resting energy expenditure and subsequent mortality risk in peritoneal dialysis patients. *Journal of the American Society of Nephrology: JASN*, *15*, 3134–3143.

Wellhoner, P., Horster, R., Jacobs, F., Sayk, F., Lehnert, H., & Dodt, C. (2011). Intranasal application of the melanocortin 4 receptor agonist MSH/ACTH(4-10) in humans causes lipolysis in white adipose tissue. *International Journal of Obesity*, *36*, 703–708.

Weyermann, P., Dallmann, R., Magyar, J., Anklin, C., Hufschmid, M., Dubach-Powell, J., et al. (2009). Orally available selective melanocortin-4 receptor antagonists stimulate food intake and reduce cancer-induced cachexia in mice. *PLoS One*, *4*, e4774.

Whitaker, K. W., & Reyes, T. M. (2008). Central blockade of melanocortin receptors attenuates the metabolic and locomotor responses to peripheral interleukin-1β administration. *Neuropharmacology*, *54*, 509–520.

Wilson, B. D., Bagnol, D., Kaelin, C. B., Ollmann, M. M., Gantz, I., Watson, S. J., et al. (1999). Physiological and anatomical circuitry between agouti-related protein and leptin signaling. *Endocrinology*, *140*, 2387–2397.

Wisse, B. E., Frayo, R. S., Schwartz, M. W., & Cummings, D. E. (2001). Reversal of cancer anorexia by blockade of central melanocortin receptors in rats. *Endocrinology*, *142*, 3292–3301.

Wren, A. M., Small, C. J., Ward, H. L., Murphy, K. G., Dakin, C. L., Taheri, S., et al. (2000). The novel hypothalamic peptide ghrelin stimulates food intake and growth hormone secretion. *Endocrinology*, *141*, 4325–4328.

Wu, R., Dong, W., Zhou, M., Zhang, F., Marini, C. P., Ravikumar, T. S., et al. (2007). Ghrelin attenuates sepsis-induced acute lung injury and mortality in rats. *American Journal of Respiratory and Critical Care Medicine*, *176*, 805–813.

Wynne, K., Giannitsopoulou, K., Small, C. J., Patterson, M., Frost, G., Ghatei, M. A., et al. (2005). Subcutaneous ghrelin enhances acute food intake in malnourished patients who receive maintenance peritoneal dialysis: A randomized, placebo-controlled trial. *Journal of the American Society of Nephrology, 16*, 2111–2118.

Xu, Y., Jones, J. E., Kohno, D., Williams, K. W., Lee, C. E., Choi, M. J., et al. (2008). 5-HT2CRs expressed by Pro-opiomelanocortin neurons regulate energy homeostasis. *Neuron, 60*, 582–589.

Yamamoto, K., Takiguchi, S., Miyata, H., Adachi, S., Hiura, Y., Yamasaki, M., et al. (2010). Randomized phase II study of clinical effects of ghrelin after esophagectomy with gastric tube reconstruction. *Surgery, 148*, 31–38.

Yamashita, J.-i, & Ogawa, M. (2000). Medroxyprogesterone acetate and cancer cachexia: Interleukin-6 involvement. *Breast Cancer, 7*, 130–135.

Yang, Q., Berthiaume, F., & Androulakis, I. P. (2011). A quantitative model of thermal injury-induced acute inflammation. *Mathematical Biosciences, 229*, 135–148.

Yoshimoto, A., Mori, K., Sugawara, A., Mukoyama, M., Yahata, K., Suganami, T., et al. (2002). Plasma ghrelin and desacyl ghrelin concentrations in renal failure. *Journal of the American Society of Nephrology: JASN, 13*, 2748–2752.

Zhang, F., Basinski, M. B., Beals, J. M., Briggs, S. L., Churgay, L. M., Clawson, D. K., et al. (1997). Crystal structure of the obese protein leptin-E100. *Nature, 387*, 206–209.

CHAPTER NINE

The Influence of Estrogen Therapies on Bone Mineral Density in Premenopausal Women with Anorexia Nervosa and Amenorrhea

Jocelyn Lebow, Leslie Sim[1]
Department of Psychiatry and Psychology, Mayo Clinic, Rochester, Minnesota, USA
[1]Corresponding author: e-mail address: sim.leslie@mayo.edu

Contents

1. Introduction 244
2. Estrogen Therapy and Bone Mass 245
3. Potential Clinical Drawbacks of Estrogen Therapy for Patients with AN 246
4. Influence of Oral Contraceptives on Bone Mineral Density 247
5. Influence of Hormone Replacement Therapy on Bone Mineral Density 248
6. The Role of Insulin-Like Growth Factor 1 and Estrogen on Bone Mineral Density 251
7. Implications 252
   7.1 Future directions 255
   7.2 Conclusion 255
References 256

Abstract

Low bone mineral density is one of the primary risks of chronic amenorrhea, and the effects of potentially long-term menstrual disruption on bone mass are serious concerns for individuals with a past or current anorexia nervosa (AN) diagnosis. As such, estrogen therapies are frequently used to address amenorrhea associated with AN. A systematic review of the literature was conducted to examine the effectiveness of estrogen therapies on bone mineral density in women with amenorrhea. Data regarding the effectiveness of oral contraceptives were of low quality and mixed, with the majority of studies finding no benefit of these treatments on bone mineral density. Hormone replacement therapy findings were also mixed, though promising results were found in a study comparing transdermal administration of physiologic estrogen, delivered in developmentally sensitive incremental doses to placebo controls. Though this study suggests a possible role for estrogen therapies in addressing bone density loss in women with AN, in general, more studies are needed. Clinical drawbacks of using these therapies in the treatment of AN, including the loss of menses resumption as a clinical

ISSN 0083-6729
http://dx.doi.org/10.1016/B978-0-12-410473-0.00009-X

marker for weight and nutritional rehabilitation, must be considered in the decision to use estrogen therapies, particularly given the uncertain effectiveness of most of these treatments.

1. INTRODUCTION

Anorexia nervosa (AN) is a dangerous condition marked by extreme weight loss and malnutrition. An estimated 1.2 million Americans are afflicted with AN, a group that predominantly comprises adolescent and young adult females. Given that this disorder is so disproportionately diagnosed in premenopausal females, amenorrhea due to AN-related weight loss is a significant concern in the medical management of the disorder. Disrupted menstrual function is a particularly pervasive consequence of AN, with even after full recovery, only 35–86% of patients regaining normal weight status and menstrual function (Herzog, Keller, & Lavori, 1988; Strober, Freeman, & Morrell, 1997).

As low bone mineral density is one of the primary risks of chronic amenorrhea, the effects of potentially long-term menstrual disruption on bone mass are serious concerns for individuals with a past or current AN diagnosis. Further, given that adolescence is both a time of significant bone mass development, as well as the most common time for AN onset, effects of AN-related amenorrhea can be exponentially deleterious in this population. In fact, after controlling for duration of amenorrhea, women who have a history of adolescent AN have been found to have lower bone mass density in adulthood as compared with women who had adult AN (Biller et al., 1989).

Comparitive studies have further confirmed that patients with AN have significantly lower bone mineral density than normal controls (Rigotti, Nussbaum, Herzog, & Neer, 1984; Ward, Brown, & Treasure, 1997). On average, approximately 50% of adolescents with AN have bone mass density *Z*-scores lower than −1 at one site at least (Misra et al., 2004; Misra, Miller, et al., 2004). Further, AN patients have been found to have a significantly higher rate of bone fractures as compared to the general population (Rigotti, Neer, Skates, Herzog, & Nussbaum, 1991). Some studies estimate that more than 40% of patients with long-term anorexia will have fracturing as a result of their low weight status and related low bone density (Herzog et al., 1993).

2. ESTROGEN THERAPY AND BONE MASS

In general, research has shown that weight restoration and successful elimination of AN symptoms are the most effective interventions in eliminating further bone density reduction (e.g., Olmos et al., 2010). Results suggest, however, that not all bone loss is effectively reversed by weight gain and that residual deficits in bone mass density can persist even following full weight restoration and recovery (e.g., Misra et al., 2008, Olmos et al., 2010). Therefore, efforts have also been made to evaluate medical interventions that could potentially serve to increase bone accrual and minimize deleterious effects of prolonged amenorrhea relatively early in the treatment process, so as to decrease the chance of prolonged negative bone mass outcomes for AN patients.

Hypoestrogenic states are a major risk factor for reduced bone mineral density (Eriksen et al., 1988; Rigotti et al., 1984). As such, estrogen replacement therapies are frequently used to attempt to increase bone mass in amenorrheic patients with AN (Haberland, Seddick, Marcus, & Bachrach, 1995). Treatment with these therapies generally regulates or restarts menstruation, and therefore is thought to potentially have a similar restorative effect on bone mineral density.

Research into this hypothesized relationship between estrogen and bone mass, however, has been far from conclusive. Animal studies conducted with skeletally immature monkeys found lower bone mineral density in those treated with oral contraceptives as compared with untreated controls (Register, Jayo, & Jerome, 1997). Studies looking at the effects of estrogen therapy on the bone mass of both healthy and anorexic premenopausal women have also had mixed results (e.g., Grinspoon, Thomas, Miller, Herzog, & Klibanski, 2002; Strokosch, Friedman, Wu, & Kamin, 2006). Inconclusive and confusing findings may be a result of the fact that only a relatively few well-designed randomized controlled trials exist that look at the effect of estrogen therapies on bone mass. Assessment is further limited by the heterogeneity of these few studies. Trials differ with respect to participant characteristics: studies include subjects from a wide range of ages, often different from the ages at which the majority of bone density increases occur. Further, some studies compare amenorrheic and perimenopausal women. Studies also vary methodologically: delivery and dosage of estrogen therapy ranges, as well as overall length of treatment and follow-up. Finally, outcome measurement and variables differ as well, with different groups using highly different technologies to assess bone mineral density and compare bone mass at different sites.

3. POTENTIAL CLINICAL DRAWBACKS OF ESTROGEN THERAPY FOR PATIENTS WITH AN

The lack of clarity regarding the effectiveness of estrogen therapies on the treatment of amenorrhea is of particular concern given the potential drawbacks of using these interventions on patients with AN. Primarily of concern, in the treatment of AN resumption of regular menstruation is a valuable clinical marker, signifying weight restoration has progressed to a point sufficient for healthy functioning. Utilizing estrogen therapies to artificially induce menstruation eliminates this indicator and thus interferes with the clinician's ability to gauge treatment progress.

Further, medical intervention resulting in the resumption of menses can inadvertently serve to undermine one of the primary messages of AN treatment, namely, that weight restoration to the point where regular menstruation is possible without intervention is, and should be, the main goal of therapy. Part of the AN symptom profile is patients' denial regarding the gravity of their severe weight loss. Therefore, a "quick fix" for amenorrhea, one of the most objective signs that one's body is not functioning optimally, may interfere with the sense of urgency that should accompany efforts toward reversing malnourishment. The overall message that weight restoration and balanced nutrition are the best way to protect against bone loss may be weakened (Grinspoon et al., 2000). In this way, employing estrogen therapies as an intervention to offset bone loss may actually impede the treatment of patients with AN. Nevertheless, if a treatment has a robust effect on mitigating bone loss, some of these potential disadvantages could be tolerated.

To examine if there are benefits of estrogen therapies on bone mineral density to offset the potential drawbacks for patients with AN, we set out to review the literature, focusing on randomized controlled trials and prospective cohort studies of estrogen therapies of patients with AN and patients with amenorrhea due to other causes. We included studies of amenorrhea regardless of AN status due to the small number of studies that met criteria, as long as the participants did not have amenorrhea due to premature ovarian failure, perimenopause, or due to not having a uterus. If, as has been hypothesized, the bone mineral density deficits in patients with AN are due to the effects of amenorrhea, we would expect to see similar effects regardless of the etiology of the amenorrhea.

4. INFLUENCE OF ORAL CONTRACEPTIVES ON BONE MINERAL DENSITY

With regard to the effectiveness of estrogen therapy administered through oral contraceptives, there were five studies, including three RCTs and two prospective cohort studies (i.e., Golden et al., 2002; Grinspoon et al., 2002; Hergenroeder et al., 1997; Munoz-Calvo et al., 2007; Strokosch et al., 2006). Across the studies, oral contraceptives were dosed at 25–35 μg of ethinyl estradiol. Of these studies, one RCT (Hergenroeder et al., 1997) found evidence that oral contraceptives significantly improved bone mass density at the lumbar spine in a very small sample ($n=24$) of adolescent and young adult women. The medication did not have any beneficial effect, however, on hip bone mass. It is possible that the relatively brief duration of the study, which followed participants for only 1 year, was responsible for the lack of meaningful changes at the hip region (Hergenroeder et al., 1997). Authors posited that the greater amount of metabolic activity at the vertebrae, due to the larger percentage of trabecular bone as compared to the femoral neck, might explain why the earliest changes were seen at the spine (Hergenroeder et al., 1997).

These findings differed from those reported by other authors. Though Strokosch et al. (2006) found some increases in spine BMD at midpoint, these improvements were no longer significant by the end of the study. Similarly, other studies concluded that, in general, oral contraceptives were insufficient to reverse bone loss in either adolescent or young adult amenorrheic patients (e.g., Golden et al., 2002; Grinspoon et al., 2002; Munoz-Calvo et al., 2007; Strokosch et al., 2006). In both randomized controlled trials and prospective cohort studies, osteopenia was persistent and, in some cases, progressive.

Although most individual studies did not find a benefit, sample sizes were small, which may have obscured findings due to low power and decreased probability of finding significant treatment effects. In addition, relatively short measurement potentially served to artificially deflate outcome data (see Tables 9.2 and 9.3 for summaries of the quality of included RCTs and cohort studies). It is possible that, though during the course of the majority of these studies estrogen therapies were not effective, over longer measurement intervals and with larger samples, the treatments in question might be found to be more effective, particularly in protecting against additional bone loss.

5. INFLUENCE OF HORMONE REPLACEMENT THERAPY ON BONE MINERAL DENSITY

Three RCTs have evaluated the effectiveness of hormone replacement therapy (HRT) in the treatment of amenorrhea-related bone loss. HRT dosing and composition varied by study and are summarized in Table 9.1. Similar to the findings regarding oral contraceptives, these studies produced somewhat discrepant results.

One RCT of amenorrheic athletes without AN (Gibson, Mitchell, Reeve, & Harries, 1999) found some gains in bone mass at both the lumbar vertebrae and hip for participants dosed with HRT. These gains were not significant, though the study's small sample size ($n=34$) and a high rate of participant attrition, likely, significantly limited the study's power (Gibson et al., 1999). In contrast, other studies found no improvement in bone mass density, outside of that which was directly related to weight gain (Gordon et al., 2002; Warren, Miller, Olson, Grinspoon, & Friedman, 2005).

Another RCT compared HRT to oral contraceptives and a placebo condition in young adult women with AN (Klibanski, Biller, Schoenfeld, Herzog, & Saxe, 1995). Participants in all groups exhibited persistent osteopenia, leading the group to conclude that both forms of estrogen therapy were equally insufficient in preventing the progression of bone loss (Klibanski et al., 1995).

In an effort to address insulin-like growth factor-1 (IGF-1) suppressant effects of relatively high doses of estrogen used in previous studies, a recent RCT used low estrogen doses titrated to mimic normative pubertal increases in the hormone (Misra et al., 2011). Further, estrogen therapy was administered transdermally, a modality which has been shown to have little to no IGF-1 suppressive effect, as compared with oral contraceptives (Weissberger, Ho, & Lazarus, 1991). The group enrolled 110 anorexic patients, aged 12–18, as well as 40 normal-weight controls. As an additional safeguard against decreasing IGF-1 levels, estrogen was dosed according to developmental phase, with girls under 15 years old receiving incremental low doses of ethinyl estradiol (doses increased from 3.5 μg daily to 11.25 μg over 18 months), at a level calculated to simulate normative pubertal increases in estrogen levels. More mature teens, aged 15 and older, received a consistent 100-μg dose of estradiol and cyclic progesterone throughout the 18-month study (Misra et al., 2011).

Table 9.1 Description of studies

Author	Study design	Description of patients	Interventions	Type of control	Outcomes	Duration of follow-up
Gibson et al. (1999)	RCT	34 Middle and long distance Caucasian runners with amenorrhea and oligomenorrhea (18–35 years)	0.5–1 mg estriol/ 1–2 mg estradiol	No medication	Femoral neck and lumbar spine DXA	12 months
Golden et al. (2002)	Cohort	50 Adolescent and young adult females with AN (13–21 years)	Combined oral contraceptive with a preparation of between 25 μg and 35 μg ethinyl estradiol (EE)	No medication	Lumbar spine and femoral neck DXA	12 months
Gordon et al. (2002)	RCT	61 Women with AN (14–28 years)	20 μg EE and 0.1 mg levonorgestrel	DHEA	Lumbar spine, femoral neck, and total body DXA	12 months
Grinspoon et al. (2002)	RCT	60 Women with AN (18–38 years)	35 μg EE and 0.4 mg norethindrone	Placebo	Lumbar spine, femoral neck, radius, and total body DXA	9 months
Hergenroeder et al. (1997)	RCT	24 Caucasian women with hypothalamic amenorrhea or oligomenorrhea (14–28 years)	35 μg EE and 0.5–1 mg of norethindrone or 10 mg of medroxyprogesterone	Placebo matched to medroxyprogesterone regimen	Lumbar spine, femoral neck, and total body DXA	12 months

Continued

Table 9.1 Description of studies—cont'd

Author	Study design	Description of patients	Interventions	Type of control	Outcomes	Duration of follow-up
Klibanski et al. (1995)	RCT	48 Women with AN (16.3–42.5 years)	0.625 mg Premarin and 5 mg Provera	No medication	Spinal CT	18 months
Misra et al. (2011)	RCT	110 Girls with AN (12–18 years)	Transdermal 17β-estradiol (100-mg patch applied twice weekly)	Placebo patch	Lumbar spine, hip DXA	18 months
Munoz-Calvo et al. (2007)	Cohort	20 Women with AN (M age = 15.3, SD = 1.5 years)	35 μg EE	No medication	Lumbar spine DXA	12 months
Strokosch et al. (2006)	RCT	146 Adolescents with AN (11–17 years)	35 μg EE and 180–250 μg norgestimate (NGM)	Placebo	Lumbar spine and femoral neck DXA	13 months
Warren et al. (2005)	RCT	24 Amenorrheic dancers from a sample of 55 dancers (M age = 22, SD = 4)	0.625 mg Premarin and 10 mg Provera	Placebo	Lumbar spine, wrist, and foot DXA	24 months

Bone mass density at both the hip and spine of all the participants receiving the intervention was significantly increased as compared to placebo controls (Misra et al., 2011). These findings are extremely promising, given that they are more robust than those from previous studies. Further, IGF-1 levels in the intervention group were not significantly different from the placebo (Misra et al., 2011).

6. THE ROLE OF INSULIN-LIKE GROWTH FACTOR 1 AND ESTROGEN ON BONE MINERAL DENSITY

As highlighted in the Misra et al. study, which used a low dose of estrogen titrated to mimic puberty to reduce the IGF-1 suppressant effects of high doses of estrogen, it has been hypothesized that oral contraceptives may have an IGF-1 suppressive effect, which, in combination with the fact that IGF-1 is already depressed in an underweight population, potentially explains the small to negligible effectiveness of these therapies (Misra & Klibanski, 2011). Inconclusive and inconsistent findings might also be an indication that hypoestrogenism is not singularly responsible for amenorrhea-related osteopenia. The lack of effectiveness of conventional estrogen therapies seems to suggest the relationship between bone loss and menses is more complex than initially hypothesized. In particular, IGF-1, a nutritionally-dependent bone trophic hormone also known as somatomedin C, has been identified as a potential contributing factor. Recombinant IGF-1 therapy has been found to increase bone formation in adolescents, and decreased IGF-1 levels have been used as an indicator of low bone mass density in individuals with AN (e.g., Misra et al., 2009). In particular, adolescent and young adult women with anorexia typically have high levels of growth hormone (GH), concurrent with low levels of IGF-1 (Misra & Klibanski, 2011). Patients who are severely malnourished have been shown to develop a resistance to GH action, which contributes to a decrease in IGF-1, thus limiting collagen synthesis and bone development (Grinspoon et al., 2002). Although a complete discussion of the role and potential impact of IGF-1 was not a focus of these studies, and is thus beyond the scope of this chapter, several authors have offered speculation about the possible confounding influence of IGF-1 on the effectiveness of estrogen therapies on an amenorrheic population (e.g., Grinspoon et al., 2002; Misra et al., 2009, 2011).

Though one group (Gordon et al., 2002) found that HRT actually increased IGF-1 levels, these findings were not borne out by other studies.

Grinspoon et al. (2002) compared the influence of recombinant IGF-1 therapy both when administered alone and when given in conjunction with oral contraceptives, to an oral contraceptive-only group as well as a placebo control group. The group found that combined treatment of both estrogen therapy and IGF-1 had a small significant improvement in lean body mass (not weight) and bone mass density as compared to other treatments, and that IGF-1 alone was better than treatments without IGF-1 (Grinspoon et al., 2002).

Additional study is needed to clarify the relationship between estrogen therapy and IGF-1. However, the discrepant findings regarding the effects of estrogen therapies on amenorrhea suggest that the relationship between AN and osteopenia is a complex one, in which many different physiological factors potentially play a role. Other areas suggested for further examination include leptin, androgen levels, and other metabolic agents.

7. IMPLICATIONS

These trials represent the strongest findings on the effectiveness of estrogen therapy in increasing bone mass in premenopausal women with amenorrhea. In general, however, the quality of evidence from these studies is low, using the GRADE system of classification (Guyatt et al., 2006) (please refer to Tables 9.2 and 9.3 for a summary of the quality of included RCTs and cohort studies). Also of concern, side effects were rarely discussed in these studies. This oversight limits direct comparison of the benefits and costs of these treatments. Given the previously discussed clinical drawbacks, the decision to use estrogen therapies in the treatment of amenorrhea is one that must be based on sound provider and patient judgment and careful consideration of the broader psychosocial clinical picture. Specifically, patients and providers must weigh the advantage of maintaining resumption of menses as an indicator of optimal weight restoration against long-term bone health. In cases where patients have had a shorter course of amenorrhea, it may be clinically indicated to postpone or avoid estrogen therapy altogether. In the early stage of the illness, it has been established that there is a lower chance of severe bone loss and a higher chance of a positive overall prognosis with early intervention (Ward et al., 1997). For patients with a more chronic, treatment-resistant course of AN, however, estrogen therapy should remain a consideration, so as to decrease the deleterious and potentially long-term consequences for bone density.

Table 9.2 Quality of randomized control trials

Author	Allocation concealment	Participants blind	Participants blind	Providers blind	Data collectors blinded	% Lost to follow-up	Trial sponsor	Sponsor medicine	Sponsor personnel
Gibson et al. (1999)	No	No	No	No	Unclear	20.6	Not for profit	No	No
Gordon et al. (2002)	Yes	Yes	No	Yes	Yes	16.4	Not for profit	No	No
Grinspoon et al. (2002)	Yes	No	No	No	Yes	11.6	Not for profit	Yes	No
Hergenroeder et al. (1997)	Yes	No	No	No	Yes	13	Mixed	Yes	No
Klibanski et al. (1995)	Yes	No	No	No	Yes	8.3	Not for profit	No	No
Misra et al. (2011)	Yes	Yes	Yes	Yes	Yes	44.5	Not for profit	No	No
Strokosch et al. (2006)	Yes	Yes	No	Yes	Yes	27.6	For profit	Yes	Yes
Warren et al. (2005)	No	Yes	No	No	Yes	45.8	Mixed	Yes	No

Table 9.3 Quality of cohort studies

Author	Representativeness of exposed cohort	Selection of nonexposed cohort	Ascertainment of exposure	Comparability of cohorts	Outcome assessment	Outcome F/U	% Lost to follow-up	Trial sponsor	Sponsor provided study medicine	Sponsor provided study personnel
Golden et al. (2002)	Representative of the average patient with AN in the community	Drawn from a different source	No description	Study controls for body weight and duration of amenorrhea	No description	Adequate length of follow-up	14	Not reported	Not reported	Not reported
Munoz-Calvo et al. (2007)	Representative of the average patient with AN in the community	Drawn from the same community as the exposed cohort	No description	Study controls for BMI	No description	Adequate length of follow-up	0	Not reported	Not reported	Not reported

Consideration must also be given to the mode of delivery and dosage schedule for estrogen treatment. Promising findings from transdermal administration of physiologic estrogen, delivered in developmentally sensitive incremental doses, recommend further research on this method of delivery. Additional study regarding the limits to the external validity of these interventions is also indicated. In particular, the majority of these studies were conducted using subjects who were racially homogenous. As such, the applicability of these findings for noncaucasian patients is unclear.

Further research must also be conducted over longer follow-up periods. In general, studies reviewed here had relatively short measurement intervals, far shorter than average AN illness duration or the length of time during which most women use oral contraceptives. As was discussed, it is possible this limitation resulted in artificially lowered treatment effects. Future trials should use longer follow-up periods, to be more consistent with real-life application of estrogen therapies.

7.1. Future directions

In short, there is a need for additional large, well-designed randomized controlled trials of diverse patient populations with longer measurement intervals. Efforts should also be taken to minimize between-study methodological discrepancies in measurement tools and outcome variables. Finally, data collection should also include information on bone fractures, as this outcome is one that has significant practical value for patients. Access to this information would facilitate more meaningful conversations between clinicians and patients on the subject of estrogen therapies, and perhaps, increase overall compliance with the interventions.

7.2. Conclusion

In general, it appears that bone loss in the lumbar spine and hip regions in adolescents and young adult women with amenorrhea can be moderately well treated through estrogen therapy. Oral contraceptives and HRT appear to be more effective than placebo and no treatment. In particular, the use of incremental doses of estrogen delivered transdermally appears to be a promising new intervention option that may be superior to other estrogen therapies. However, conclusions are limited by the small amount of relatively low quality evidence that is available for all types of estrogen therapies. Larger, methodologically rigorous trials are needed to conclusively determine whether the benefits of using estrogen therapy are worth the clinical drawbacks of treating amenorrhea with medical interventions in patients with AN and amenorrhea due to other causes.

REFERENCES

Biller, B., Saxe, V., Herzog, D., Rosenthal, D., Holzman, S., & Klibanski, A. (1989). Mechanisms of osteoporosis in adult and adolescent women with anorexia nervosa. *The Journal of Clinical Endocrinology and Metabolism, 68*, 548–554.

Eriksen, E. F., Colvard, D. S., Berg, N. J., Graham, M. L., Mann, K. G., Spelsberg, T. C., et al. (1988). Evidence of estrogen receptors in normal human osteoblast like cells. *Science, 241*, 84–86.

Gibson, J. H., Mitchell, A., Reeve, J., & Harries, M. G. (1999). Treatment of reduced bone mineral density in athletic amenorrhea: A pilot study. *Osteoporosis International, 10*, 284–289.

Golden, N. H., Lanzkowsky, L., Schebendach, J., Palestro, C. J., Jacobson, M. S., & Shenker, L. R. (2002). The effect of estrogen-progestin treatment on bone mineral density in anorexia nervosa. *Journal of Pediatric and Adolescent Gynecology, 15*, 135–143.

Gordon, C. M., Grace, E., Emans, S., Feldman, H., Goodman, E., Becker, K., et al. (2002). Effects of oral dehydroepiandrosterone on bone density in young women with anorexia nervosa: A randomized trial. *The Journal of Clinical Endocrinology and Metabolism, 87*, 4935–4941.

Grinspoon, S., Thomas, E., Miller, K., Herzog, D., & Klibanski, A. (2002). Effects of recombinant human IGF-I and oral contraceptive administration on bone density in anorexia nervosa. *The Journal of Clinical Endocrinology and Metabolism, 87*, 2883–2891.

Grinspoon, S. K., Thomas, E., Pitts, S., Gross, E., Mickley, D., MIller, K., et al. (2000). Prevalence and predictive factors for regional osteopenia in women with anorexia nervosa. *Annals of Internal Medicine, 133*, 790–794.

Guyatt, G., Vist, G., Falck-Ytter, Y., Kunz, R., Magrini, N., & Schunemann, H. (2006). An emerging consensus on grading recommendations? *ACP Journal Club, 144*, A8–A9.

Haberland, C. A., Seddick, D., Marcus, R., & Bachrach, L. (1995). A physician survey of therapy for exercise associated amenorrhea: A brief report. *Clinical Journal of Sport Medicine, 5*, 246–250.

Hergenroeder, A. C., Smith, E. O. B., Shypailo, R., Jones, L. A., Klish, W. J., & Ellis, K. (1997). Bone mineral changes in young women with hypothalamic amenorrhea treated with oral contraceptives, medroxyprogesterone, or placebo over 12 months. *American Journal of Obstetrics and Gynecology, 176*, 1017–1025.

Herzog, D. B., Keller, M. B., & Lavori, P. W. (1988). Outcome in anorexia nervosa and bulimia nervosa: A review of the literature. *The Journal of Nervous and Mental Disease, 176*, 131–143.

Herzog, W., MInne, H., Deter, C., Leidig, G., Schellberg, D., Wuster, C., et al. (1993). Outcome ofbone mineral density in anorexia nervosa patients 11.7 years after first admission. *Journal of Bone and Mineral Research, 8*, 597–605.

Klibanski, A., Biller, B. M. K., Schoenfeld, D. A., Herzog, D. B., & Saxe, V. C. (1995). The effects of estrogen administration on trabecular bone loss in young women with anorexia nervosa. *The Journal of Clinical Endocrinology and Metabolism, 80*, 898–904.

Misra, M., Aggarwal, A., Miller, K., Almaxan, C., Worley, M., Soyka, L., et al. (2004). Effects of anorexia nervosa on clinical, hematologic, biochemical, and bone density parameters in community-dwelling adolescent girls. *Pediatrics, 114*, 1574–1583.

Misra, M., & Klibanski, A. (2011). The neuroendocrine basis of anorexia nervosa and its impact on bone metabolism. *Neuroendocrinology, 93*, 65–73.

Misra, M., Miller, K. K., Almazan, C., Ramaswamy, K., Lapcharoensap, W., Worley, M., et al. (2004). Alterations in cortisol secretory dynamics in adolescent girls with anorexia nervosa and effects on bone metabolism. *The Journal of Clinical Endocrinology and Metabolism, 89*, 4972–4980.

Misra, M., Prabhakaran, R., Miller, K., Goldstein, M., Mickley, D., Clauss, L., et al. (2008). Weight gain and restoration of menses as predictors of bone mineral density change in adolescent girls with anorexia nervosa-1. *The Journal of Clinical Endocrinology and Metabolism, 93*, 1231–1237.

Misra, M., McGrane, J., MIller, K., Goldstein, M., Ebrahimi, S., Weigel, T., et al. (2009). Effects of rhIGF-1 administration on surrogate markers of bone turnover in adolescents with anorexia nervosa. *Bone, 45*, 493–498.

Misra, M., Katzman, D., MIller, K., Mendes, N., Snelgrove, D., Russell, M., et al. (2011). Physiologic estrogen replacement increases bone density in adolescent girls with anorexia nervosa. *Journal of Bone and Mineral Research, 26*, 2430–2438.

Munoz-Calvo, M. T., Barrios, V., De Alvaro, M. T. G., Lefort, M., Mendez-Davila, C., Argente, J., et al. (2007). Maintained malnutrition produces a progressive decrease in (OPG)/RANKL ratio and leptin levels in patients with anorexia nervosa. *Scandinavian Journal of Clinical and Laboratory Investigation, 67*, 387–393.

Olmos, J. M., Valero, C., Gomez del Barrio, A., Amado, J., Hernandez, J., Menendez-Arango, J., et al. (2010). Time course of bone loss in patients with anorexia nervosa. *The International Journal of Eating Disorders, 43*, 537–542.

Register, T. C., Jayo, M. J., & Jerome, C. P. (1997). Oral contraceptive treatment inhibits the normal acquisition of bone mineral in skeletally immature young adult female monkeys. *Osteoporosis International*, 7, 348–353.

Rigotti, N. A., Neer, R. M., Skates, S. J., Herzog, D. B., & Nussbaum, S. R. (1991). The clinical course of osteoporosis in anorexia nervosa. *Journal of the American Medical Association, 265*, 1133–1138.

Rigotti, N. A., Nussbaum, S. R., Herzog, D. B., & Neer, R. M. (1984). Osteoporosis in women with anorexia nervosa. *The New England Journal of Medicine, 311*, 1601–1606.

Strober, M., Freeman, R., & Morrell, W. (1997). The long-term course of severe anorexia nervosa in adolescents: Survival of recovery, relapse, and outcome predictors over 10-15 years in a prospective study. *The International Journal of Eating Disorders, 22*, 339–360.

Strokosch, G. R., Friedman, A. J., Wu, S. C., & Kamin, M. (2006). Effects of an oral contraceptive (norgestimate/ethinyl estradiol) on bone mineral density in adolescent females with anorexia nervosa: A double-blind, placebo-controlled study. *The Journal of Adolescent Health, 39*, 819–827.

Ward, A., Brown, J., & Treasure, J. (1997). Persistent osteopenia after recovery from anorexia nervosa. *The International Journal of Eating Disorders, 22*, 71–75.

Warren, M. P., Miller, K. K., Olson, W. H., Grinspoon, S. K., & Friedman, A. J. (2005). Effects of an oral contraceptive (norgestimate/ethinyl estradiol) on bone mineral density in women with hypothalamic amenorrhea and osteopenia: An open-label extension of a double-blind, placebo-controlled study. *Contraception, 72*, 206–211.

Weissberger, A. J., Ho, K. K., & Lazarus, L. (1991). Contrasting effects of oral and transdermal routes of estrogen replacement therapy on 24-hour growth hormone (GH) secretion, insulin-like growth factor 1, and GH-binding protein in postmenopausal women. *The Journal of Clinical Endocrinology and Metabolism, 72*, 374–381.

CHAPTER TEN

Clinical and Hormonal Variables Related to Bone Mass Loss in Anorexia Nervosa Patients

María Luisa Fernández-Soto[*,1], **Amalia González-Jiménez**[†], **Marta Chamorro-Fernández**[‡], **Socorro Leyva-Martínez**[*]

[*]Eating Disorders Unit, Department of Endocrinology and Clinical Nutrition, University Hospital San Cecilio, Granada, Spain
[†]Department of Medicine, University of Granada, Granada, Spain
[‡]Department of Psychiatry, University Hospital Carlos Haya, Málaga, Spain
[1]Corresponding author: e-mail address: mlfernan@ugr.es; marisafsoto@gmail.com

Contents

1. Introduction 260
2. Materials and Methods 261
   2.1 Subject selection 261
   2.2 Experimental protocol 261
   2.3 Biochemical assessment 262
   2.4 Statistical analysis 262
3. Results 263
4. Discussion 265
Acknowledgments 267
References 267

Abstract

A better understanding of the prognostic factors of low bone mass in anorexia nervosa (AN) and development of effective therapeutic strategies is critical. In order to determine which clinical, biochemical, and/or hormonal parameters could be related to bone mineral density (BMD), 47 female AN patients were classified according to the WHO osteoporosis criteria at lumbar spine (LS). This was a cross-sectional study of 16 AN women with osteoporosis criteria and 31without. Control group was 25 healthy, normal-weight, age-matched women. We assessed BMD using dual-energy X-ray absorptiometry at the LS and body composition. We measured serum fasting cortisol, estradiol, insulin-like growth factor-1 (IGF-1), leptin, sex hormone-binding globulin, albumin and retinol binding protein levels. The prevalence of osteoporosis was 34% and osteopenia 19% at the LS. The AN group with osteoporosis had lower IGF-1 and estradiol levels (both $p<0.001$), lower serum leptin ($p<0.02$), and higher cortisolemia ($p<0.03$) levels compared with AN group without osteoporosis. The BMD and *T*-score at LS was inversely related to the duration of amenorrhea ($p<0.02$) and directly related

ISSN 0083-6729
http://dx.doi.org/10.1016/B978-0-12-410473-0.00010-6

to body mass index (BMI, $p < 0.002$), total fat mass ($p < 0.03$), serum IGF-1 ($p < 0.01$), and estradiol levels ($p < 0.001$) in AN patients. We conclude that AN women with a significant BMD loss have a high risk of developing osteoporosis. A low BMD is a consequence of hormonal alterations which include hypoestrogenism, hypoleptinemia, hypercortisolism, and decreases in IGF-1 levels, as well as a low BMI and fat mass.

1. INTRODUCTION

Anorexia nervosa (AN) is a common disorder that has increased in prevalence over the last decade and 0.2–4% of all adolescent girls suffer from this disorder, according to our results (García-Gil, Ortiz-Gómez, & Fernández-Soto, 2007). Since the disorder goes undiagnosed as much as 50% of the time, the true prevalence is probably even higher. Osteopenia and osteoporosis are well-established complications of AN and an onset of disease during adolescence is associated with more severe bone mineral density (BMD) reduction (Audí et al., 2002; Soyka et al., 1999). Whereas adult women with AN have an uncoupling of bone turnover markers with increased bone reabsorption and decreased bone formation markers, adolescents with AN have an overall decreased bone turnover (Fernández-Soto, González-Jiménez, & Varsavsky, 2010; Misra & Klibanski, 2006). More than 50% of the women with previous AN will suffer a bone fracture by approximately 40 years of age, and the risk of osteoporosis-related fracture after menopause among these women is triple that of women without AN (Lucas, Melton, Crowson, & O´Fallon, 1999). The duration of AN is a predictor of low bone mass. In fact, a relationship exists between vertebral BMD and the time during which body mass index (BMI) is below 15 kg/m^2 (Hotta, Shibasaki, Sato, & Demura, 1998). In addition, the duration of amenorrhea is necessarily to be considered as a factor closely related to bone mass loss (Jayasinghe, Grover, & Zacharin, 2008). It is known that low levels of estradiol are associated with a low bone mass. Nevertheless, oral estrogen does not increase BMD or prevent bone loss in AN (Karlsson, Weigall, Duan, & Seeman, 2000). Weight restoration is an effective way to attenuate and sometimes impede further BMD loss (Baker, Roberts, & Towell, 2000; Rigotti, Neer, & Skates, 1991). Growth hormone (GH) and insulin-like growth factor-1 (IGF-1), which are maximally secreted during puberty, continue to play a role in the acquisition and maintenance of bone mass and the determination of body composition in adulthood. In AN adult women, low IGF-1 levels and high GH values have been demonstrated and are attributed to a nutritionally acquired GH resistance

(Argente et al., 1997). However, currently, the pathogenic role of decline in the activity of the GH–IGF axis in AN osteoporotic adolescents is less conclusive (Giustina, Mazziotti, & Canalis, 2008). Over recent years, several other hormonal changes have been observed in AN patients, such as serum testosterone, leptin, vitamin D, sex hormone-binding globulin, and cortisol (Fernández-García et al., 2009; Turner et al., 2001). The specific contribution of these factors to bone remodeling is not completely understood, and the development of effective therapeutic strategies is critical. This is particularly so for adolescents, who are in the process of accruing peak bone mass, and in whom a failure to attain peak bone mass may occur in AN, in addition to loss of already established bone.

The objective of the study was to examine whether anthropometric and hormonal variables provide insight into the underlying mechanisms related to bone mass loss in AN patients.

2. MATERIALS AND METHODS

2.1. Subject selection

We selected 47 out-patients in a cross-sectional study. All of them were Caucasian women with restrictive AN diagnosed according to the Diagnostic and Statistical Manual of Mental Disorders (DSM-IV) (1994). Mean age (±SD) was 21.3 ± 2.5 years and ranged between 18 and 24. The mean illness duration was 43.3 ± 12.2 months (range 2–58 months), and the mean treatment time was 12.6 ± 12.3 months. The mean BMI was 16.8 ± 3.4 kg/m^2 and ranged from 15 to 21 kg/m^2. The control group included 25 healthy, Caucasian women aged 19.3 ± 1.6, who were postmenarchal with regular menstrual period and no history of eating disorders.

2.2. Experimental protocol

Conditions other than AN, drugs which might affect bone metabolism and past history of estrogen replacement therapy excluded subjects from study participation. Height was measured in triplicate on a single stadiometer and averaged and weight was measured on a single electronic scale in a fasting state. BMI was calculated as the ratio of weight to square height (kg/m^2). Morning fasting samples of venous blood were collected for analysis of albumin, retinol binding protein (RBP), cortisol, estradiol, IGF-1, leptin, and sex hormone-binding globulin (SHBG) levels.

A dual-energy X-ray absorptiometry (QDR-4500 W, Hologic, Inc., Waltham, MA, USA) evaluation for BMD (g/cm^2) at the lumbar spine (LS) as well as the *T*-score at LS was done. The coefficient of variation was lower than 2% at different sites of measurement. According to the WHO criteria (2003), the diagnosis of osteoporosis is when the *T*-score is ≥ -2.5 SD and osteopenia when *T*-score is > -1 SD and < -2.5 SD. Total body fat mass and lean body mass were quantified using the impedanciometer using specific equations for BMI <18.5 kg/m^2 (Tanita, Hologic®). The study was performed in accordance with the Helsinki Declaration (1975) and was approved by the Research Committee of the University Hospital, San Cecilio (Granada, Spain).

2.3. Biochemical assessment

Serum IGF-1 levels were measured by RIA (Nichols Institute Diagnostics, Inc.), with a lower detection limit of 10 μg/l. The intraassay and interassay coefficients of variation were less than 6%. The reference values for subjects between 18 and 40 years old were 90–360 μg/l. The RIA was used to measure serum estradiol (Diagnostic Systems Laboratories, Inc., Webster, TX; limit of detection, 2.2 pg/ml, and CV 6.5–8.9%). SHBG was measured by chemiluminescent immunometric assay (IMMULITE 2000, SIEMENS) and the values for women (not pregnant) were 18–114 nmol/l with limit of detection 0.02 nmol/l. RBP was measured by nephelometry and the reference values were 3–6 mg/dl. Serum albumin levels were measured by photometry in a Roche Modular ACN 413 with reference values of 3.4–4.8 g/dl, limit of detection of 0.2 g/dl, and a coefficient variation of 0.39–1.71%. Serum cortisol levels were measured by electrochemiluminescence Immunoassay "ECLIA" (Roche Elecys 1010/2010); reference values at 7–10 am were 6.2–19.4 μg/dl, a limit of detection of 0.018 μg/dl, and a coefficient of variation of 1.7–2.2%. Serum leptin was measured by RIA (Nichols Institute Diagnostics, Inc.), reference values for a normal BMI (18.5–25 kg/m^2) were 3.6–11.2 μg/l.

2.4. Statistical analysis

For the descriptive analysis, all values are presented as mean values and standard deviations (±SD). Two-tailed unpaired Student *t*-test was used to calculate differences between groups. Simple linear regression analysis was employed to study the relationship among variables. A BMD variable was used in two categories using the osteoporosis densitometric criteria

(T-score ≥ -2.5 SD) as a cutoff. Statistical analysis was carried out using SPSS 15.0 package for Windows (SPSS, Inc., Chicago, IL, USA). $p < 0.05$ was considered as statistically significant.

3. RESULTS

According to the WHO criteria, 16/47 AN women met osteoporosis criteria (34%) and 9/47 (19%) showed osteopenia at LS. Table 10.1 shows the clinical characteristics of the study population. The control group had a significant higher BMI, fat mass, and lean body mass than the AN patients with ($p < 0.01$) and without osteoporosis ($p < 0.05$) after adjusting for age, height, and age at menarche. Those patients with osteoporosis had a significantly lower BMI ($p < 0.01$), total fat mass ($p < 0.001$), lean body mass ($p < 0.05$), and a higher duration of amenorrhea ($p < 0.01$) compared to AN patients without osteoporosis. No significant differences were found between the two groups for chronological age and the age at menarche.

The nutritional and hormonal variables are detailed in Table 10.2. The mean serum IGF-1 and estradiol levels were significantly lower in women with osteoporosis compared to those without (both $p < 0.001$). The first AN group had significantly higher serum cortisol levels ($p < 0.03$) and significant lower leptin levels ($p < 0.02$) compared to the latter. No significant

Table 10.1 Clinical characteristics of the study population

	Control group	AN-OTP	AN-non-OTP	p*
Chronological age (years)	19.3 ± 1.6	21.5 ± 3.6	19.6 ± 3.1	NS
Height (cm)	160.5 ± 5.5	159.3 ± 5.7	160 ± 5.6	NS
Age at menarche (years)	13.1 ± 1.5	12.5 ± 1.1	12.4 ± 1.0	NS
Amenorrhea duration (months)	–	18.7 ± 5.4	10.1 ± 4.8	<0.01
BMI (kg/m^2)	21.8 ± 0.9	16.8 ± 1.5*	19.1 ± 2.0**	<0.01
Total BMD (g/cm^2)	1.4 ± 0.3	0.8 ± 0.1	1.2 ± 0.2	<0.01
Total fat mass (kg)	17.4 ± 5.2	9.3 ± 3.1*	13.5 ± 3.2**	<0.001
Lean body mass (kg)	45.1 ± 4.7	36.4 ± 4.1*	40.2 ± 3.5**	<0.05

AN, anorexia nervosa; AN-OTP, AN group with osteoporosis; AN-non-OTP, AN group without osteoporosis; BMD, bone mineral density. Mean values ± standard deviations.
p^*, unpaired Student t-test (AN-OTP vs. AN-non-OTP patients).
Difference when we compared AN-OTP and AN-non-OTP with control group $^*p < 0.01$, $^{**}p < 0.05$.

Table 10.2 Nutritional and hormonal parameters

	Control group	AN-OTP	AN-non-OTP	p^*
IGF-1 (ng/ml)	309.2 ± 56.4	123.4 ± 32.5*	220.6 ± 16.4	<0.001
RBP (mg/dl)	12.6 ± 4.8	8.7 ± 1.6	9.2 ± 7.1	NS
Albumin (g/dl)	4.3 ± 2.2	4.3 ± 1.2	4.7 ± 1.2	NS
SHBG (nmol/l)	145.3 ± 7.3	75.7 ± 5.7*	105.8 ± 9.3	NS
Estradiol (pg/ml)	92.6 ± 7.8	14.5 ± 3.0**	32.4 ± 12.3**	<0.001
Cortisol (μg/dl)	20.5 ± 3.6	13.4 ± 3.8**	8.7 ± 3.0**	<0.03
Leptin (μg/l)	6.1 ± 4.8	2.4 ± 1.52**	5.6 ± 4.9	<0.02

AN, anorexia nervosa; AN-OTP, AN group with osteoporosis; AN-non-OTP, AN group without osteoporosis; IGF-1, insulin-like growth factor-1; RBP, retinol binding protein; SHBG, sex hormone-binding globulin. Mean values ± standard deviations.
p^* unpaired Student *t*-test (AN-OTP vs. AN-non-OTP patients).
Difference from control group $^*p<0.05$, $^{**}p<0.01$.

Table 10.3 Relationships between biological variables and bone parameters in patients with AN

	BMD LS (g/m^2)		*T*-Score LS	
	r	p^*	*r*	p^*
Body weight (kg)	0.41	<0.04	0.43	<0.03
BMI (kg/m^2)	0.58	<0.002	0.58	<0.002
Amenorrhea duration (months)	−0.44	<0.02	−0.45	<0.02
Estradiol (pg/ml)	0.99	<0.001	0.99	<0.001
IGF-1 (ng/ml)	0.61	<0.01	0.69	<0.01
Total fat mass (kg)	0.57	<0.03	0.60	<0.01

BMD LS, bone mineral density in the lumbar spine; p^*, correlation analysis by Pearson's test.

differences were found in RBP, SHBG, and albumin concentrations between groups. The control group had a significant higher estradiol, cortisol, and leptin levels ($p<0.01$) and IGF-1 ($p<0.05$) compared to AN-OTP. Estradiol and cortisol levels were significatively lower compared with AN-non-OTP patients ($p<0.01$).

Bivariate analysis (Table 10.3) showed a significant positive correlation between BMD LS and *T*-score LS to body weight ($r=0.41$, $p<0.04$ and $r=0.43$, $p<0.03$, respectively), BMI ($r=0.58$, $p<0.002$), total fat mass

($r=0.57$, $p<0.03$ and $r=0.60$, $p<0.01$, respectively), IGF-1 ($r=0.61$ and 0.69, $p<0.01$, respectively), and a highly significant correlation, related to estradiol ($r=0.99$, $p<0.001$). Significant negative correlation was demonstrated with amenorrhea duration ($r=-0.44$, $p<0.02$). There was no significant correlation between cortisol, leptin, or SHBG levels with bone parameters.

4. DISCUSSION

Low bone mass is a relevant complication of AN. It has been estimated that osteoporosis is present in 20–50% of women with an increased risk of fracture particularly at nonvertebral sites. Thus, bone mass loss is a major clinical concern in AN patients, justifying systematic evaluation (Trombetti, Richert, & Rizzoli, 2007). In a 2000 article about the prevalence of osteopenia and osteoporosis, Grinspoon established percentages similar to those obtained in the present study (Grinspoon, Thomas, Pitts, & Gross, 2000). More than half had osteopenia at the spine and almost a quarter had osteoporosis at the spine. Over 90% of women had abnormally low bone density at one or more sites in the skeleton. The pathogenesis of osteoporosis in AN remains unclear. Although it has been demonstrated that the duration of amenorrhea is an important risk factor in the development of osteoporosis, other authors have associated the diagnosis of the disease in peripubertal ages, at a time when bone mass accrual is critical for reaching a peak bone mass (Soyka et al., 2002). These results reveal that there is a significant loss of bone mass at the level of the LS, which would indicate a result of estrogen deficiency related to an inadequate mineralization of trabecular bone. These results demonstrated that patients with osteoporosis have levels of estradiol significantly lower than those not suffering from this condition. The loss of bone mass can be more severe depending on whether the amenorrhea present is primary or itoccurred before the age of 14–15 years, the latter being an important stage in the female reproduction life cycle and provides a major contribution to the bone mass peak. These results are similar to those outlined in other studies, which concluded that the duration of the amenorrhea and the levels of estradiol are inversely proportional to the DMO measurement (Misra et al., 2008).

In relation to IGF-1 levels, several researchers have demonstrated its role in women's skeletal integrity with postmenopausal osteoporosis (Muñoz-Torres et al., 2001) and in women with AN (Argente et al., 1997). Recently, their role has been demonstrated in an experimental and clinical phase; even alterations in bone microarchitecture may explain the risk of fracture independent of BMI (Lawson et al., 2010), being beneficial in bone metabolism since the short-term administration of rhIGF-1 causes an increase in a surrogate bone formation marker in girls with AN without significant side effects (Misra et al., 2009). The results showed significant lower IGF-1 levels in AN women with osteoporosis compared to those without, and there was an excellent correlation with BMD at the lumbar site. Because bone mass accrual in adolescence depends greatly on rising levels of IGF-1 and estrogen, maximal increases in bone density would be expected when IGF-1 levels increase as weight improves and levels of estradiol increase.

The majority of the studies carried out confirm that body weight is one of the most important factors of reversible or irreversible osteoporosis in the locations studied (Compston et al., 2006). BMD does not increase until a BMI of 17–18 kg/m^2 is achieved and does not reach a normal enclosed range until several years after a full recovery (Misra et al., 2003). This study confirmed the significant association between BMD, BMI, and fat mass at the LS. Besides, AN patients with osteoporosis have lower total body weight, and lean, and fat mass compared with those without.

Leptin exerts a critical role in the regulation of the body energy balance and as a protective factor inhibiting bone reabsorption (Herpertz, Albers, & Wagner, 2000). However, the exact mechanism underlying the effect of variation in this adipokine on bone anomalies in patients with AN is still unclear. According to Ducy et al. (2000), the intracerebroventricular infusion of leptin produced loss of bone mass in mice ob/ob deficient in leptin. It has therefore been suggested that leptin modulates indirectly the loss of bone mass across a central effect, and the deficiency of leptin is associated with a decrease of the bone mass. Equally, it has been demonstrated that the decrease of leptin in AN is directly related to the percentage of fat mass. This study corroborates these remarks by finding leptin levels significantly lower in AN patients with osteoporosis compared with those without. The decrease in leptin levels observed in AN patients with osteoporosis could contribute to BMD loss due to the reduction in bone formation (Muñoz & Argente, 2002). Conversely, a significant correlation between leptin and BMD at LS has yet to be demonstrated.

The alterations in different hormonal axes also contribute in an important way to the modifications of the BMD. Between them, the increased secretion of cortisol seems to be a direct consequence of malnutrition and it has been demonstrated that the levels are higher in patients with both AN and osteoporosis than those who do not suffer from osteoporosis.

Investigations published recently corroborate these results, finding disturbance in the dynamics of secretion of cortisol and an inverse association with bone formation markers (Lawson et al., 2009). The osteoporotic process of these patients may be reversible on the conditions that the psychiatric disorder evolves favorably, resulting in mineral bone content reaching near-normal values (Misra, 2008; Nakahara et al., 2006).

To conclude, the present results are consistent with data suggesting that the degree of underweight and low body fat mass together with low serum estradiol, are the most important predictors of low BMD. This alteration is also related to biochemical and hormonal parameters that include hypercortisolism, hypoleptinemia, and decreases in IGF-1, a bone trophic factor related to malnutrition. The treatment of underlying psychiatric disorder, the improvement of caloric intake together with the consistent increase in weight, calcium and vitamin D supplements, and the recovery of menstruation, are amongst the factors to be taken into consideration in the restoration of bone health.

ACKNOWLEDGMENTS

The authors wish to thank Jacqueline Anne Taylor, the freelance translator, and the proofreader for meticulous work in the preparation of this final draft.

REFERENCES

American Psychiatric Association, (1994). *Diagnostic and statistical manual for mental disorders.* Washington, DC: APA Press.

Argente, J., Caballo, N., Barrios, V., Muñoz, M. T., Pozo, J., & Chowen, J. A. (1997). Multiple endocrine abnormalities in the growth hormone (GH) and insulin-like growth factor (IGF) axes in patients with anorexia nervosa. Effect of a short and long-term weight recuperation. *Journal of Clinical Endocrinology and Metabolism, 82,* 2084–2092.

Audí, L., Vargas, D. M., Gussinyé, M., Yeste, D., Martí, G., & Carrascosa, A. (2002). Clinical and biochemical determinants of bone metabolism and bone mass in adolescent female patients with anorexia nervosa. *Pediatric Research, 51,* 497–504.

Baker, D., Roberts, R., & Towell, T. (2000). Factors predictive of bone mineral density in eating-disordered women: A longitudinal study. *International Journal of Eating Disorders, 27,* 29–35.

Compston, J. E., McConachie, C., Stott, C., Hannon, R. A., Kaptoge, S., Debiram, I., et al. (2006). Changes in bone mineral density, body composition and biochemical markers of bone turnover during weight gain in adolescents with severe anorexia nervosa: A 1-year prospective study. *Osteoporosis International, 17,* 77–84.

Ducy, P., Amling, M., Takeda, S., Priemel, M., Schilling, A. F., & Beil, F. T. (2000). Leptin inhibits bone formation through a hypothalamic relay: A central control of bone mass. *Cell, 100,* 197–204.

Fernández-García, D., Rodríguez, M., García Alemán, J., García-Almeida, J. M., Picón, M. J., Fernández-Aranda, F., et al. (2009). Thin healthy women have a similar low bone mass to women with anorexia nervosa. *British Journal of Nutrition, 3,* 1–7.

Fernández-Soto, M. L., González-Jiménez, A., & Varsavsky, M. (2010). Mineral metabolism and the risk of fractures in anorexia nervosa. *Medicina Clínica (Barc)*, *135*, 274–279.

García-Gil, E., Ortiz-Gómez, T., & Fernández-Soto, M. L. (2007). Social profiles, diet and prediction of eating disorders in Andalusian urban adolescents. *Atención Primaria*, *39*, 7–13.

Giustina, A., Mazziotti, G., & Canalis, E. (2008). Growth hormone, insulin-like growth factors and the skeleton. *Endocrine Reviews*, *29*, 535–559.

Grinspoon, S., Thomas, E., Pitts, S., & Gross, E. (2000). Prevalence and predictive factors for regional osteopenia in women with anorexia nervosa. *Annals of Internal Medicine*, *133*, 790–794.

Herpertz, S., Albers, N., & Wagner, R. (2000). Longitudinal changes of circadian leptin, insulin and cortisol plasma levels and their correlation during refeeding in patients with anorexia nervosa. *European Journal of Endocrinology*, *142*, 373–379.

Hotta, M., Shibasaki, T., Sato, K., & Demura, H. (1998). The importance of body weight history in the occurrence and recovery of osteoporosis in patients with anorexia nervosa: Evaluation by dual X-ray absorptiometry and bone metabolic markers. *European Journal of Endocrinology*, *139*, 276–283.

Jayasinghe, Y., Grover, S. R., & Zacharin, M. (2008). Current concepts in bone and reproductive health in adolescents with anorexia nervosa. *Journal of Obstetrics and Ginecology*, *115*, 304–315.

Karlsson, M. K., Weigall, S. J., Duan, Y., & Seeman, E. (2000). Bone size and volumetric density in women with anorexia nervosa receiving estrogen replacement therapy and in women recovered from anorexia nervosa. *Journal of Clinical Endocrinology and Metabolism*, *85*, 3177–3182.

Lawson, E. A., Donoho, D., Miller, K. K., Misra, M., Meenaghan, E., Lydecker, J., et al. (2009). Hypercortisolemia is associated with severity of bone loss and depression in hypothalamic amenorrhea and anorexia nervosa. *Journal of Clinical Endocrinology and Metabolism*, *94*, 4710–4716.

Lawson, E. A., Miller, K. K., Bredella, M. A., Phan, C., Misra, M., Meenaghan, E., et al. (2010). Hormone predictors of abnormal bone microarchitecture in women with anorexia nervosa. *Bone*, *46*, 458–463.

Lucas, A., Melton, J., Crowson, C., & O´Fallon, M. (1999). Long-term fracture risk among women with anorexia nervosa. *Mayo Clinic Proceedings*, *74*, 972–977.

Misra, M. (2008). Long-term skeletal effects of eating disorders with onset in adolescence. *Annals of the New York Academy of Sciences*, *1135*, 212–218.

Misra, M., & Klibanski, A. (2006). Anorexia nervosa and osteoporosis. *Reviews in Endocrine & Metabolic Disorders*, *7*, 91–99.

Misra, M., McGrane, J., Miller, K. K., Goldstein, M. A., Ebrahimi, S., Weigel, T., et al. (2009). Effects of rhIGF-1 administration on surrogate markers of bone turnover in adolescents with anorexia nervosa. *Bone*, *45*, 493–498.

Misra, M., Prabhakaran, R., Miller, K., Goldstein, M., Mickley, D., Clauss, L., et al. (2008). Weight gain and restoration of menses as predictors of bone mineral density change in adolescent girls with anorexia nervosa. *Journal of Clinical Endocrinology and Metabolism*, *93*, 1231–1237.

Misra, M., Soyka, L., Miller, K., Grinspoon, S., Levitsky, L., & Klibanski, A. (2003). Regional body composition in adolescents with anorexia nervosa and changes with weight recovery. *American Journal of Clinical Nutrition*, *77*, 1361–1367.

Muñoz, M. T., & Argente, J. (2002). Anorexia nervosa in female adolescents: Endocrine and bone mineral density disturbances. *European Journal of Endocrinology*, *147*, 275–286.

Muñoz-Torres, M., Mezquita-Raya, P., López-Rodríguez, F., Torres-Vela, E., Luna, J. D., & Escobar-Jiménez, F. (2001). The contribution of IGF-1 to skeletal integrity in postmenopausal women. *Clinical Endocrinology*, *55*, 759–767.

Nakahara, T., Nagai, N., Tanaka-Muranaga, T., Kojima, S., Nozoe, S., & Naruo, T. (2006). The effects of bone therapy on tibial bone loss in young women with anorexia nervosa. *International Journal of Eating Disorders, 39*, 20–26.
Rigotti, N. A., Neer, R. M., & Skates, S. J. (1991). The clinical course of osteoporosis in anorexia nervosa. *Journal of the American Medical Association, 265*, 1133–1138.
Soyka, L. A., Grinspoon, S., Levitsky, L. L., Herzog, D. B., Misra, M., & Klibanski, A. (1999). The effects of anorexia nervosa on bone metabolism in female adolescents. *Journal of Clinical Endocrinology and Metabolism, 84*, 4489–4496.
Soyka, L., Misra, M., Frenchman, A., Miller, K., Grinspoon, S., Schoenfeld, D., et al. (2002). Abnormal bone mineral accrual in adolescent girls with anorexia nervosa. *Journal of Clinical Endocrinology and Metabolism, 87*, 4177–4185.
Trombetti, A., Richert, L., & Rizzoli, R. (2007). Anorexia nervosa and its consequences on bone: A therapeutic challenge. *Revue Médicale Suisse, 115*, 1502–1505.
Turner, J. M., Bulsara, M. K., McDermott, B. M., Byrne, G. C., Prince, R. L., & Forbes, D. A. (2001). Predictors of low bone density in young adolescent females with anorexia nervosa and other dieting disorders. *International Journal of Eating Disorders, 30*, 245–251.
WHO Scientific Group (2003). *Prevention and management of osteoporosis*. WHO Technical Report Series 921. Geneva.

CHAPTER ELEVEN

Mechanism-Based Therapeutic Approaches to Cachexia

Fabio Penna, Gabriella Bonelli, Francesco M. Baccino, Paola Costelli[1]
Department of Clinical and Biological Sciences, University of Torino, Turin, Italy
[1]Corresponding author: e-mail address: paola.costelli@unito.it

Contents

1. Introduction 272
2. Body and Tissue Wasting 273
3. Anorexia 274
4. Inflammation 275
5. Tissue Wasting in Cachexia: Hypoanabolism or Hypercatabolism? 279
6. From Mechanistic Alterations to Therapeutic Strategies 281
7. Nutritional Interventions 281
8. Anti-Inflammatory Strategies 283
9. Inhibition of Cytokine Production 284
10. Interference with Cytokine-Receptor Interaction 285
11. Strategies to Correct Metabolic Alterations 286
12. Conclusions 290
References 290

Abstract

Cachexia is a multifactorial syndrome characterized by body weight loss, depletion of adipose tissue and skeletal muscle mass, and marked alterations in the metabolic homeostasis. The occurrence of cachexia significantly impinges on patients' morbidity and mortality, and on quality of life. Inflammation, anorexia/malnutrition, alterations of protein and lipid metabolism are among the main mechanisms involved in the development of cachexia. While anorexia and malnutrition have long been known to be contributing factors, the mechanisms leading to inflammation and metabolic alterations were clarified much later. On these premises, several therapeutic approaches were proposed. Most of them are in the preclinical phase, but some have already reached the clinical experimentation stage. This review focuses on treatment options proposed on the basis of mechanistic alterations. In this regard, in addition to nutritional and anti-inflammatory strategies, approaches based on perturbation of specific signal transduction pathways are taken into consideration.

Vitamins and Hormones, Volume 92
ISSN 0083-6729
http://dx.doi.org/10.1016/B978-0-12-410473-0.00011-8

1. INTRODUCTION

Chronic pathologies such as diabetes, cancer, congestive heart failure, autoimmune, or neurological diseases result in a significant impairment of patients' quality of life. Indeed, in addition to features specific to each disease, patients often show marked alterations in whole-body homeostasis, which ultimately result in tissue wasting, impaired nutritional status, and reduced ability to perform daily activities. This condition, termed cachexia, is often disregarded until it becomes clinically evident. Unfortunately, at this point, it is barely responsive to the few treatments available, most of which, however, are merely symptomatic. In this regard, early targeted interventions have been proposed to be helpful in preventing the progression of cachexia from a "latent" to an "overt" condition. Indeed, once a sort of a point of no return is reached, the balance among several components contributing to disease-induced derangement is likely to get lost, and no intervention can be successful anymore. These observations highlight the urgent need of biomarkers suitable for the detection of the condition of "latent" cachexia.

A few years ago, a couple of papers reported a definition of cachexia (Evans et al., 2008; Muscaritoli et al., 2010): "*Cachexia may be defined as a multifactorial syndrome characterized by severe body weight, fat, and muscle loss, and increased protein catabolism due to underlying disease(s). Cachexia is clinically relevant since it increases patients' morbidity and mortality. Contributory factors to the onset of cachexia are anorexia and metabolic alterations, i.e. increased inflammatory status, increased muscle proteolysis, impaired carbohydrate, protein, and lipid metabolism*" (quoted from Muscaritoli et al., 2010). Such efforts in defining cachexia are particularly relevant especially in view of identifying populations of patients in whom the syndrome is more likely to develop. In this regard, a three-stage classification of cachexia has been recently proposed: precachexia, cachexia, and refractory cachexia (Fearon et al., 2011). Due to the complex etiology of this syndrome, the assessment of cachexia should include several parameters, such as the occurrence of anorexia and malnutrition, the loss of body weight, the depletion of adipose tissue, the loss of muscle mass and strength, the activation of hypercatabolism, the presence of a chronic inflammatory state, and last, but not least, the impact that cachexia exerts on the patient.

2. BODY AND TISSUE WASTING

The loss of body weight is one of the hallmarks of cachexia. While its pathogenesis may be different, ranging from simple caloric restriction to the profound derangements observed in cancer patients, its occurrence often associates with worse prognosis and poor tolerance to therapies. This is particularly evident in cancer patients, where weight loss has been reported in about 50–70% of new diagnoses (Muscaritoli, Bossola, Aversa, Bellantone, & Rossi Fanelli, 2006). Neoplastic patients presenting with weight loss before the beginning of treatment often show poor tolerance to surgery, chemotherapy, and radiotherapy. By contrast, a good performance status correlates positively with tolerance and response rates to chemotherapy and radiotherapy and with survival (Tan & Fearon, 2008). In this regard, particular attention should be given to patients in whom body weight loss could be masked, such as those presenting with water retention (cancer, liver cirrhosis, heart or renal failure) or obesity.

Body weight loss results mainly from reduced adipose tissue and/or skeletal muscle mass. The latter should be regarded as the main feature of ongoing cachexia for the following reasons: first, muscle mass below 50% of body weight is not compatible with survival (Wolfe, 2006, and references therein), and, second, the adipose tissue may not be affected early, at least in neoplastic patients. Consequently, obese cancer patients often show significant muscle depletion in face of elevated body mass index and maintenance of adipose tissue mass (sarcopenic obesity; Prado et al., 2008; Stenholm et al., 2008). Not only this, the increase in fat in obese subjects masks the occurrence of lean body mass, in particular in the early stages of the disease, thus delaying the adoption of specific metabolic interventions. The different kinetic characteristics of depletion in muscle and fat, however, should not divert the attention from the latter. Indeed, many years ago, Argilés, López-Soriano, Almendro, Busquets, and López-Soriano (2005) proposed the existence of a cross-talk between the two tissue compartments. This hypothesis has been clearly demonstrated in a recent report (Das et al., 2011), showing that inhibition of lipolysis in tumor-bearing mice by genetic ablation of lipolytic enzymes prevents not only hyperlipidemia and adipose mass depletion but also skeletal muscle wasting.

Irrespective of the underlying disease, skeletal muscle, which accounts for approximately half of the body protein mass, is severely affected in cachexia. It is a very heterogeneous tissue, in charge of several biological functions such as movement, stability, heat production, and cold tolerance. Considered in the past as merely a protein reservoir, it is now recognized to release cytokines and other humoral factors (Pedersen & Febbraio, 2008). Since the skeletal muscle plays a pivotal role in the overall energy balance, regulating lipid flux, plasma glucose storage, and insulin sensitivity, it participates in the control of whole-body metabolism, also acting in concert with the adipose tissue. The main factor regulating skeletal muscle mass is protein content, which strictly depends on the balance between synthesis and degradation rates. Physiologically, in the adult individual, protein synthesis does not exceed degradation, and vice versa, allowing the maintenance of the skeletal muscle mass. Generally speaking, modulations of both sides of turnover eventually converge to produce a new steady state. In this regard, enhanced protein synthesis, which responds earlier than degradation to the inducing stimuli, mainly results in muscle hypertrophy, while protein hypercatabolism leads to muscle depletion.

3. ANOREXIA

Defined as a reduced desire to eat and early satiety, anorexia leads to a decreased number of meals during the day and a reduction in the amount of food consumed at each meal. It is a common feature of chronic pathologies; however, it is often not recognized and is left untreated, and as a result contributes significantly to malnutrition. In this regard, food intake in patients should be accurately and routinely monitored, in order to immediately identify a change from the usual habit. At least in cancer patients, tools such as the Functional Assessment of Anorexia/Cachexia Therapy and the North Central Cancer Treatment Group Anorexia/Cachexia can provide a qualitative and quantitative assessment of anorexia (Muscaritoli et al., 2010).

In addition to alterations in the central control of eating, secondary causes of reduced food intake may be constipation, stomatitis, pain, and depression. From a therapeutic point of view, the mechanisms underlying anorexia in the different patients should be readily identified, in order to adopt the most correct approach. To recognize the occurrence of anorexia may be relevant also in view of the fact that early satiety correlates with worse outcome, at least in cancer patients (Walsh, Rybicki, Nelson, & Donnelly, 2002).

The altered control of eating behavior depends mainly on proinflammatory cytokines (TNF-α, IL-6, and IL-1). Such mediators modify appetite and metabolic rate directly, or indirectly through modulations of the physiological levels of several neuropeptides (leptin, neuropeptide Y, melanocortin, agouti-related peptides). More specifically, cytokine bioactivity results in induction of anorexigenic pathways and inhibition of the orexigenic ones, leading to appetite loss and increased satiety (Grossberg, Scarlett, & Marks, 2010).

The occurrence of anorexia may contribute to explain the loss of body weight that characterizes patients affected by chronic diseases. However, weight loss, at least in cancer cachexia, generally differs from that due to simple food deprivation. Indeed, during caloric restriction, glucose and amino acids are initially mobilized from the liver, fat becoming the primary energy source later on, in order to preserve tissue protein. By contrast, patients with cancer cachexia fail to turn metabolism into a protein-sparing setting, which results in a persistently negative nitrogen balance that defies a purely nutritional correction (Laviano, Meguid, & Rossi Fanelli, 2003a, 2003b).

4. INFLAMMATION

Inflammation is a tightly regulated mechanism aimed at protecting the organism against alterations in homeostasis due to different stimuli such as biological, physical, or chemical agents on one side, and damaged, infected, or neoplastic cells on the other. The inflammatory response is generally endowed with self-regulation properties, achieved through a complex network including both inflammatory/immune cells and humoral mediators that regulates the equilibrium between pro- and anti-inflammatory stimuli. When the balance between pro- and anti-inflammatory response is persistently lost, chronic inflammation occurs. This was suggested to significantly contribute to the pathogenesis of several chronic illnesses such as autoimmune and neurodegenerative diseases, diabetes and its complications, cancer, AIDS, obesity. In this regard, all these pathological states are associated with increased circulating levels of proinflammatory mediators. As an example, IL-6, TNFα, and TNF soluble receptors are detectable in patients affected by chronic heart or renal failure (Li, Lu, Wang, Zhang, & Shen, 2011; Niewczas et al., 2012). In the latter, increased levels of acute-phase reactants correlate with increased mortality (Noori et al., 2011). Similarly, proinflammatory cytokines such as TNFα, IL-6, γ-INF, and LIF are also increased in cachectic neoplastic patients (reviewed by Seruga, Zhang, Bernstein, & Tannock, 2008).

The link between cancer and inflammation had already been proposed by Virchow in the nineteenth century (the Virchow hypothesis; Durham, Dillon, & Sheffield-Moore, 2009), and again after the discovery of the first cytokines (see Winfield et al., 2008). Prehn (1972) demonstrated that immune cells in tumor stroma, such as M2 macrophages, Treg lymphocytes, and dendritic cells, promote tumor growth. Indeed, inflammation plays a dual role: it is involved not only in carcinogenesis and tumor progression but also in the metabolic derangements induced in the patient by the presence of the tumor. Recently, the relation between the acute-phase response (systemic inflammation) and cancer cachexia was proposed from the observation that enhanced liver protein synthesis could drive muscle protein hypercatabolism contributing to the elevated resting energy expenditure (Durham et al., 2009). Not only this, the skeletal muscle itself was proposed as a source of acute-phase reactants, likely diverting amino acids from the synthesis of structural proteins to that of acute-phase mediators (Bonetto et al., 2011). It is of interest to note that acute-phase proteins are further increased by nutritional supplementation, suggesting that anti-inflammatory treatments should be included in the therapeutic protocol (Stephens, Skipworth, & Fearon, 2008). Systemic inflammation appears correlated with reduced survival. Indeed, cancer patients with high CRP levels survive less than those with low/normal levels (Stephens et al., 2008). In some studies, survival is more accurately predicted by CRP levels than by tumor stage (Stephens et al., 2008). In this regard, CRP is used to provide scores suitable for clinical use, such as the Glasgow prognostic score that couples increased CRP ($\geq$10 mg/l) and hypoalbuminemia ($\leq$35 mg/l); CRP and white blood cells; CRP ($\geq$10 mg/l), body weight loss ($\geq$10%), and reduced food intake ($\leq$1500 kcal/day; Fearon, Voss, Hustead, & Cancer Cachexia Study Group, 2006).

Another good example of inflammation-driven disease is diabetes. Hyperglycemia, indeed, leads to the production and accumulation of advanced glycation end-products (AGE), known to induce inflammatory reactions. AGE accumulation leads to oxidative stress, increasing the risk of diabetes complications such as hypertension, neuropathy, nephropathy, and retinopathy, as well as the risk of cancer development (Nienhuis et al., 2009). In addition, diabetes, at least type II diabetes, is often associated with obesity, another proinflammatory condition (de Heredia, Gómez-Martínez, & Marcos, 2012).

Over the last several years, a number of signaling pathways, directly or indirectly activated by proinflammatory cytokines, were proposed to contribute to the development of cachexia, with particular reference to those involved in causing anorexia (see earlier), lipid depletion, and skeletal muscle wasting.

Proinflammatory cytokines, together with altered production/release of classical hormones and/or growth factors, result in a complex network that exerts an inhibitory effect on anabolic and/or anticatabolic signals, in favor of lipolysis and proteolysis. As an example, muscle wasting, increased ubiquitin expression, and proteasome enzymatic activity are induced in healthy animals by administration of TNFα or IL-1 (reviewed in Tisdale, 2008). Consistently, at least in cancer cachexia, a few studies demonstrated many years ago the crucial role played by cytokines in the onset of muscle wasting, showing that loss of muscle mass, protein hypercatabolism, and ubiquitin hyperexpression could be prevented by treatment of tumor-bearing animals with antibodies directed against IL-6, TNFα, or IFNγ (Costelli et al., 1993; Matthys, Heremans, Opdenakker, & Billiau, 1991; Strassmann et al., 1993). Altered cytokine homeostasis, which positively correlated with disease progression and mortality rates, was also reported in cancer patients (Attard-Montalto et al., 1998; Nakashima et al., 1998). Cancer cachexia apart, proinflammatory cytokines contribute to muscle wasting in other chronic diseases such as sepsis or AIDS, as well as in aging (see Späte & Schulze, 2004).

Proinflammatory mediators are likely also involved in pathological states where muscle depletion results from the coexistence of protein hypercatabolism and impaired activation of the regenerative response. In this regard, TNFα was shown to impinge on myogenesis with opposite outcomes: increased circulating levels appear to inhibit myogenesis (Coletti, Moresi, Adamo, Molinaro, & Sassoon, 2005; Coletti, Yang, Marazzi, & Sassoon, 2002; Guttridge, Mayo, Madrid, Wang, & Baldwin, 2000), while high local concentrations promote regeneration in injured muscles (Chen et al., 2005). Reduced stem cell recruitment may contribute to impaired myogenesis (Nicolas, Marazzi, Kelley, & Sassoon, 2005), and TNFα was proposed to abrogate satellite cell function, resulting in delayed or impaired muscle regeneration in mice after injury (Moresi et al., 2008). Recently, a TNFα-dependent, p38α-regulated epigenetic control of Pax7 expression was identified, which directly linked TNFα action to the inhibition of satellite cell proliferation (Palacios et al., 2010).

In addition to protein turnover, several cytokines significantly affect lipid metabolism. TNFα, IL-6, LIF, and γ-INF are known to downregulate lipoprotein lipase (LPL) activity, thus reducing triglyceride storage in adipose tissue, resulting in hyperlipidemia. TNFα, in particular, interferes with the synthesis of adipocyte lipogenic enzymes and stimulates triglyceride degradation by activating the hormone-sensitive lipase (HSL; van de Woestijne,

Monajemi, Kalkhoven, & Visseren, 2011). The relevance of these enzymes to the genesis of tissue depletion, at least in cancer cachexia, was recently demonstrated by Das et al. (2011), showing that tumor growth in mice null for the adipose triglyceride lipase (ATGL) or HSL fails to induce both adipose tissue and skeletal muscle wasting. In contrast with the effects exerted on the adipose tissue, TNFα increases hepatic lipogenesis, contributing to the hyperlipidemia that characterizes cachexia (van de Woestijne et al., 2011).

Finally, the adipose tissue itself produces and releases a huge number of cytokines, termed adipokines; they are involved in several physiological processes including the regulation of lipid metabolism and were also shown to play a role in the pathogenesis of several diseases (Trayhurn & Wood, 2004). Among adipokines, leptin and adiponectin deserve particular attention. The former, produced and secreted proportionally to the adipose tissue mass, interferes with the regulation of both food intake and energy consumption, by acting on the central control of eating (Shan & Yeo, 2011). Physiologically, leptin levels are low and increase in the fasted or fed state, respectively. Other factors, such as inflammation and the mediators involved, may impinge on this regulation; in particular, leptin synthesis is increased during acute responses, while it is decreased in chronic inflammation (Popa et al., 2005). It is of interest to note that leptin itself may act as a proinflammatory cytokine (Lago, Dieguez, Gómez-Reino, & Gualillo, 2007). As for adiponectin, it is known to potentiate fatty acid oxidation and to reduce liver gluconeogenesis, and appears to correlate with body mass index and insulin resistance (Lago et al., 2007). In this regard, adiponectin appears to play a role not only in protecting against excess adipose tissue deposition, but also in other pathological states characterized by an inflammatory component. Consistently, adiponectin secretion is inhibited by proinflammatory cytokines (Bruun et al., 2003). However, at least in cancer cachexia, the involvement of adipokines appears unlikely. Indeed, leptin plasma levels and expression in the adipose tissue were reported to decrease in tumor-bearing animals even in the absence of fat depletion and anorexia (López-Soriano, Carbó, Tessitore, López-Soriano, & Argilés, 1999). Similarly, in gastric cancer patients, neither fat loss nor anorexia seems to be regulated by leptin (Wallace, Sattar, & McMillan, 1998). Such observations have been confirmed by recent evidence showing the lack of correlation between adipokines and markers of inflammation such as CRP and IL-6 in patients with non-small cell lung cancer (NSCLC) (Gulen et al., 2012). However, a different view is reported by Kerem et al. (2008).

5. TISSUE WASTING IN CACHEXIA: HYPOANABOLISM OR HYPERCATABOLISM?

The reduction of both adipose tissue and skeletal muscle mass may depend on reduced deposition, increased mobilization, or both. In other words, this means that increased rates of lipid/protein degradation, reduced rates of synthesis, or both are responsible for the changes in tissue mass that characterize cachexia in chronic diseases. Increased lipolysis and enhanced protein breakdown are generally accepted as hallmarks of cachexia. However, the possible role played by a condition of hypoanabolism is less clear. In this regard, for example, muscle protein synthesis rates were reported to be reduced, unaltered, or even enhanced in cancer patients (see Pisters & Pearlstone, 1993).

Increased lipid mobilization was shown to play a central role in adipose tissue depletion associated with cachexia. As an example, high rates of lipolysis (glycerol and free fatty acid turnover, lipid oxidation), also in the presence of hyperglycemia, occur in cachectic cancer patients (Körber, Pricelius, Heidrich, & Müller, 1999; Sakurai & Klein, 1998). In this regard, both expression and activity levels of two lipases (HSL and ATGL) are increased in experimental and human cancer cachexia (Agustsson et al., 2007). In cancer patients, in particular, lipase expression is inversely correlated with body mass index (see Bing, 2011). Finally, genetic manipulations aimed at deleting each of the two lipases result in restoration of normal adipose tissue mass in tumor-bearing mice (Das et al., 2011; see earlier). Lipolysis-derived fatty acids, through the action of the adipocyte-specific gene cell death-inducing DNA fragmentation factor-[alpha]-like effector A (CIDEA), may serve as substrates for energy production through oxidation (Laurencikiene et al., 2008).

On the other side, the role played by impaired adipogenesis in cachexia is still to be determined. Generally speaking, the occurrence of reduced lipogenesis is generally inferred by the observation that the activity of LPL is often inhibited in cachexia (Nara-Ashizawa, Akiyama, Maruyama, Tsukada, & Yamaguchi, 2001). Similarly, reduced expression of the fatty acid synthase, an enzyme that plays a crucial role in *de novo* lipogenesis, was reported in rats with adjuvant-induced arthritis, in the absence of increased lipolysis (Martín et al., 2008).

As for protein metabolism, intracellular proteolysis in the skeletal muscle is operated by several systems (see Bonetto et al., 2009). The autophagic-lysosomal and the proteasomal ones are able to degrade proteins into amino acids or small peptides. By contrast, both the Ca^{2+}-dependent and the caspase pathways, characterized by a restricted catabolic specificity, lead to only a limited proteolysis of their substrates. As reported earlier, several proinflammatory cytokines were proposed to mediate the induction of protein hypercatabolism. On the other side, anabolism is regulated by a complex interplay among amino acids and hormones/growth factors such as insulin and IGF-1. In this regard, amino acids, in addition to be necessary for the synthesis of new proteins, were shown to interfere with the regulation of mRNA translation (Kadowaki & Kanazawa, 2003). The stimulation of protein synthesis by anabolic signals such as insulin or IGF-1 results from a transduction pathway involving several kinases such as Akt, phosphoinositide-3-kinase (PI3K), glycogen synthase kinase (GSK)-3β, mammalian target of rapamycin (mTOR), and p70 ribosomal S6 kinase ($p70^{S6K}$). The pivotal role that this pathway plays in the skeletal muscle results clear from observations showing that experimental conditions aimed at enhancing Akt activity, in cultured myocytes or in the whole muscle, lead to a hypertrophic phenotype (Lai et al., 2004; Rommel et al., 2001). The other way round, inhibition of this pathway was reported in conditions characterized by muscle wasting such as denervation, aging, disuse, or glucocorticoid treatment, and its restoration by means of IGF-1 administration or IGF-1 local hyperexpression is able to prevent or correct muscle depletion (reviewed in Glass, 2010). An exception, in this regard, is experimental cancer cachexia, where the PI3K/Akt/mTOR pathway is not downregulated (Acharyya et al., 2005; Penna, Bonetto, et al., 2010), and muscle atrophy cannot be prevented by IGF-1 administration or its hyperexpression in the skeletal muscle (Costelli et al., 2006; Penna, Bonetto, et al., 2010).

On the whole, the observations reported earlier could support the concept that, cancer cachexia apart, hypoanabolism is a relevant factor contributing to muscle depletion. However, besides inducing protein synthesis, the PI3K/Akt signaling pathway also downregulates protein catabolism by maintaining the inactive conformation transcription factors of the FoxO family. FoxO3, in particular, regulates both the expression of molecules involved in proteasomal degradation, namely the muscle-specific ubiquitin ligase atrogin-1 (Sandri et al., 2004; Stitt et al., 2004) and the lipidation of LC3, an essential actor in autophagic-lysosomal proteolysis (Zhao et al., 2007). Consistently, FoxO3 deletion results in protection against muscle wasting in experimental models of fasting and denervation atrophy (Zhao et al., 2007).

Taking these considerations into account, the question arises as to whether hypoanabolism is a crucial actor in muscle wasting or just a "side effect" of the marked hypercatabolic state. The question is still more compelling for adipose tissue depletion, since most of the studies address the lipolytic side of metabolism, without taking into account the anabolic processes.

6. FROM MECHANISTIC ALTERATIONS TO THERAPEUTIC STRATEGIES

Studies performed on different experimental models have begun to unravel the causative factors and the pathophysiological perturbations that underlie cachexia, providing information useful to devise novel antagonist tools. The vast majority of the research in the field of new therapies is centered on the treatment of cancer-related cachexia. For this reason, the following paragraphs summarize the state of the art in terms of therapeutic strategies proposed to counteract this specific form of body wasting.

While it is obvious, although not precisely an easy task, that the best treatment for cancer cachexia would be tumor eradication, to reverse or at least delay cachexia should be one of the main goals of therapeutic protocols. Indeed, the occurrence of such a syndrome markedly worsens patients' quality of life, increases morbidity and mortality, and reduces tolerance to antiblastic treatments (Fallowfield, 2002).

7. NUTRITIONAL INTERVENTIONS

The maintenance of a good nutritional status in cancer patients is the main goal. Indeed, well-nourished patients will recover and will tolerate the side effects of antineoplastic treatments better than malnourished ones (Ross et al., 2004).

Anorexia is the most effectively treatable cachexia-contributing factor (Laviano et al., 2003a, 2003b). In this regard, different orexigenic drugs have been proposed (Laviano, Meguid, Inui, Muscaritoli, & Rossi Fanelli, 2005), among which megestrol acetate is the most widely used, although it improves appetite but not global quality of life (Lopez et al., 2004). A comparable effect was shown for corticosteroids, which also control pain and reduce nausea and asthenia (Loprinzi, Kruger, & Sloan, 1999), likely in view of their ability to inhibit the release of anorexia-inducing cytokines (Patra & Arora, 2012). More recently, dronabinol and other cannabinoids were proposed to stimulate appetite (Fide, Bregman, & Kirkham, 2005), through a direct action on the endocannabinoid receptors as well as an indirect one on anorexigenic cytokines (Fide et al., 2005; Klein, Lane, Newton, & Friedman, 2000). Finally, gastric cell-derived ghrelin was shown to improve appetite and also to interfere with insulin/IGF-1-dependent pathways (see earlier); it is interesting to note that only anorexic cancer patients benefit from ghrelin administration (Neary et al., 2004).

However, anorexia is just one of the factors contributing to the nutritional status of cancer patients. In this regard, several tools (fortified normal food, sip food, integrators, nutritional supplements, enteral or parenteral nutrition) aimed at supplementing patients' normal diet are actually available (Rivadaneira, Evoy, Fahey, Lieberman, & Daly, 1998). Nutritional supports generally include functional compounds, such as ω-3 polyunsaturated fatty acids (PUFAs; eicosapentaenoic (EPA) and docosahexaenoic (DHA) acids), also endowed with anti-inflammatory properties, antioxidants, and amino acids. In this regard, the branched -chain amino acids (BCAAs) leucine, isoleucine, and valine, were shown to exert clinically relevant metabolic effects (Bianchi, Marzocchi, Agostini, & Marchesini, 2005). The administration of BCCAs to cancer patients is reported to result in improvements in anorexia and energy intake, likely in view of their ability to modulate the synthesis of serotonin in the hypothalamus (Cangiano, Laviano, & Meguid, 1996).

Finally, a few years ago, an interesting "nutritional modulation" approach, based on a rationale somewhat contrary to that described earlier, and for this reason, not easily accepted by the clinician community, was proposed by Raffaghello et al. (2008, 2010). In order to counteract the side effects of chemotherapeutic treatments, the authors proposed to face the metabolic stress occurring after chemotherapy administration by "preparing" the organism with a few days of complete starvation (1–2 days before chemotherapy assumption, and 1–2 days after). The study reports that cancer patients voluntarily undergoing starvation report a marked reduction of side effects such as fatigue, weakness, nausea, vomiting, diarrhea (Raffaghello et al., 2010). In addition, the same group in a recent report shows that starvation renders tumor cells more prone to the cytotoxic effects of chemotherapeutic drugs and that fasting cycles result in delayed tumor growth (Lee et al., 2012). The approach proposed would thus result in improved effectiveness of antiblastic treatments in face of reduced whole-body toxicity. Such a strategy, although not directly aimed at counteracting cachexia, could also prove helpful in this regard, since chemotherapy toxicity is now recognized to worsen body wasting in cancer patients (Prado, Antoun, Sawyer, & Baracos, 2011).

8. ANTI-INFLAMMATORY STRATEGIES

Interference with the chronic inflammation associated with cachexia was developed on different levels: approaches aimed to downregulate the inflammatory response in a rather unspecific way (corticosteroids, ω-3 PUFAs, cycloxygenase inhibitors, antioxidants) or strategies targeting specific steps of cytokine-dependent signaling (cytokine production, cytokine-receptor interaction).

Among the unspecific approaches, the most relevant is probably the one based on the use of ω-3 PUFAs. EPA and DHA acid, in particular, are endowed with anti-inflammatory properties, being able to reduce the production of proinflammatory cytokines, of molecules deriving from the arachidonic acid cascade (prostaglandins and leukotrienes), and of acute-phase reactants such as CRP (Laviano et al., 2005; Muscaritoli et al., 2006). Tumor-bearing animals treated with EPA show improved body and skeletal muscle weight loss and reduced muscle proteasome enzymatic activity. Of interest, EPA treatment also results in impaired tumor growth and metastasis (Beck et al., 1991; Kimura & Sumiyoshi, 2005). Most of the EPA effects are ascribed to its ability to antagonize the effects of supposed procachectic factors, namely, the lipid mobilizing factor and the proteolysis inducing factor (Tisdale, 2008). Consistently, EPA administration to malnourished patients has been shown to improve body weight loss and to reduce urinary PIF levels (Barber & Fearon, 2001). These observations, however, were not confirmed by a multicenter study on pancreatic cancer patients (Fearon et al., 2003), while another report showed that the weight gain induced by administration of megestrol acetate is more marked than that obtained with EPA (Jatoi et al., 2004) Despite these results, a recent systematic review shows the beneficial effects of ω-3 PUFAs supplementation in cancer, surgical oncology, and critical care patients (van der Meij, van Bokhorst-de van der Schueren, Langius, Brouwer, & van Leeuwen, 2011). In particular, ω-3 PUFAs appear to be effective mainly in terms of quality of life, performance status, and physical activity in patients with NSCLC (van der Meij et al., 2011). Finally, EPA-containing nutritional supplements may be useful to increase perioperative lean body mass in patients with head and neck cancer (Weed et al., 2011).

Another class of compounds endowed with anti-inflammatory properties is represented by statins, drugs widely used to treat hypercholesterolemia because of their ability to inhibit the hydroxy-methyl glutaryl CoA reductase (Ikeda & Shimada, 1999). Despite this putative anti-inflammatory effect, however, simvastatin administration to tumor-bearing animals was unable to correct cancer-induced body and tissue wasting (Muscaritoli et al., 2003).

As reported earlier, specific anticytokine strategies may target cytokine synthesis and release or their interaction with cell surface receptors.

9. INHIBITION OF CYTOKINE PRODUCTION

Cytokine production can be blocked by destabilizing their mRNA or by directly interfere with their synthesis or release.

Thalidomide, known in the past mainly because of its teratogenicity, affects proinflammatory cytokine mRNA stability (Haslett, 1998), although more recently, a direct effect on the transcritpion factor NF-κB was also proposed (Wilkes & Freeman, 2006). A number of clinical trials were set up to test thalidomide effectiveness in the management of cancer cachexia. Patients with metastatic cancer receiving thalidomide showed improvement in quality of life (Bruera et al., 1999), weight loss (Gordon et al., 2005, Khan et al., 2003), lean body mass, and physical functions (Gordon et al., 2005). Finally, a large randomized trial including cachectic cancer patients showed that thalidomide alone is less effective than its combination with other treatments (Mantovani et al., 2010). More recently, an experimental study reported that thalidomide inhibits an E3 ubiquitin ligase complex involved in embryonal development (Ito et al., 2010), leading to the hypothesis that thalidomide effectiveness on muscle wasting in cancer hosts could be achieved through inhibition of muscle-specific ubiquitin ligases.

However, in addition to teratogenicity, thalidomide has several side effects such as deep venous thrombosis and peripheral neuropathy, constipation, vomiting, and drowsiness (BNF, 2009). In this regard, a recent report that systematically reviews data on thalidomide treatment in cancer cachexia clearly shows that the data available are still much too scanty for any significant conclusion to be drawn (Reid et al., 2012).

Several phosphodiesterase inhibitors were proposed in order to inhibit cytokine synthesis in cachexia, among which pentoxifylline. This drug, in the past used as a hemorheological agent, exerts marked anti-inflammatory actions, leading to beneficial effects on cerebral malaria and chronic sarcoidosis (Das et al., 2003; Zabel, Entzian, Dalhoff, & Schlaak, 1997). More recently, it was proposed as a tool to treat diabetes (Bryson, 2008). By contrast, data regarding the use of pentoxifylline to treat cachexia are quite conflicting. Its administration to tumor-bearing animals prevents muscle atrophy, mainly by inhibiting the induction of protein hypercatabolism (Combaret, Ralliere, Taillandier,

Tanaka, & Attaix, 1999; Costelli et al., 2002). On the other side, a double-blind, placebo-controlled study showed that pentoxifylline administration neither improves anorexia nor induces weight gain (Goldberg et al., 1995).

Atractylenolide I, a compound isolated from largehead atractylodes rhizome, used by Chinese traditional medicine to improve nausea, vomiting, and anorexia, was proposed to exert anti-inflammatory effects by inhibiting cytokine production (Li et al., 2007). A few years ago, it was evaluated as an anticachectic agent in a randomized pilot study that included gastric cancer patients. Both body weight and mid-arm muscle circumference significantly increased with respect to the control group, while circulating IL-1 markedly decreased (Liu, Jia, Dong, Wang, & Qiu, 2008). Finally, OHR118, a drug endowed with immunomodulatory and cytoprotective properties, is also able to inhibit the synthesis of proinflammatory chemokines and cytokines. On this basis, a pilot clinical trial was designed to assess its usefulness in the management of cancer cachexia. Of the 21 patients who enrolled, only 11 completed the 2-week study. The results show significant improvements in appetite and depression scores, as well as in weight-gain maintenance (Chasen, Hirschman, & Bhargava, 2011).

Some proinflammatory cytokines are synthesized as inactive precursors. This is well known for both interlukin (IL)-1 and TNFα, proteolytically activated by the IL1-converting enzyme (better known as caspase 1; Thornberry et al., 1992) and the TNFα-converting enzyme (TACE, or ADAM17; Moss et al., 1997), respectively. Provided that IL-1 is not the most relevant cytokine in the pathogenesis of cachexia, most of the studies have concentrated on the search for inhibitors to TACE, in order to prevent dangerous increases of TNFα levels. TACE inhibitors, however, never passed phase II clinical trials (for review, see Murumkar, DasGupta, Chandani, Giridhar, & Yadav, 2010), and despite a couple of them were patented for the treatment of cachexia, no supporting literature is available.

10. INTERFERENCE WITH CYTOKINE-RECEPTOR INTERACTION

The cytokine-receptor engagement can be disrupted by means of cytokine blocking agents (monoclonal antibodies, soluble receptors) or receptor inactivating molecules (receptor antagonists or antireceptor antibodies). Both groups include molecules commonly used in clinical practice to reduce the inflammatory response in chronic pathologies such as rheumatoid arthritis or Crohn disease (anti-TNFα monoclonal antibodies, different formulations of soluble TNFα-receptor 1 or 2, IL-1β receptor antagonist; reviewed in Ghezzi & Cerami, 2005). The literature reports data on the effectiveness of such treatments in preventing body wasting in chronic inflammatory diseases. As an example, etanercept (chimeric soluble TNFα receptor 2) or infliximab (anti-TNFα monoclonal antibody) was reported to increase body weight and lean body mass in patients with rheumatoid arthritis (Briot, Garnero, Le Henanff, Dougados, & Roux, 2005). However, this observation was not confirmed by a different study (Marcora, Chester, Mittal, Lemmey, & Maddison, 2006). Only few data are actually available on the effectiveness of such kinds of drugs in preventing or delaying cancer cachexia. In this regard, anti-TNFα antibodies, though not antagonists of IL-1 receptor, proved effective in reducing anorexia, body weight loss, and protein hypercatabolism in tumor-bearing rats (Costelli et al., 1993; Costelli et al., 1995). More recently, a clinical trial performed on advanced cancer patients receiving etanercept showed no significant improvement in weight loss, anorexia, and survival rate (Jatoi et al., 2007). Another clinical trial showed that lean body mass, performance status, quality of life, and progression-free and overall survival are not different between pancreatic cancer patients receiving gemcitabine alone or gemcitabine plus infliximab (Kishimoto, 1996).

Other compounds are actually reaching the clinical experimentation. In this regard, an anti-IL-6 antibody resulted in increased hemoglobinemia and albuminemia in a small phase I trial including patients with advanced cancer. CRP levels also tended to reduction, while an apparent improvement of hand grip strength and fatigue was reported (Clarke, Gebbie, Sweeney, Olzewski, & Smith, 2009). These preliminary results were confirmed by a phase II trial that included NSCLC patients receiving the anti-IL-6 antibody at different doses (Bayliss, Smith, Schuster, Dragnev, & Rigas, 2011). An anti-IL-6 receptor antibody is also available (Ohtori et al., 2012); however, no data are shown in the literature on its effectiveness in both experimental and human cancer cachexia. By contrast, another inhibitor of the interaction between IL-6 and its receptor, 20S,21-epoxy-resibufogenin-3 acetate, appears to prevent carcass weight loss in tumor-bearing mice (Enomoto et al., 2004).

11. STRATEGIES TO CORRECT METABOLIC ALTERATIONS

Derangements of both protein and lipid metabolism play a crucial role in cachexia, since they are directly responsible for the profound tissue wasting that ultimately leads to patient death. In this regard, strategies aimed at targeting such alterations, irrespective of the trigger(s) responsible for their occurrence (cytokines, anorexia, oxidative stress), are being actively pursued.

As for the skeletal muscle, the data collected over the last decade point to deregulation of signaling pathways such as those dependent on insulin/IGF-1, MAP-kinases (p38, JNK, and ERK), and AMP-kinase as crucial in the onset of the protein hypercatabolic response. The insulin/IGF-1-dependent signaling, in particular, impinges on both the anabolic and the catabolic side of protein turnover (see earlier). In this regard, induction of this pathway would result in inhibition of protein breakdown and stimulation of protein synthesis, likely restoring the normal protein content in the wasted muscle. Such a strategy appears to work perfectly well in several experimental models of muscle wasting including denervation, amyotrophic lateral sclerosis, disuse (reviewed in Glass, 2010). However, it is useless in experimental cancer cachexia, where, despite the occurrence of high protein breakdown rates, the insulin/IGF-1 pathway is not downregulated, protein synthesis rates are only slightly reduced or even unchanged, and protein synthetic signaling is poised into the activated state (Aversa et al., 2012; Costelli et al., 1993; Penna, Bonetto, et al., 2010).

Increased activation of the MAPKs was reported in different conditions presenting with muscle wasting, including aging, diabetes, and inflammatory myopathies (reviewed in Glass, 2010). In particular, p38 phosphorylation was shown to induce the expression of the ubiquitin ligases atrogin-1 and MuRF1, both *in vitro* and *in vivo* (Li et al., 2005; Liu et al., 2011; Romanello et al., 2010). Activation of p38 was also shown to occur in response to mechanical or electrical stimulation and functional overload of the skeletal muscle (Boppart, Hirshman, Sakamoto, Fielding, & Goodyear, 2001; Huey, 2006; Sakamoto, Aschenbach, Hirshman, & Goodyear, 2003), suggesting that this kinase plays a role in both anabolic and catabolic responses. Among the targets of p38 is MAPK-kinase 2 (MKK2). Its phosphorylation at T317 allows MKK2 nuclear export in a complex containing p38 itself (Meng et al., 2002). Phosphorylation of heat shock protein 27 (HSP27), a substrate of MKK2, is increased in skeletal muscle hypertrophy and decreased during atrophy (Huey, 2006; Kawano et al., 2007), while HSP27 hyperexpression reduces disuse-induced muscle depletion (Dodd, Hain, Senf, & Judge, 2009). Finally, MKK2 expression is also reduced in denervation-induced atrophy (Norrby & Tågerud, 2010). The occurrence of a cross-talk between MKK2/p38 and PI3K/Akt/mTOR pathways was proposed. In this regard, the MKK2/p38 complex exported from the nucleus appears to interact with a cytoplasmic HSP27/Akt complex (Wu et al., 2007). Similar to Akt, also MKK2 impinges on both protein synthesis and catabolism, by phosphorylating molecules involved in the two pathways (reviewed in Rosner, Hanneder, Siegel, Valli, & Hengstschläger, 2008). However, despite p38 appears involved in the pathogenesis of muscle wasting, no studies demonstrate that its pharmacological inhibition may result in muscle mass preservation. Preliminary data show that tumor-bearing mice treated with the p38 inhibitor SB203580 are not significantly different from untreated animals in terms of muscle force, food intake, and tumor mass (Penna et al., 2012).

The other MAPK possibly involved in modulating muscle protein content is ERK, although its role is still quite controversial. Its inactivation in experimental animals results in muscle atrophy (Shi et al., 2009). Not only this, it appears able to counteract the anabolic stimuli induced by treatment with β_2-adrenergic agonists or IGF-1 (Haddad & Adams, 2004; Shi et al., 2007). Consistently, reduced levels of active ERK were reported in sarcopenia of aging (Carlson et al., 2009). ERK inhibition seems required to increase ubiquitin ligase expression in cultured murine myocytes (Shi et al., 2008). By contrast, in the same model system, ERK activation results in reduced myotube size (Rommel et al., 1999), while its inhibition leads to a hypertrophic phenotype (Rommel et al., 1999). Also the IGF-1 protective effects against oxidative-stress myotube damage would involve ERK activity (Yang et al., 2010). Finally, muscle atrophy due to immobilization by hindlimb suspension was associated with increased levels of phosphorylated ERK (Kato, Ito, Kamei, Iwamoto, & Inaguma, 2002). As IGF-1, also ERK plays a role in myogenesis, being able to enhance the regenerative capacity of human satellite cells isolated from both young and old subjects (Carlson et al., 2009). Treatment of mice bearing the C26 colon carcinoma with the ERK inhibitor PD98059 partially but significantly protects tumor hosts from the onset of body weight loss and muscle mass depletion (Penna, Bonetto, et al., 2010; Penna, Costamagna, et al., 2010). ERK inhibition also results in normalization of atrogin-1 hyperexpression, independently from the state of activation of Akt. In addition, Pax7 expression, a marker of activated satellite cells, is significantly increased in the muscle of C26 hosts with respect to controls, while myogenin levels, indicative of an ongoing differentiative process, are reduced. Such a pattern likely reflects an impairment of muscle regeneration, suggesting that the accumulation of activated satellite cells in the muscle of tumor hosts may derive from enhanced proliferation, impaired differentiation, or both. However, when tumor bearers are treated with PD98059, Pax7 and myogenin expression is restored to control values. These observations suggest that ERK activation likely plays a role in maintaining satellite cells in an undifferentiated state, thus contributing with an additional mechanism to muscle depletion (Penna, Bonetto, et al., 2010; Penna, Costamagna, et al., 2010).

Finally, AMPK, which mainly works as a sensor of intracellular energetic balance, is also involved in the regulation of protein turnover (Mihaylova & Shaw, 2011). AMPK may affect protein synthesis mainly in view of its ability to inhibit mTOR-dependent signaling (Mihaylova & Shaw, 2011); however, it was also shown to modulate protein degradation rates, acting on atrogin-1 expression through a FoxO-dependent mechanism (Nakashima & Yakabe, 2007; Romanello et al., 2010). Of interest, increased AMPK activation is detectable in the skeletal muscle of tumor-bearing animals (Penna, Bonetto, et al., 2010; White et al., 2011), where it is associated with marked alterations of mitochondrial morphology (Penna et al., unpublished observations).

As a conclusion, protein turnover modulations in the skeletal muscle could also be counteracted by tools aimed at directly inhibiting the intracellular proteolytic systems. In this regard, however, despite encouraging initial observations obtained by treating tumor-bearing animals with inhibitor of lysosomal proteases (Ruff & Secrist, 1984; Tessitore, Costelli, & Baccino, 1994), no significant data were obtained.

Proteasome inhibitors (bortezomib), currently used for the treatment of some hematologic malignancies, have severe side effects, and preliminary data show that they are ineffective in preventing muscle wasting in tumor-bearing rats (P. Costelli and M. Muscaritoli, unpublished data). Similar observations were obtained by treating tumor-bearing animals with inhibitors of the Ca^{2+}-dependent proteolytic system (dantrolene; P. Costelli and M. Muscaritoli, unpublished data) or with an inhibitor of serine proteases (gabexate mesilate; M. Muscaritoli, unpublished observations). The possible explanation for such negative results is that when inhibiting a specific proteolytic system, the others likely compensate, eventually resulting in a pattern of muscle wasting. Not only a note of care should be introduced in view of administering inhibitors of the lysosomal proteolysis to cachectic subjects. Indeed, tumor-bearing mice with advanced cachexia cannot cope a treatment with colchicine, suggesting that the autophagic flux blocked by the inhibitor represents a survival mechanism (Penna et al., unpublished data).

While strategies aimed at blocking muscle protein breakdown are extensively studied, little is done in terms of correction of the altered lipid metabolism. This likely arises from the notion that skeletal muscle mass is the limiting factor for patient survival (see earlier). This concept, however, should be promptly revised, in view of the results showing that inhibition of lipolytic enzymes in tumor-bearing mice reverses the loss in muscle mass, in addition to restoring normal adipose depots (Das et al., 2011; see earlier).

Few results are available in the literature on the use of inhibitors of lipolysis. Recently, YC-1, used as an agent against platelet aggregation, was shown to stimulate preadipocyte differentiation, to inhibit TNFα-induced lipolysis *in vitro*, and to restore normal circulating level of free fatty acids in tumor-bearing mice (Chung, Yen-Ping Kuo, Chen, & Huang, 2011).

12. CONCLUSIONS

The different options proposed to treat cachexia were built up taking into account the results obtained from experimental and clinical studies, showing that this syndrome is characterized by marked metabolic alterations, mainly due to mediators of both tumor and host origin. In addition, such metabolic perturbations are now recognized to occur very early in the course of the disease, well before any evidence of general wasting. A number of drugs selected because of their effectiveness in preventing experimental cachexia, mostly the cancer-related one, are either in the preclinical phase, or reaching the clinical experimentation stage. Of particular relevance, in this regard, appears the adoption of anticytokine strategies, although the results available point to combination protocols as the best choice to address the different aspects of cachexia (e.g., both lipid and protein mass depletion). Moreover, since cachexia often becomes clinically evident at a rather advanced disease stage, the detection of early subclinical perturbations that may be indicative of a situation of "latent cachexia" (precachexia) is important in order to prevent the onset of overt cachexia. The definition of effective therapeutic strategies will also be useful in improving patient management and quality of life.

REFERENCES

Acharyya, S., Butchbach, M. E., Sahenk, Z., Wang, H., Saji, M., Carathers, M., et al. (2005). Dystrophin glycoprotein complex dysfunction: A regulatory link between muscular dystrophy and cancer cachexia. *Cancer Cell*, *8*, 421–432.

Agustsson, T., Rydén, M., Hoffstedt, J., van Harmelen, V., Dicker, A., Laurencikiene, J., et al. (2007). Mechanism of increased lipolysis in cancer cachexia. *Cancer Research*, *67*, 5531–5537.

Argilés, J. M., López-Soriano, J., Almendro, V., Busquets, S., & López-Soriano, F. J. (2005). Cross-talk between skeletal muscle and adipose tissue: A link with obesity? *Medicinal Research Reviews*, *25*, 49–65.

Attard-Montalto, S. P., Camacho-Hubner, C., Cotteril, A. M., D'Souza-Li, L., Bartlett, K., Halliday, D., et al. (1998). Changes in protein turnover, IGF-I and IGF binding proteins in children with cancer. *Acta Pediatrica*, *87*, 54–60.

Aversa, Z., Bonetto, A., Penna, F., Costelli, P., Di Rienzo, G., Lacitignola, A., et al. (2012). Changes in myostatin signaling in non-weight-losing cancer patients. *Annals of Surgical Oncology*, *19*, 1350–1356.

Barber, M. D., & Fearon, K. C. (2001). Tolerance and incorporation of a high-dose eicosapentaenoic acid diester emulsion by patients with pancreatic cancer cachexia. *Lipids*, *36*, 347–351.

Bayliss, T. J., Smith, J. T., Schuster, M., Dragnev, K. H., & Rigas, J. R. (2011). A humanized anti-IL-6 antibody (ALD518) in non-small cell lung cancer. *Expert Opinion on Biological Therapy*, *11*, 1663–1668.

Beck, S. A., Smith, K. L., & Tisdale, M. J. (1991). Anticachectic and antitumor effect of eicosapentaenoic acid and its effect on protein turnover. *Cancer Research*, *51*, 6089–6093.

Bianchi, G., Marzocchi, R., Agostini, F., & Marchesini, G. (2005). Update on nutritional supplementation with branched-chain amino acids. *Current Opinion in Clinical Nutrition and Metabolic Care*, *8*, 83–87.

Bing, C. (2011). Lipid mobilization in cachexia: Mechanisms and mediators. *Current Opinion in Supportive and Palliative Care*, *5*, 356–360.

British National Formulary. Vol. 58, London: British Medical Association, September 2009.

Bonetto, A., Aydogdu, T., Kunzevitzky, N., Guttridge, D. C., Khuri, S., Koniaris, L. G., et al. (2011). STAT3 activation in skeletal muscle links muscle wasting and the acute phase response in cancer cachexia. *PLoS One*, *6*, e22538.

Bonetto, A., Penna, F., Minero, V. G., Reffo, P., Bonelli, G., Baccino, F. M., et al. (2009). Deacetylase inhibitors modulate the myostatin/follistatin axis without improving cachexia in tumor-bearing mice. *Current Cancer Drug Targets*, *9*, 608–616.

Boppart, M. D., Hirshman, M. F., Sakamoto, K., Fielding, R. A., & Goodyear, L. J. (2001). Static stretch increases c-Jun NH2-terminal kinase activity and p38 phosphorylation in rat skeletal muscle. *American Journal of Physiology. Cell Physiology*, *280*, C352–C358.

Briot, K., Garnero, P., Le Henanff, A., Dougados, M., & Roux, C. (2005). Body weight, body composition, and bone turnover changes in patients with spondyloarthropathy receiving anti-tumour necrosis factor alpha treatment. *Annals of the Rheumatic Diseases*, *64*, 1137–1140.

Bruera, E., Neumann, C. M., Pituskin, E., Calder, K., Ball, G., & Hanson, J. (1999). Thalidomide in patients with cachexia due to terminal cancer: Preliminary report. *Annals of Oncology*, *10*, 857–859.

Bruun, J. M., Lihn, A. S., Verdich, C., Pedersen, S. B., Toubro, S., Astrup, A., et al. (2003). Regulation of adiponectin by adipose tissue-derived cytokines: in vivo and in vitro investigations in humans. *American Journal of Physiology. Endocrinology and Metabolism*, *285*, E527–E533.

Bryson, N. (2008). Combination for treatment of diabetes mellitus. WO2008151415.

Cangiano, C., Laviano, A., & Meguid, M. M. (1996). Effects of administration of oral branched-chain amino acids on anorexia and caloric intake in cancer patients. *Journal of the National Cancer Institute*, *88*, 550–552.

Carlson, M. E., Suetta, C., Conboy, M. J., Aagaard, P., Mackey, A., Kjaer, M., et al. (2009). Molecular aging and rejuvenation of human muscle stem cells. *EMBO Molecular Medicine*, *1*, 381–391.

Chasen, M., Hirschman, S. Z., & Bhargava, R. (2011). Phase II study of the novel peptide-nucleic acid OHR118 in the management of cancer-related anorexia/cachexia. *Journal of the American Medical Directors Association*, *12*, 62–67.

Chen, S. E., Gerken, E., Zhang, Y., Zhan, M., Mohan, R. K., Li, A. S., et al. (2005). Role of TNF-{alpha} signaling in regeneration of cardiotoxin-injured muscle. *American Journal of Physiology. Cell Physiology*, *289*, C1179–C1187.

Chung, T. H., Yen-Ping Kuo, M., Chen, J. K., & Huang, D. M. (2011). YC-1 rescues cancer cachexia by affecting lipolysis and adipogenesis. *International Journal of Cancer*, *9*, 2274–2283.

Clarke, S., Gebbie, C., Sweeney, C., Olzewski, N., & Smith, J. (2009). A phase I, pharmacokinetic (PK) and preliminary efficacy assessment of ALD518, a humanized anti-IL-6 antibody, in patients with advanced cancer. In *5th cachexia conference, Barcelona 5-8 December 2009* Abstracts p.53.

Coletti, D., Moresi, V., Adamo, S., Molinaro, M., & Sassoon, D. (2005). Tumor necrosis factor-alpha gene transfer induces cachexia and inhibits muscle regeneration. *Genesis*, *43*, 120–128.

Coletti, D., Yang, E., Marazzi, G., & Sassoon, D. (2002). TNFalpha inhibits skeletal myogenesis through a PW1-dependent pathway by recruitment of caspase pathways. *The EMBO Journal*, *21*, 631–642.

Combaret, L., Ralliere, C., Taillandier, D., Tanaka, K., & Attaix, D. (1999). Manipulation of the ubiquitin-proteasome pathway in cachexia: Pentoxifylline suppresses the activation of 20S and 26S proteasomes in muscles from tumor-bearing rats. *Molecular Biology Reports*, *26*, 95–101.

Costelli, P., Bossola, M., Muscaritoli, M., Grieco, G., Bonelli, G., Bellantone, R., et al. (2002). Anticytokine treatment prevents the increase in the activity of ATP-ubiquitin- and $Ca2^{+}$-dependent proteolytic systems in the muscle of tumor-bearing rats. *Cytokine*, *19*, 1–5.

Costelli, P., Carbó, N., Tessitore, L., Bagby, G. J., Lopez-Soriano, F. J., Argilès, J. M., et al. (1993). Tumour necrosis factor-α mediates changes in tissue protein turnover in a rat cancer cachexia model. *The Journal of Clinical Investigation*, *92*, 2783–2789.

Costelli, P., Llovera, M., Carbó, N., García-Martínez, C., López-Soriano, F. J., & Argilés, J. M. (1995). Interleukin-1 receptor antagonist (IL-1ra) is unable to reverse cachexia in rats bearing an ascites hepatoma (Yoshida AH-130). *Cancer Letters*, *95*, 33–38.

Costelli, P., Muscaritoli, M., Bossola, M., Penna, F., Reffo, P., Bonetto, A., et al. (2006). IGF-1 is downregulated in experimental cancer cachexia. *American Journal of Physiology. Regulatory, Integrative and Comparative Physiology*, *291*, R674–R683.

Das, S. K., Eder, S., Schauer, S., Diwoky, C., Temmel, H., Guertl, B., et al. (2011). Adipose triglyceride lipase contributes to cancer-associated cachexia. *Science*, *333*, 233–238.

Das, B. K., Mishra, S., Padhi, P. K., Manish, R., Tripathy, R., Sahoo, P. K., et al. (2003). Pentoxifylline adjunct improves prognosis of human cerebral malaria in adults. *Tropical Medicine & International Health*, *8*, 680–684.

de Heredia, F. P., Gómez-Martínez, S., & Marcos, A. (2012). Obesity, inflammation and the immune system. *The Proceedings of the Nutrition Society*, *20*, 1–7.

Dodd, S. L., Hain, B., Senf, S. M., & Judge, A. R. (2009). Hsp27 inhibits IKKbeta-induced NF-kappaB activity and skeletal muscle atrophy. *The FASEB Journal*, *23*, 3415–3423.

Durham, W. J., Dillon, E. L., & Sheffield-Moore, M. (2009). Inflammatory burden and amino acid metabolism in cancer cachexia. *Current Opinion in Clinical Nutrition and Metabolic Care*, *12*, 72–77.

Enomoto, A., Rho, M. C., Fukami, A., Hiraku, O., Komiyama, K., & Hayashi, M. (2004). Suppression of cancer cachexia by 20S,21-epoxy-resibufogenin-3-acetate-a novel non-peptide IL-6 receptor antagonist. *Biochemical and Biophysical Research Communications*, *323*, 1096–1102.

Evans, W. J., Morley, J. E., Argilès, J., Bales, C., Baracos, V., Guttridge, D., et al. (2008). Cachexia: A new definition. *Clinical Nutrition*, *27*, 793–799.

Fallowfield, L. (2002). Quality of life: A new perspective for cancer patients. *Nature Reviews. Cancer*, *2*, 873–879.

Fearon, K., Strasser, F., Anker, S. D., Bosaeus, I., Bruera, E., Fainsinger, R. L., et al. (2011). Definition and classification of cancer cachexia: An international consensus. *The Lancet Oncology*, *12*, 489–495.

Fearon, K. C., von Meyenfeldt, M. F., Moses, A. G., Van Geenen, R., Roy, A., Gouma, D. J., et al. (2003). Effect of a protein and energy dense N-3 fatty acid enriched oral supplement on loss of weight and lean tissue in cancer cachexia: A randomised double blind trial. *Gut*, *52*, 1479–1486.

Fearon, K. C., Voss, A. C., Hustead, D. S., & Cancer Cachexia Study Group, (2006). Definition of cancer cachexia: Effect of weight loss, reduced food intake, and systemic inflammation on functional status and prognosis. *The American Journal of Clinical Nutrition*, *83*, 1345–1350.

Fide, E., Bregman, T., & Kirkham, T. C. (2005). Endocannabinoids and food intake: Newborn suckling and appetite regulation in adulthood. *Experimental Biology and Medicine*, *230*, 225–234.

Ghezzi, P., & Cerami, A. (2005). Tumor necrosis factor as a pharmacological target. *Molecular Biotechnology*, *31*, 239–244.

Glass, D. J. (2010). Signaling pathways perturbing muscle mass. *Current Opinion in Clinical Nutrition and Metabolic Care*, *13*, 225–229.

Goldberg, R. M., Loprinzi, C. L., Mailliard, J. A., O'Fallon, J. R., Krook, J. E., Ghosh, C., et al. (1995). Pentoxifylline for treatment of cancer anorexia and cachexia? A randomized, double-blind, placebo-controlled trial. *Journal of Clinical Oncology*, *13*, 2856–2859.

Gordon, J. N., Trebble, T. M., Ellis, R. D., Duncan, H. D., Johns, T., & Goggin, P. M. (2005). Thalidomide in the treatment of cancer cachexia: A randomised placebo controlled trial. *Gut*, *54*, 540–545.

Grossberg, A. J., Scarlett, J. M., & Marks, D. L. (2010). Hypothalamic mechanisms in cachexia. *Physiology & Behavior*, *100*, 478–489.

Gulen, S. T., Karadag, F., Karul, A. B., Kilicarslan, N., Ceylan, E., Kuman, N. K., et al. (2012). Adipokines and systemic inflammation in weight-losing lung cancer patients. *Lung*, *190*, 327–332.

Guttridge, D. C., Mayo, M. W., Madrid, L. V., Wang, C. Y., & Baldwin, A. S., Jr. (2000). NFkappaB-induced loss of MyoD messenger RNA: Possible role in muscle decay and cachexia. *Science*, *289*, 2363–2366.

Haddad, F., & Adams, G. R. (2004). Inhibition of MAP/ERK kinase prevents IGF-I-induced hypertrophy in rat muscles. *Journal of Applied Physiology*, *96*, 203–210.

Haslett, P. A. (1998). Anticytokine approaches to the treatment of anorexia and cachexia. *Seminars in Oncology*, *25*, 53–57.

Huey, K. A. (2006). Regulation of HSP25 expression and phosphorylation in functionally overloaded rat plantaris and soleus muscles. *Journal of Applied Physiology*, *100*, 451–456.

Ikeda, U., & Shimada, K. (1999). Statins and monocytes. *Lancet*, *353*, 2070.

Ito, T., Ando, H., Suzuki, T., Ogura, T., Hotta, K., Imamura, Y., et al. (2010). Identification of a primary target of thalidomide teratogenicity. *Science*, *327*, 1345–1350.

Jatoi, A., Dakhil, S. R., Nguyen, P. L., Sloan, J. A., Kugler, J. W., Rowland, K. M., Jr., et al. (2007). A placebo-controlled double blind trial of etanercept for the cancer anorexia/weight loss syndrome: Results from N00C1 from the North Central Cancer Treatment Group. *Cancer*, *110*, 1396–1403.

Jatoi, A., Rowland, K., Loprinzi, C. L., Sloan, J. A., Dakhil, S. R., MacDonald, N., et al. (2004). An eicosapentaenoic acid supplement versus megestrol acetate versus both for patients with cancer-associated wasting: A North Central Cancer Treatment Group and National Cancer Institute of Canada collaborative effort. *Journal of Clinical Oncology*, *22*, 2469–2476.

Kadowaki, M., & Kanazawa, T. (2003). Amino acids as regulators of proteolysis. *The Journal of Nutrition, 133*, 2052S–2056S.

Kato, K., Ito, H., Kamei, K., Iwamoto, I., & Inaguma, Y. (2002). Innervation-dependent phosphorylation and accumulation of alphaB-crystallin and Hsp27 as insoluble complexes in disused muscle. *The FASEB Journal, 16*, 1432–1434.

Kawano, F., Matsuoka, Y., Oke, Y., Higo, Y., Terada, M., Wang, X. D., et al. (2007). Role (s) of nucleoli and phosphorylation of ribosomal protein S6 and/or HSP27 in the regulation of muscle mass. *American Journal of Physiology. Cell Physiology, 293*, C35–C44.

Kerem, M., Ferahkose, Z., Yilmaz, U. T., Pasaoglu, H., Ofluoglu, E., Bedirli, A., et al. (2008). Adipokines and ghrelin in gastric cancer cachexia. *World Journal of Gastroenterology, 14*, 3633–3641.

Khan, Z. H., Simpson, E. J., Cole, A. T., Holt, M., MacDonald, I., Pye, D., et al. (2003). Oesophageal cancer and cachexia: The effect of short-term treatment with thalidomide on weight loss and lean body mass. *Alimentary Pharmacology & Therapeutics, 17*, 677–682.

Kimura, Y., & Sumiyoshi, M. (2005). Antitumor and antimetastatic actions of eicosapentaenoic acid ethylester and its by-products formed during accelerated stability testing. *Cancer Science, 96*, 441–450.

Kishimoto, C. (1996). Chugai Pharmaceutical Co LTD. Therapeutic agent for disease due to IL-6 production. JP8169846.

Klein, T. W., Lane, B., Newton, C. A., & Friedman, H. (2000). The cannabinoid system and cytokine network. *Proceedings of the Society for Experimental Biology and Medicine, 225*, 1–8.

Körber, J., Pricelius, S., Heidrich, M., & Müller, M. J. (1999). Increased lipid utilization in weight losing and weight stable cancer patients with normal body weight. *European Journal of Clinical Nutrition, 53*, 740–745.

Lago, F., Dieguez, C., Gómez-Reino, J., & Gualillo, O. (2007). The emerging role of adipokines as mediators of inflammation and immune responses. *Cytokine & Growth Factor Reviews, 18*, 313–325.

Lai, K.-M., Gonzalez, M., Poueymirou, W. T., Kline, W. O., Na, E., Zlotchenko, E., et al. (2004). Conditional activation of akt in adult skeletal muscle induces rapid hypertrophy. *Molecular and Cellular Biology, 24*, 9295–9304.

Laurencikiene, J., Stenson, B. M., Arvidsson Nordström, E., Agustsson, T., Langin, D., Isaksson, B., et al. (2008). Evidence for an important role of CIDEA in human cancer cachexia. *Cancer Research, 68*, 9247–9254.

Laviano, A., Meguid, M. M., Inui, A., Muscaritoli, M., & Rossi Fanelli, F. (2005). Therapy insight: Cancer anorexia-cachexia syndrome—When all you can eat is yourself. *Nature Clinical Practice. Oncology, 2*, 158–165.

Laviano, A., Meguid, M. M., & Rossi Fanelli, F. (2003). Improving food intake in anorectic cancer patients. *Current Opinion in Clinical Nutrition and Metabolic Care, 6*, 421–426.

Laviano, A., Meguid, M. M., & Rossi-Fanelli, F. (2003). Cancer anorexia: Clinical implications, pathogenesis, and therapeutic strategies. *The Lancet Oncology, 4*, 686–694.

Lee, C., Raffaghello, L., Brandhorst, S., Safdie, F. M., Bianchi, G., Martin-Montalvo, A., et al. (2012). Fasting cycles retard growth of tumors and sensitize a range of cancer cell types to chemotherapy. *Science Translational Medicine, 4*, 124ra27.

Li, Y. P., Chen, Y., John, J., Moylan, J., Jin, B., Mann, D. L., et al. (2005). TNF-α acts via p38 MAPK to stimulate expression of the ubiquitin ligase atrogin1/MAFbx in skeletal muscle. *The FASEB Journal, 19*, 362–370.

Li, J. P., Lu, L., Wang, L. J., Zhang, F. R., & Shen, W. F. (2011). Increased serum levels of S100B are related to the severity of cardiac dysfunction, renal insufficiency and major cardiac events in patients with chronic heart failure. *Clinical Biochemistry, 44*, 984–988.

Li, H. H., Willis, M. S., Lockyer, P., Miller, N., McDonough, H., Glass, D. J., et al. (2007). Atrogin-1 inhibits Akt-dependent cardiac hypertrophy in mice via ubiquitin-dependent coactivation of Forkhead proteins. *The Journal of Clinical Investigation, 117*, 3211–3223.

Liu, Y., Jia, Z., Dong, L., Wang, R., & Qiu, G. (2008). A randomized pilot study of atractylenolide I on gastric cancer cachexia patients. *Evidence-Based Complementary and Alternative Medicine: eCAM, 5*, 337–344.

Liu, Q., Xu, W. G., Luo, Y., Han, F. F., Yao, X. H., Yang, T. Y., et al. (2011). Cigarette smoke-induced skeletal muscle atrophy is associated with up-regulation of USP-19 via p38 and ERK MAPKs. *Journal of Cellular Biochemistry, 112*, 2307–2316.

Lopez, A. P., Roque Figuls, M., Cuchi, G. U., Berenstein, E. G., Pasies, B. A., Alegre, M. B., et al. (2004). Systematic review of megestrol acetate in the treatment of anorexia-cachexia syndrome. *Journal of Pain and Symptom Management, 27*, 360–369.

López-Soriano, J., Carbó, N., Tessitore, L., López-Soriano, F. J., & Argilés, J. M. (1999). Leptin and tumor growth in rats. *International Journal of Cancer, 81*, 726–729.

Loprinzi, C. L., Kruger, J. W., & Sloan, J. A. (1999). Randomized comparison of megestrol acetate versus dexamethasone versus fluoxymesterone for the treatment of cancer anorexia/cachexia. *Journal of Clinical Oncology, 17*, 3299–3306.

Mantovani, G., Macciò, A., Madeddu, C., Serpe, R., Massa, E., Dessì, M., et al. (2010). Randomized phase III clinical trial of five different arms of treatment in 332 patients with cancer cachexia. *The Oncologist, 15*, 200–211.

Marcora, S. M., Chester, K. R., Mittal, G., Lemmey, A. B., & Maddison, P. J. (2006). Randomized phase 2 trial of anti-tumor necrosis factor therapy for cachexia in patients with early rheumatoid arthritis. *The American Journal of Clinical Nutrition, 84*, 1463–1472.

Martín, A. I., Castillero, E., Granado, M., López-Menduiña, M., Villanúa, M. A., & López-Calderón, A. (2008). Adipose tissue loss in adjuvant arthritis is associated with a decrease in lipogenesis, but not with an increase in lipolysis. *The Journal of Endocrinology, 197*, 111–119.

Matthys, P., Heremans, H., Opdenakker, G., & Billiau, A. (1991). Anti-interferon-gamma antibody treatment, growth of Lewis lung tumours in mice and tumour-associated cachexia. *European Journal of Cancer, 27*, 182–187.

Meng, W., Swenson, L. L., Fitzgibbon, M. J., Hayakawa, K., Ter Haar, E., Behrens, A. E., et al. (2002). Structure of mitogen-activated protein kinase-activated protein (MAPKAP) kinase 2 suggests a bifunctional switch that couples kinase activation with nuclear export. *The Journal of Biological Chemistry, 277*, 37401–37405.

Mihaylova, M. M., & Shaw, R. J. (2011). The AMPK signalling pathway coordinates cell growth, autophagy and metabolism. *Nature Cell Biology, 13*, 1016–1023.

Moresi, V., Pristera, A., Scicchitano, B. M., Molinaro, M., Teodori, L., Sassoon, D., et al. (2008). Tumor necrosis factor-alpha inhibition of skeletal muscle regeneration is mediated by a caspase-dependent stem cell response. *Stem Cells, 26*, 997–1008.

Moss, M. L., Jin, S. L., Milla, M. E., Bickett, D. M., Burkhart, W., Carter, H. L., et al. (1997). Cloning of a disintegrin metalloproteinase that processes precursor tumour-necrosis factor-alpha. *Nature, 385*, 733–736.

Murumkar, P. R., DasGupta, S., Chandani, S. R., Giridhar, R., & Yadav, M. R. (2010). Novel TACE inhibitors in drug discovery: A review of patented compounds. *Expert Opinion on Therapeutic Patents, 20*, 31–57.

Muscaritoli, M., Anker, S. D., Argilés, J., Aversa, Z., Bauer, J. M., Biolo, G., et al. (2010). Consensus definition of sarcopenia, cachexia and pre-cachexia: Joint document elaborated by Special Interest Groups (SIG) "cachexia-anorexia in chronic wasting diseases" and "nutrition in geriatrics". *Clinical Nutrition, 29*, 154–159.

Muscaritoli, M., Bossola, M., Aversa, Z., Bellantone, R., & Rossi Fanelli, F. (2006). Prevention and treatment of cancer cachexia: New insights into an old problem. *European Journal of Cancer, 42*, 31–41.

Muscaritoli, M., Costelli, P., Bossola, M., Grieco, G., Bonelli, G., Bellantone, R., et al. (2003). Effects of simvastatin administration in an experimental model of cancer cachexia. *Nutrition, 19*, 936–939.

Nakashima, J., Tachibana, M., Ueno, M., Miyajima, A., Baba, S., & Murai, M. (1998). Association between tumor necrosis factor in serum and cachexia in patients with prostate cancer. *Clinical Cancer Research, 4*, 1743–1748.

Nakashima, K., & Yakabe, Y. (2007). AMPK activation stimulates myofibrillar protein degradation and expression of atrophy-related ubiquitin ligases by increasing FOXO transcription factors in C2C12 myotubes. *Bioscience, Biotechnology, and Biochemistry, 71*, 1650–1656.

Nara-Ashizawa, N., Akiyama, Y., Maruyama, K., Tsukada, T., & Yamaguchi, K. (2001). Lipolytic and lipoprotein lipase (LPL)-inhibiting activities produced by a human lung cancer cell line responsible for cachexia induction. *Anticancer Research, 21*, 3381–3387.

Neary, N. M., Small, C. J., Wren, A. M., Lee, J. L., Druce, M. R., Palmieri, C., et al. (2004). Ghrelin increases energy intake in cancer patients with impaired appetite: Acute, randomized, placebo-controlled trial. *The Journal of Clinical Endocrinology and Metabolism, 89*, 2832–2836.

Nicolas, N., Marazzi, G., Kelley, K., & Sassoon, D. (2005). Embryonic deregulation of muscle stress signaling pathways leads to altered postnatal stem cell behavior and a failure in postnatal muscle growth. *Developmental Biology, 281*, 171–183.

Nienhuis, H. L., Westra, J., Smit, A. J., Limburg, P. C., Kallenberg, C. G., & Bijl, M. (2009). AGE and their receptor RAGE in systemic autoimmune diseases: An inflammation propagating factor contributing to accelerated atherosclerosis. *Autoimmunity, 42*, 302–304.

Niewczas, M. A., Gohda, T., Skupien, J., Smiles, A. M., Walker, W. H., Rosetti, F., et al. (2012). Circulating TNF receptors 1 and 2 predict ESRD in type 2 diabetes. *Journal of the American Society of Nephrology, 23*, 507–515.

Noori, N., Kovesdy, C. P., Dukkipati, R., Feroze, U., Molnar, M. Z., Bross, R., et al. (2011). Racial and ethnic differences in mortality of hemodialysis patients: Role of dietary and nutritional status and inflammation. *American Journal of Nephrology, 33*, 157–167.

Norrby, M., & Tågerud, S. (2010). Mitogen-activated protein kinase-activated protein kinase 2 (MK2) in skeletal muscle atrophy and hypertrophy. *Journal of Cellular Physiology, 223*, 194–201.

Ohtori, S., Miyagi, M., Eguchi, Y., Inoue, G., Orita, S., Ochiai, N., et al. (2012). Efficacy of epidural administration of anti-interleukin-6 receptor antibody onto spinal nerve for treatment of sciatica. *European Spine Journal, 21*, 2079–2084.

Palacios, D., Mozzetta, C., Consalvi, S., Caretti, G., Saccone, V., Proserpio, V., et al. (2010). TNF/p38α/polycomb signaling to Pax7 locus in satellite cells links inflammation to the epigenetic control of muscle regeneration. *Cell Stem Cell, 7*, 455–469.

Patra, S. K., & Arora, S. (2012). Integrative role of neuropeptides and cytokines in cancer anorexia-cachexia syndrome. *Clinica Chimica Acta, 413*, 1025–1034.

Pedersen, B. K., & Febbraio, M. A. (2008). Muscle as an endocrine organ: Focus on muscle-derived interleukin-6. *Physiological Reviews, 88*, 1379–1406.

Penna, F., Bonetto, A., Muscaritoli, M., Costamagna, D., Minero, V. G., Bonelli, G., et al. (2010). Muscle atrophy in experimental cancer cachexia: Is the IGF-1 signaling pathway involved? *International Journal of Cancer, 127*, 1706–1717.

Penna, F., Costamagna, D., Camperi, A., Muscaritoli, M., Baccino, F. M., & Bonelli, G. (2012). Protein kinases in the pathogenesis of muscle wasting. In G. Da Silva Xavier (Ed.), *Protein Kinases/Book 2*. Rijeka, Croatia: InTech in press.

Penna, F., Costamagna, D., Pin, F., Camperi, A., Fanzani, A., Chiarpotto, E.M., et al. (2013). Autophagic Degradation Contributes to Muscle Wasting in Cancer Cachexia. *American Journal of Pathology*, doi:pii: S0002-9440(13)00033-3. 10.1016/j.ajpath.2012.12.023. [Epub ahead of print]

Penna, F., Costamagna, D., Fanzani, A., Bonelli, G., Baccino, F. M., & Costelli, P. (2010). Muscle wasting and impaired myogenesis in tumor bearing mice are prevented by ERK inhibition. *PLoS One*, *5*, e13604.

Pisters, P. W., & Pearlstone, D. B. (1993). Protein and amino acid metabolism in cancer cachexia: Investigative techniques and therapeutic interventions. *Critical Reviews in Clinical Laboratory Sciences*, *30*, 223–272.

Popa, C., Netea, M. G., Radstake, T. R., van Riel, P. L., Barrera, P., & van der Meer, J. W. (2005). Markers of inflammation are negatively correlated with serum leptin in rheumatoid arthritis. *Annals of the Rheumatic Diseases*, *64*, 1195–1198.

Prado, C. M., Antoun, S., Sawyer, M. B., & Baracos, V. E. (2011). Two faces of drug therapy in cancer: Drug-related lean tissue loss and its adverse consequences to survival and toxicity. *Current Opinion in Clinical Nutrition and Metabolic Care*, *14*, 250–254.

Prado, C. M., Lieffers, J. R., McCargar, L. J., Reiman, T., Sawyer, M. B., Martin, L., et al. (2008). Prevalence and clinical implications of sarcopenic obesity in patients with solid tumours of the respiratory and gastrointestinal tracts: A population-based study. *The Lancet Oncology*, *9*, 629–635.

Prehn, R. T. (1972). The immune reaction as a stimulator of tumor growth. *Science*, *176*, 170–171.

Raffaghello, L., Lee, C., Safdie, F. M., Wei, M., Madia, F., Bianchi, G., et al. (2008). Starvation-dependent differential stress resistance protects normal but not cancer cells against high-dose chemotherapy. *Proceedings of the National Academy of Sciences of the United States of America*, *105*, 8215–8220.

Raffaghello, L., Safdie, F., Bianchi, G., Dorff, T., Fontana, L., & Longo, V. D. (2010). Fasting and differential chemotherapy protection in patients. *Cell Cycle*, *9*, 4474–4476.

Reid, J., Mills, M., Cantwell, M., Cardwell, C. R., Murray, L. J., & Donnelly, M. (2012). Thalidomide for managing cancer cachexia. *Cochrane Database of Systematic Reviews*, *4*, CD008664.

Rivadaneira, D. E., Evoy, D., Fahey, T. J., 3rd., Lieberman, R. D., & Daly, J. M. (1998). Nutritional support of the cancer patient. *CA: A Cancer Journal for Clinicians*, *48*, 69–80.

Romanello, V., Guadagnin, E., Gomes, L., Roder, I., Sandri, C., Petersen, Y., et al. (2010). Mitochondrial fission and remodelling contributes to muscle atrophy. *The EMBO Journal*, *29*, 1774–1785.

Rommel, C., Bodine, S. C., Clarke, B. A., Rossman, R., Nunez, L., Stitt, T. N., et al. (2001). Mediation of IGF-1-induced skeletal myotube hypertrophy by PI(3)K/Akt/mTOR and PI(3)K/Akt/GSK3 pathways. *Nature Cell Biology*, *3*, 1009–1013.

Rommel, C., Clarke, B. A., Zimmermann, S., Nunez, L., Rossman, R., Reid, K., et al. (1999). Differentiation stage-specific inhibition of the Raf-MEK-ERK pathway by Akt. *Science*, *286*, 1738–1741.

Rosner, M., Hanneder, M., Siegel, N., Valli, A., & Hengstschläger, M. (2008). The tuberous sclerosis gene products hamartin and tuberin are multifunctional proteins with a wide spectrum of interacting partners. *Mutation Research*, *658*, 234–246.

Ross, P. J., Ashley, S., Norton, A., Priest, K., Waters, J. S., Eisen, T., et al. (2004). Do patients with weight loss have a worse outcome when undergoing chemotherapy for lung cancers? *British Journal of Cancer*, *90*, 1905–1911.

Ruff, R. L., & Secrist, D. (1984). Inhibitors of prostaglandin synthesis or cathepsin B prevent muscle wasting due to sepsis in the rat. *The Journal of Clinical Investigation*, *73*, 1483–1486.

Sakamoto, K., Aschenbach, W. G., Hirshman, M. F., & Goodyear, L. J. (2003). Akt signaling in skeletal muscle: Regulation by exercise and passive stretch. *American Journal of Physiology. Endocrinology and Metabolism*, *285*, E1081–E1088.

Sakurai, Y., & Klein, S. (1998). Metabolic alterations in patients with cancer: Nutritional implications. *Surgery Today*, *28*, 247–257.

Sandri, M., Sandri, C., Gilbert, A., Skurk, C., Calabria, E., Picard, A., et al. (2004). Foxo transcription factors induce the atrophy-related ubiquitin ligase atrogin-1 and cause skeletal muscle atrophy. *Cell, 117*, 399–412.

Seruga, B., Zhang, H., Bernstein, L. J., & Tannock, I. F. (2008). Cytokines and their relationship to the symptoms and outcome of cancer. *Nature Reviews. Cancer, 8*, 887–899.

Shan, X., & Yeo, G. S. (2011). Central leptin and ghrelin signalling: Comparing and contrasting their mechanisms of action in the brain. *Reviews in Endocrine & Metabolic Disorders, 12*, 197–209.

Shi, H., Scheffler, J. M., Pleitner, J. M., Zeng, C., Park, S., Hannon, K. M., et al. (2008). Modulation of skeletal muscle fiber type by mitogen-activated protein kinase signaling. *The FASEB Journal, 22*, 2990–3000.

Shi, H., Scheffler, J. M., Zeng, C., Pleitner, J. M., Hannon, K. M., Grant, A. L., et al. (2009). Mitogen-activated protein kinase signaling is necessary for the maintenance of skeletal muscle mass. *American Journal of Physiology. Cell Physiology, 296*, C1040–C1048.

Shi, H., Zeng, C., Ricome, A., Hannon, K. M., Grant, A. L., & Gerrard, D. E. (2007). Extracellular signal-regulated kinase pathway is differentially involved in beta-agonist-induced hypertrophy in slow and fast muscles. *American Journal of Physiology. Cell Physiology, 292*, C1681–C1689.

Späte, U., & Schulze, P. C. (2004). Proinflammatory cytokines and skeletal muscle. *Current Opinion in Clinical Nutrition and Metabolic Care*, 7, 265–269.

Stenholm, S., Harris, T. B., Rantanen, T., Visser, M., Kritchevsky, S. B., & Ferrucci, L. (2008). Sarcopenic obesity: Definition, cause and consequences. *Current Opinion in Clinical Nutrition and Metabolic Care, 11*, 693–700.

Stephens, N. A., Skipworth, R. J., & Fearon, K. C. (2008). Cachexia, survival and the acute phase response. *Current Opinion in Supportive and Palliative Care, 2*, 267–274.

Stitt, T. N., Drujan, D., Clarke, B. A., Panaro, F., Timofeyva, Y., Kline, W. O., et al. (2004). The IGF-1/PI3K/Akt pathway prevents expression of muscle atrophy-induced ubiquitin ligases by inhibiting FOXO transcription factors. *Molecular Cell, 14*, 395–403.

Strassmann, G., Fong, M., Freter, C. E., Windsor, S., D'Alessandro, F., & Nordan, R. P. (1993). Suramin interferes with interleukin-6 receptor binding in vitro and inhibits colon-26-mediated experimental cancer cachexia in vivo. *The Journal of Clinical Investigation, 92*, 2152–2159.

Tan, B. H., & Fearon, K. C. (2008). Cachexia: Prevalence and impact in medicine. *Current Opinion in Clinical Nutrition and Metabolic Care, 11*, 400–407.

Tessitore, L., Costelli, P., & Baccino, F. M. (1994). Pharmacological interference with tissue protein hypercatabolism in tumor-bearing rats. *The Biochemical Journal, 299*, 71–78.

Thornberry, N. A., Bull, H. G., Calaycay, J. R., Chapman, K. T., Howard, A. D., Kostura, M. J., et al. (1992). A novel heterodimeric cysteine protease is required for interleukin-1 beta processing in monocytes. *Nature, 356*, 768–7674.

Tisdale, M. J. (2008). Catabolic mediators of cancer cachexia. *Current Opinion in Supportive and Palliative Care, 2*, 256–261.

Trayhurn, P., & Wood, I. S. (2004). Adipokines: Inflammation and the pleiotropic role of white adipose tissue. *The British Journal of Nutrition, 92*, 347–355.

van de Woestijne, A. P., Monajemi, H., Kalkhoven, E., & Visseren, F. L. (2011). Adipose tissue dysfunction and hypertriglyceridemia: Mechanisms and management. *Obesity Reviews, 12*, 829–840.

van der Meij, B. S., van Bokhorst-de van der Schueren, M. A., Langius, J. A., Brouwer, I. A., & van Leeuwen, P. A. (2011). n-3 PUFAs in cancer, surgery, and critical care: A systematic review on clinical effects, incorporation, and washout of oral or enteral compared with parenteral supplementation. *The American Journal of Clinical Nutrition, 94*, 1248–1265.

Wallace, A. M., Sattar, N., & McMillan, D. C. (1998). Effect of weight loss and the inflammatory response on leptin concentrations in gastrointestinal cancer patients. *Clinical Cancer Research*, *4*, 2977–2979.

Walsh, D., Rybicki, L., Nelson, K. A., & Donnelly, S. (2002). Symptoms and prognosis in advanced cancer. *Supportive Care in Cancer*, *10*, 385–388.

Weed, H. G., Ferguson, M. L., Gaff, R. L., Hustead, D. S., Nelson, J. L., & Voss, A. C. (2011). Lean body mass gain in patients with head and neck squamous cell cancer treated perioperatively with a protein- and energy-dense nutritional supplement containing eicosapentaenoic acid. *Head & Neck*, *33*, 1027–1033.

White, J. P., Baynes, J. W., Welle, S. L., Kostek, M. C., Matesic, L. E., Sato, S., et al. (2011). The regulation of skeletal muscle protein turnover during the progression of cancer cachexia in the Apc(Min/+) mouse. *PLoS One*, *6*, e24650.

Wilkes, E. A., & Freeman, J. G. (2006). Thalidomide: An effective anabolic agent in gastrointestinal cancer cachexia. *Alimentary Pharmacology and Therapeutics*, *23*, 445–446.

Winfield, R. D., Delano, M. J., Pande, K., Scumpia, P. O., Laface, D., & Moldawer, L. L. (2008). Myeloid-derived suppressor cells in cancer cachexia syndrome: A new explanation for an old problem. *Journal of Parenteral and Enteral Nutrition*, *32*, 651–655.

Wolfe, R. R. (2006). The underappreciated role of muscle in health and disease. *The American Journal of Clinical Nutrition*, *84*, 475–482.

Wu, R., Kausar, H., Johnson, P., Montoya-Durango, D. E., Merchant, M., & Rane, M. J. (2007). Hsp27 regulates Akt activation and polymorphonuclear leukocyte apoptosis by scaffolding MK2 to Akt signal complex. *The Journal of Biological Chemistry*, *282*, 21598–21608.

Yang, S. Y., Hoy, M., Fuller, B., Sales, K. M., Seifalian, A. M., & Winslet, M. C. (2010). Pretreatment with insulin-like growth factor I protects skeletal muscle cells against oxidative damage via PI3K/Akt and ERK1/2 MAPK pathways. *Laboratory Investigation*, *90*, 391–401.

Zabel, P., Entzian, P., Dalhoff, K., & Schlaak, M. (1997). Pentoxifylline in treatment of sarcoidosis. *American Journal of Respiratory and Critical Care Medicine*, *155*, 1665–1669.

Zhao, J., Brault, J. J., Schild, A., Cao, P., Sandri, M., Schiaffino, S., et al. (2007). FoxO3 coordinately activates protein degradation by the autophagic/lysosomal and proteasomal pathways in atrophying muscle cells. *Cell Metabolism*, *6*, 472–483.

CHAPTER TWELVE

Cisplatin-Induced Anorexia and Ghrelin

Tomohisa Hattori[*,1], **Koji Yakabi**[†], **Hiroshi Takeda**[‡,§]
[*]Tsumura Research Laboratories, Tsumura & Co., Yoshiwara, Ami-machi, Inashiki-gun, Ibaraki, Japan
[†]Department of Gastroenterology and Hepatology, Saitama Medical Center, Saitama Medical University, Tsujido-machi, Kamoda, Kawagoe, Saitama, Japan
[‡]Pathophysiology and Therapeutics, Hokkaido University, Faculty of Pharmaceutical Sciences, Kita-ku, Sapporo, Japan
[§]Department of Gastroenterology and Hematology, Graduate School of Medicine, Hokkaido University, Kita-ku, Sapporo, Japan
[1]Corresponding author: e-mail address: hattori_tomohisa@mail.tsumura.co.jp

Contents

1. Introduction 302
2. Cisplatin-Induced Overproduction of 5-HT 303
3. Cisplatin, 5-HT-Induced Ghrelin Regulation 307
4. Treatment of Ghrelin- and Ghrelin Enhancer-Based, Cisplatin-Caused Dyspepsia 311
5. Conclusion 315
References 315

Abstract

Cisplatin, a formidable anticancer treatment, is used for several varieties of cancer. There are, however, many cases in which treatment must be abandoned due to a decrease in the patient's quality of life from loss of appetite associated with vomiting and nausea. There is a moderate degree of improvement in prevention of cisplatin-induced nausea and vomiting when serotonin (5-HT) 3 receptor antagonists, neurokinin 1 receptor antagonists, and steroids—either alone or in combination—are administered. The mechanism of action for anorexia, which continues during or after treatment, is, however, still unclear. This anorexia is, similar to the onset of vomiting and nausea, caused by the action of large amounts of 5-HT released as a result of cisplatin administration on tissue 5-HT receptors. Among the 5-HT receptors, the activation of 5-HT2b and 5-HT2c receptors, in particular, seems to play a major role in cisplatin-induced anorexia. Following activation of these two receptors, there is reduced gastric and hypothalamic secretion of the appetite-stimulating hormone ghrelin. There is ample evidence of the usefulness of exogenous ghrelin, synthetic ghrelin agonists, and the endogenous ghrelin signal-enhancer *rikkunshito*, which are expected to play significant roles in the clinical treatment and prevention of anorexia in future.

Vitamins and Hormones, Volume 92
ISSN 0083-6729
http://dx.doi.org/10.1016/B978-0-12-410473-0.00012-X

1. INTRODUCTION

Developed in the late 1970s, cisplatin (*cis*-diamminedichloro-platinum (II), *cis*-$[PtCl_2(NH_3)_2]$) is one of the main drugs used for solid cancer chemotherapy in the ovarian, testicular, cervical, lung, head, neck, and bladder regions (Fig. 12.1). Multiple mechanisms have been suggested to cause cisplatin-induced cytotoxicity. Examining the mechanism of action at the microlevel, DNA is the proven primary target of cisplatin, and cisplatin adduct formation affects many DNA-dependent cellular functions, including inhibition of replication and transcription, cell cycle arrest, and DNA damage, leading to cell death and apoptosis (Chaney, Campbell, Bassertt, & Wu, 2005; Zdraveski, Mello, Farinelli, Essigmann, & Marinus, 2002). While these effects markedly suppress proliferation of cancer cells, they also cause cisplatin dose-limiting side effects. While representative side effects of cisplatin include nephrotoxicity, neurotoxicity, and ototoxicity, the most distressing for cancer patients are vomiting, nausea, and simultaneous or delayed appetite loss. These cisplatin-induced gastrointestinal disturbances decrease patient quality of life (QOL) and can lead to abandonment of treatment.

Many neurotransmitter abnormalities are known to participate in cisplatin-induced gastrointestinal disturbances. Of these, the most important factors are serotonin (5-HT) and neurokinin-1 (NK1). Combined treatment with antiemetic NK1 or 5-HT3 receptor antagonists and chemotherapeutic agents has led to partial mitigation of QOL reduction in many cancer patients (Roila & Fatigoni, 2006). Acute vomiting caused by moderate emetogenic chemotherapy is 80–90% blocked by concomitant administration of a 5-HT3 receptor antagonist and dexamethasone. Administration of the NK1 antagonist MK-869 blocks delayed as well as acute vomiting. Thus, we have been able to control chemotherapy-induced nausea and vomiting to a certain extent. Use of the formidable anticancer agent cisplatin induces anorexia in addition to vomiting and nausea. Anorexia was found in approximately half the patients undergoing chemotherapy, with concomitant administration of cisplatin and vinorelbine or irinotecan, in both North

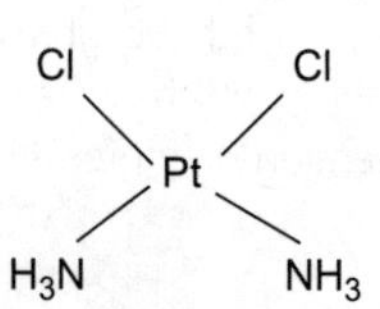

Figure 12.1 Chemical structure of cisplatin.

America (Winton et al., 2005) and Asia (Hong et al., 2006). Chemotherapy-induced anorexia, even in the absence of vomiting, is a major issue from the perspective of adequate patient nutrition, and persistent cases are common. The mechanism of this anorexia has yet to be a focus of research, and there is still no effective therapeutic agent to treat it.

There have recently been a few reported research results on the mechanism of chemotherapy-induced anorexia. The trigger in these results is excessive serotonin release followed by abnormal ghrelin dynamics. Ghrelin is an appetite-stimulating hormone discovered in 1999 as an endogenous ligand of growth hormone secretagogue receptor (GHSR) (Kojima et al., 1999), which is also reported to exhibit a range of pharmacological effects outside of its appetite-stimulating effects. In this review, we focus on the mechanism of cisplatin-induced anorexia and whether ghrelin and its signal enhancer can have a positive effect on the reduced QOL associated with chemotherapy.

2. CISPLATIN-INDUCED OVERPRODUCTION OF 5-HT

Cisplatin characteristically tends to be distributed in tissues with rapid cell proliferation. Particularly, large amounts of 5-HT are stored in the enterochromaffin cells of the gastrointestinal tract and are released into the tissue or circulation following cisplatin treatment. After being stimulated by the released 5-HT in the gastrointestinal tract, the afferent vagus nerve sends signals to the nucleus of the solitary tract within the medulla oblongata. Cisplatin also directly activates 5-HT receptors in the central nervous system (CNS) through a number of routes. 5-HT released into the blood may directly stimulate 5-HT receptors in the area postrema (Minami, Endo, Hamaue, & Sertonin, 2004). Levels of 5-HT, and its metabolite 5-hydroxyindole-acetic acid, are noted to increase in the hypothalamus, hippocampus, and medulla oblongata following cisplatin administration (Liu, Hamaue, Endo, Hirafuji, & Minami, 2003). In addition, increases in the brainstem 5-HT concentration may also cause 5-HT to bind to its receptor.

Fourteen 5-HT receptor subtypes have been found to date. Of these, the activation of the 5-HT3 receptor plays a crucial role in vomiting and nausea following cisplatin treatment. Vomiting and nausea are caused by stimulation of the vomiting center in the nucleus of the solitary tract of the medulla oblongata. This stimulation results from activation of the vagus nerve or the chemoreceptor trigger zone in the medulla oblongata by stimulation of the 5-HT3 receptor. In addition, activation of the 5-HT3 receptor reduces gastric solid body emptying. Intraperitoneal administration of the 5-HT3 receptor antagonists granisetron or ondansetron clearly suppresses cisplatin-induced delayed gastric emptying in rats (Fig. 12.2A). It is extremely interesting that these agents have no observable effect on cisplatin-induced decreases in food intake (Fig. 12.2B). Accordingly, factors other than 5-HT3 receptors must affect cisplatin-induced decreased food intake.

The activation of 5-HT1b, 5-HT2b, and 5-HT2c receptors plays a role in suppressing feeding behavior (De Vry & Schreiber, 2000; Halford, Harrold, Boyland, Lawton, & Blundell, 2007; Tecott, 2007). Administration of the respective agonists for the 5-HT1b, 5-HT2b, and 5-HT2c receptors causes clear reductions in feeding behavior in basic research studies using normal rats. As shown in Fig. 12.3, intraperitoneal administration of 5-HT2b (BW723C86) or 5-HT2c (*m*-CPP) receptor agonists to rats causes obvious decreases in food intake (Fig. 12.3A), as does intraperitoneal administration of 5-HT1b agonist (CGS-12066A) stimulants to guinea pigs (Fig. 12.3B).

5-HT1b/5-HT2c receptors are widely distributed in areas of the CNS, including the medulla oblongata and hypothalamus. 5-HT2c receptors are localized on corticotropin-releasing factor neurons and pro-opiomelanocortin (POMC) neurons, and 5-HT1b receptors on Neuropeptide Y/Agouti-related peptide (NpY/AgRP) neurons (Nonogaki, 2008). 5-HT2b receptors, however, are localized to smooth muscle of the gastrointestinal tract and vasculature, including the stomach, intestine, pulmonary smooth muscle, and myocardium (Choi and Maroteaux, 1996). 5-HT1b and 5-HT2c receptor genes expressed in the CNS are upregulated during fasting conditions and conversely decreased during fed conditions (Nonogaki, 2008). The 5-HT receptors varied in tissue distribution and it was not completely evident by what mechanism they suppress feeding behavior. The food intake of cisplatin-administered rats was significantly reduced compared to that of saline-administered control rats when subjected to appetite evaluation based on food intake for fixed periods of time. Oral administration of the 5-HT2c receptor antagonist SB242084 or 5-HT2b receptor antagonist SB215505, however, significantly mitigated this reduction in food intake (Takeda et al., 2008). Intraventricular administration of SB242084 also significantly mitigated cisplatin-induced reductions in food intake (Yakabi, Kurosawa, et al., 2010; Yakabi, Sadakane, et al., 2010). The activation of 5-HT2b and 5-HT2c receptors distributed across different sites can be said to negatively control feeding behavior in cases of cisplatin-induced anorexia.

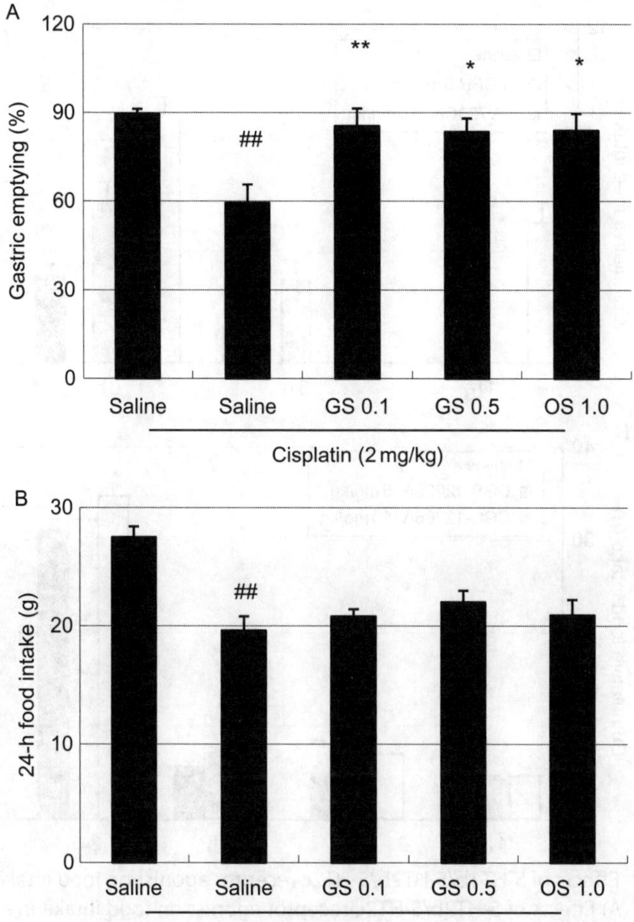

Figure 12.2 Effects of 5-HT3 receptor antagonist on delayed gastric emptying or decreased food intake in cisplatin-treated rats. The granisetron at doses of 0.1, 0.5 mg/kg, i.p., or ondansetron at a dose of 1.0 mg/kg was administered concomitantly with cisplatin (2.0 mg/kg, i.p.). (A) Effects on delayed gastric emptying. The test drugs were administered to 24-h fasted rats, and food intake was measured 24 h after the administration. (B) Effects on food intake. The test drugs were administered to 24-h fed rats and solid gastric emptying was measured 3 h after the administration. GS, glanisetron; OS, ondansetron; 0.1, 0.1 mg/kg, i.p.; 0.5, 0.5 mg/kg, i.p.; 1.0, 1.0 mg/kg, i.p.; ##, $p < 0.01$ versus saline-treated group; * and **, $p < 0.05$ and 0.01 versus cisplatin-treated group.

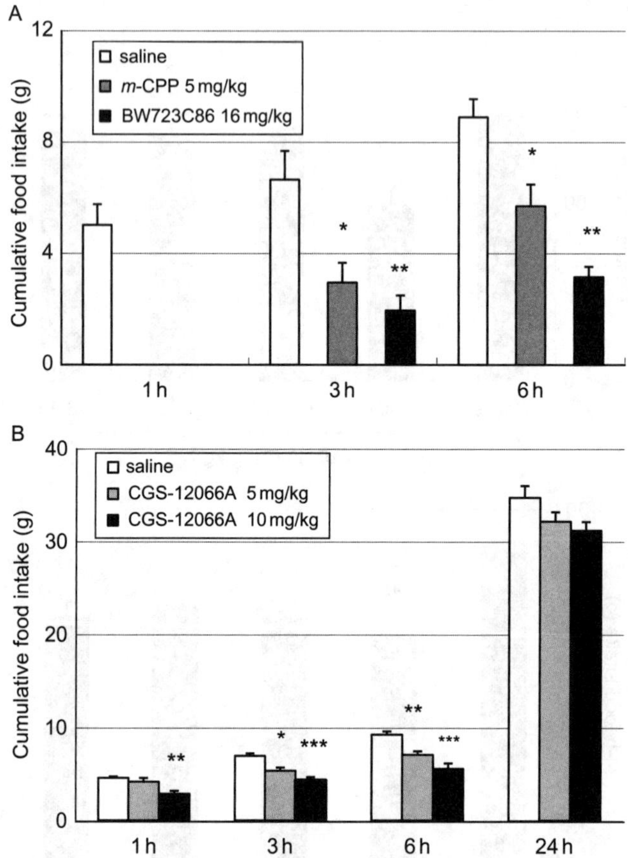

Figure 12.3 Effects of 5-HT1b/5-HT2b/5-HT2c receptor agonist on food intake in rats or guinea pig. (A) Effects of 5-HT2b/5-HT2c receptor agonist on food intake in nontreated rats. The administration of 5-HT2b receptor agonist BW723C86 or 5-HT2c receptor agonist 1-(*m*-chlorophenyl)piperazine (*m*-CPP) was performed and the food intake was measured at 1, 3, and 6 h after the treatment. (B) Effect of 5-HT1b receptor agonist on food intake in nontreated guinea pig. The administration of CGS-12066A at dose of 5 or 10 mg/kg, i.p. was performed, and the food intake was measured at 1, 3, 6, and 24 h after the treatment. *, **, and ***: $p < 0.05$, 0.01, and 0.001, respectively, versus saline-treated group by Dunnett analysis.

Mice with 5-HT2c receptor deficiency exhibit hyperphagia and obesity (Nonogaki, Stack, Dallman, & Tecott, 1998). Activation of the 5-HT2c receptor, located on the POMC neuron, promotes production of the α-melanocyte-stimulating hormone (Xu et al., 2008), which binds with melanocortin 4 receptors in the paraventricular nucleus. This results in blockage of the effects of the feeding behavior-promoting peptides NpY and AgRP. Located axonally on NpY/AgRP neurons, 5-HT1b receptors are thought to secondarily stimulate POMC neurons (Halford et al., 2007).

The stomach fundus of rats is rich in 5-HT2b receptors, which are mainly located in smooth muscle. In the *in vitro* study using the stomach fundus strip of rats, stimulation of 5-HT2b receptors caused contractions accompanied by Ca^{2+} release, mediated by phospholipase C (Cox and Cohen, 1996). The 5-HT2b receptor stimulation-induced suppression mechanism for feeding behavior is, however, unclear in relation to 5-HT1b and 5-HT2c receptors. While it may be that activation of the 5-HT2b receptor directly causes contraction of the stomach, suppressing the accommodation function of the stomach, potential 5-HT2b receptor activation-induced direct action on the stomach is no more than speculation.

3. CISPLATIN, 5-HT-INDUCED GHRELIN REGULATION

While over 90% of ghrelin is localized to the stomach, it is also present in trace quantities in the gastrointestinal tract, pancreas, placenta, and hypothalamus. Ghrelin is mainly secreted from the stomach, and acts on GHS-R1, which is localized to the afferent vagus nerve terminal of the gastric mucosa, and conveys a negative stimulus to the vagal nerve (Date et al., 2002). There are also the compounds acyl ghrelin, with octanoic acid bound to the third serine residue, and des-acyl ghrelin with no bound fatty acids (Fig. 12.4). At present, while it seems that acyl ghrelin performs the functions of ghrelin, the function of des-acyl ghrelin on appetite is unclear. Suppression of afferent vagus nerve firing counteracts the effects of cholecystokinin. These peripheral signals are induced by feeding-related hormones and are conveyed to the hypothalamus via the nucleus of the solitary tract. The A2 noradrenaline cell group of the nucleus of the solitary tract projects to the hypothalamic arcuate nucleus (Sawchenko & Swanson, 1981), with the possible involvement of α1- and β2-adrenergic

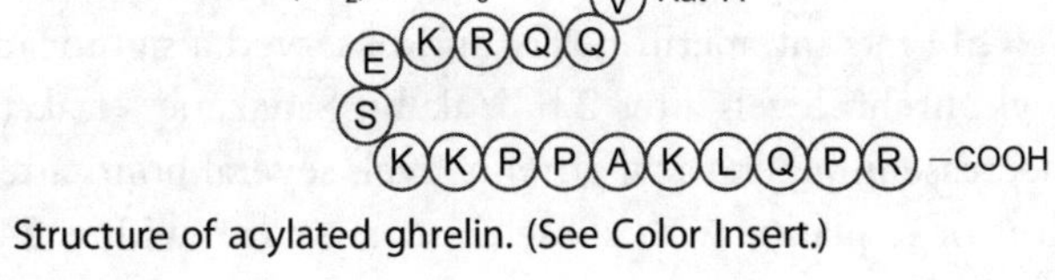

Figure 12.4 Structure of acylated ghrelin. (See Color Insert.)

receptors in signal transmission (Date et al., 2006). And also, the hypothalamus itself also produces ghrelin. Intraventricular administration of ghrelin clearly promotes feeding, causing feeding behavior independently of adrenergic neurons. This is confirmed by the fact that this promotion of feeding behavior is not canceled by intraventricular administration of α1- or β2-adrenergic receptor antagonists (Date et al., 2006). The physiological role of hypothalamus-produced ghrelin on feeding behavior has, however, yet to be fully clarified. Because the effect of ghrelin on anorexia is being examined from a number of perspectives, including reduced food intake related to cachexia (Akamizu & Kangawa, 2011; Fujitsuka et al., 2011), stress (Saegusa et al., 2011; Yakabi et al., 2011) and functional dyspepsia (Akamizu & Kangawa, 2011), networks and roles of peripheral and central ghrelin on appetite will be clear in the near future.

In terms of a clinical approach to clarify the relationship between ghrelin and chemotherapy, evaluation of cisplatin-induced peripheral ghrelin levels was conducted in advanced esophageal cancer patients (Hiura et al., 2011). The total plasma ghrelin level of cisplatin-administered patients was compared to a baseline (140 ± 54 fmol/mL), which fell to 107 ± 46 fmol/mL after 3 days, 82 ± 32 fmol/mL on the 8th day, and 126 ± 43 fmol/mL on the 28th day. Meanwhile, there were no changes in plasma leptin levels. There was significant correlation between nutritional parameters in the blood, average food intake, and VAS score and plasma ghrelin level. Looking at the relationship between total ghrelin level and grade of adverse effects, while there was a significant correlation with anorexia and neutropenia, there was no correlation with nausea and vomiting. Ohno et al. (2011) found that the plasma acyl ghrelin level 3 h after administration of cisplatin was lower than prior to administration in S-1 + cisplatin chemotherapy. While in cisplatin-based chemotherapy ghrelin has the qualities of a hormone within fixed range of individual variation in patient blood levels, QOL is reduced from a nutritional perspective with decreases in plasma ghrelin levels. Markedly low levels of ghrelin involve a pronounced decrease in appetite.

There are a few reported cases of basic research using rodents, which differ by cisplatin dosage, measurement method for peripheral ghrelin levels, and timing of blood sampling. Takeda et al. (2008) administered 2 mg/kg of cisplatin to SD rats intraperitoneally and observed a significant decrease in plasma acyl ghrelin levels after 2 h. Yakabi, Sadakane, et al. (2010) also detected a decrease in plasma acyl ghrelin levels several hours after 4 mg/kg administration of cisplatin, with subsequent recovery within 24 h. Garcia et al. measured total plasma ghrelin levels by a protocol based on intraperitoneal administration of 0.5 mg/kg of cisplatin for 3 successive days, observing an increase 24 h after the last administration of cisplatin (Garcia, Cata, Dougherty, & Smith, 2008). Malik et al. measured plasma acyl ghrelin levels 48 h after intraperitoneal administration of 6 mg/kg of cisplatin, reporting an increasing trend compared to administration of saline. It is well known that plasma ghrelin levels increase with decreases in food intake and body weight. These adaptive ghrelin increases which were demonstrated by Garcia and Malik may be mediated by reduced food intake and decreases in body weight.

The mechanism for cisplatin-induced reduction in peripheral ghrelin levels is also being investigated. Takeda et al. found reduced plasma acyl ghrelin (active ghrelin) levels 2 h after administration in SD rats administered with cisplatin (2 mg/kg), accompanied by a significant reduction in food intake. Large amounts of 5-HT, which the gastrointestinal tract contains in large quantities, were released into the body following cisplatin administration. Intraperitoneal administration of exogenous 5-HT, given to mimic this state, also led to reduced plasma ghrelin levels. Plasma acyl ghrelin reduction in cisplatin-administered rats was almost completely blocked by administration of 5-HT2b or 5-HT2c receptor antagonists, with concurrent mitigation of reduced appetite. There was no effect on plasma ghrelin levels from intraperitoneal administration of 5-HT3 receptor antagonists ondansetron or granisetron (cisplatin + saline, 36.0 ± 6.3 fmol/mL; cisplatin + granisetron 0.1 mg/kg, 31.4 ± 5.2 fmol/mL; cisplatin + granisetron 0.5 mg/kg, 38.5 ± 6.3 fmol/mL; cisplatin + ondansetron 1.0 mg/kg, 35.8 ± 1.6 fmol/mL). These findings suggest that reduced plasma acyl ghrelin levels in cisplatin-administered rats are mediated by stimulation of 5-HT2b or 5-HT2c receptors. We found in pharmacological studies using agonists that although stimulation of 5-HT2b and 5-HT2c receptors reduced acyl ghrelin levels, stimulation of 5-HT3 or 5-HT4 receptors had no effect (Takeda et al., 2008). On investigating the effects of 5–10 mg/kg intraperitoneal administration of the 5-HT1b receptor agonist CGS-12066A on plasma acyl ghrelin levels, it was found that activation of 5-HT1b receptors at this dosage did not affect plasma acyl ghrelin levels (control: 41.1 ± 6.1 fmol/mL vs. CGS: 33.4 ± 4.1 fmol/mL). These results show that among the 5-HT receptors involved in appetite control, activation of 5-HT2b and 5-HT2c receptors reduces plasma acyl ghrelin levels. One might wonder by what mechanism cisplatin-induced activation of 5-HT2b and 5-HT2c receptors reduces blood ghrelin concentrations. At the time of administration of 5-HT2b and 5-HT2c receptor agonists, stomach acyl or des-acyl ghrelin protein is conversely increased, with no change in pre-proghrelin mRNA expression (Takeda et al., 2008), indicating that the ghrelin secretory ability of the stomach is suppressed.

A small amount of ghrelin is produced in the CNS. The relationship between this ghrelin production and appetite has yet to be clarified. The model for cisplatin-induced anorexia involves acute reduction in plasma acyl ghrelin for 2–6 h after administration, followed by recovery to normal levels and then increases within 48 h (Malik et al., 2008; Yakabi, Sadakane, et al., 2010), although reduced food intake continues for 48 h. These results only pertain to the reduction in plasma acyl ghrelin and do not explain cisplatin-induced anorexia. Yakabi et al. examined ghrelin secretion in the hypothalamus of cisplatin-administered rats. The hypothalami of rats which were fasted for 48 h were compared to those of free-feeding rats and found to exhibit significantly increased ghrelin secretion. Ghrelin secretion from the hypothalamus was significantly reduced in cisplatin-administered rats 24 and 48 h after administration. Interestingly, while there was no effect from administration of 5-HT1b and 5-HT2b receptor agonists, only the administration of 5-HT2c receptor agonist recreated the same decreased ghrelin secretion from the hypothalamus produced with cisplatin administration. In addition, this decreased ghrelin secretion from the hypothalamus could not be controlled by administration of 5-HT2b and 5-HT3 receptor antagonists to cisplatin-administered rats. The decreased ghrelin secretion could only be controlled by administration of the 5-HT2c receptor antagonist SB242084 (Yakabi, Sadakane, et al., 2010). These findings suggest that decreased ghrelin secretion from the hypothalamus affects delayed-onset cisplatin-induced anorexia, with the 5-HT2c receptor antagonist involved in the mechanism of action. A detailed explanation of the mechanism for ghrelin secretion in the CNS and appetite control is a topic for future examination.

The ghrelin receptor GHSR is produced in the vagus nerve ganglion, axonally transported, and then localized to the peripheral vagal nerve terminals. Changes in GHSR protein synthesis and amounts in the stomach during cisplatin administration have not been adequately investigated. While some have reported that GHSR mRNA expression is significantly promoted in the distal stomach 48 h after cisplatin administration (Malik et al., 2008), other reports have not shown large changes. Evaluating gene expression of GHSR synthesized in ganglia using stomach samples may be affecting the interpretation of results. On the other hand, while GHSR1 gene expression in the hypothalamus was significantly reduced by feeding condition 6 h after cisplatin administration compared to saline-administration in rats (Yakabi, Kurosawa, et al., 2010), there was, conversely, a significant increase after 48 h (Malik et al., 2008). In addition, there was a significant increase in rats in the starved state after 48 h of fasting in parallel with peripheral ghrelin levels (Yakabi, Kurosawa, et al., 2010). There is still much room for debate regarding the effects on GHSR synthesis in cisplatin-administered rats. The differences in these results may be related to differences in time of measurements or cisplatin dosage. In addition to reduced food intake and body weight, the starved state signal may begin in rats 48 h after cisplatin administration.

Ghrelin-mediated orexigenic mechanisms in cisplatin-induced anorexia may focus on the periphery in the acute stage and on the CNS in the delayed stage.

4. TREATMENT OF GHRELIN- AND GHRELIN ENHANCER-BASED, CISPLATIN-CAUSED DYSPEPSIA

Efforts have begun to develop ghrelin as a therapeutic agent for various forms of anorexia including cachexia and functional dyspepsia (Akamizu, Iwakura, Ariyasu, & Kangawa, 2010; Akamizu & Kangawa, 2011; Tack & Janssen, 2011). In addition, clinical trials are underway for the ghrelin receptor agonists TZP-101 and TZP-102. While examination of the clinical effects of ghrelin on chemotherapy-induced dyspepsia is a field with much potential, we can examine a range of evidence, on the basis of basic evaluations highlighting the usefulness of ghrelin.

The anti-dyspepsia effects of ghrelin in the cisplatin-induced anorexia model have been reported. Reduction in food intake was significantly improved by cisplatin administration with simultaneous intraperitoneal (Garcia et al., 2008; Takeda et al., 2008) or intraventricular administration of ghrelin (Yakabi, Sadakane, et al., 2010). In addition, food intake reduction was significantly mitigated by ghrelin administration, even when administered 24–48 h after cisplatin administration (Lin et al., 2006; Yakabi, Sadakane, et al., 2010). Although not using appetite as an index, ghrelin administration also controlled cisplatin-induced vomiting in ferrets (Rudd et al., 2006). These results indicate that administration of exogenous ghrelin mitigates cisplatin-induced dyspepsia symptoms and highlight the potential of ghrelin-based hormone therapy as a treatment. While the effects of ghrelin receptor agonists, including TZP-101, on reduced food intake in cisplatin-administered rats are yet to be investigated, chemically modified synthetic substances may prove to be effective in overcoming the drawback of the ghrelin peptide short serum half-life.

Recently, attention has focused on notable reports that the Japanese traditional kampo medicine *rikkunshito* (RKT) directly augments ghrelin receptor signaling (Fujitsuka et al., 2011) by promoting secretion of endogenous ghrelin (Fujitsuka et al., 2009; Takeda et al., 2008; Yakabi, Sadakane, et al., 2010). While the effectiveness of RKT on dysmotility-type functional dyspepsia symptoms has already been shown in multicenter, double blind-based evaluations and its particular effectiveness in anorexia is known (Hattori, 2010), the mechanism of action is still unclear. Recently, it has been reported that RKT administration (7.5 g/day) significantly improves the amount of oral intake and grade of anorexia in cisplatin-administered patients, and although significant improvement was not observed for nausea and vomiting, there were positive trends (Ohno et al., 2011). RKT has been found to promote plasma ghrelin secretion in rats (Takeda et al., 2008; Yakabi, Sadakane, et al., 2010), mice (Matsumura et al., 2010), dogs, and humans (Matsumura et al., 2010). Two-week oral administration of RKT to healthy human volunteers and administration to mice via mixed feeds significantly increased plasma acyl ghrelin levels (Matsumura et al., 2010). Furthermore, RKT significantly suppresses reductions in plasma acyl ghrelin level after administration of cisplatin in rats when they have been either free-feeding or fasting for 24 h, and controls the reduction in food intake and body weight (Takeda et al., 2008). As shown in Fig. 12.5, plasma acyl ghrelin levels were significantly decreased 6 h after cisplatin administration and reductions in plasma acyl ghrelin levels resulting from the administration of either 500 or 1000 mg/kg doses of RKT improved. In contrast, leptin levels only exhibited a declining trend. While the effects of RKT on plasma acyl ghrelin levels in cisplatin-administered patients were enhanced (Ohno et al., 2011), further verification with a larger number of cases may be necessary. Concomitant medication must also be paid special attention when measuring plasma ghrelin during chemotherapy. The steroid hormone dexamethasone, in particular, further significantly reduces cisplatin-induced plasma ghrelin levels (Malik et al., 2008). More detailed clinical studies on RKT will no doubt be published in the near future.

RKT contains flavonoids including heptamethoxyflavone, hesperidin, and isoliquiritigenin and exhibits an antagonism for 5-HT2b or 5-HT2c receptors. 5-HT is released in large amounts by cisplatin, reducing acyl ghrelin secretion from the stomach by binding to 5-HT2b and 5-HT2c receptors. RKT blocks reduction of peripheral ghrelin secretion by blocking

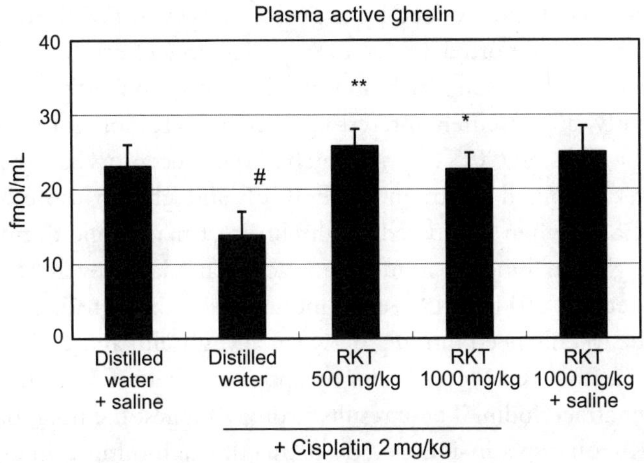

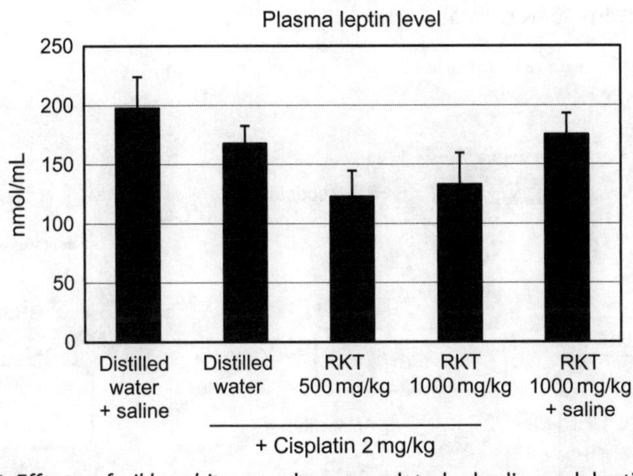

Figure 12.5 Effects of *rikkunshito* on plasma acylated ghrelin and leptin levels in cisplatin-treated rats. The administration of *rikkunshito* was performed 2 h before cisplatin treatment and blood was collected 6 h after cisplatin treatment. #: $p < 0.05$ versus saline-treated rats by Student's *t*-test. * and **: $p < 0.05$ and 0.01 versus saline-treated group by Dunnett analysis.

5-HT2b and 5-HT2c receptor signals through these constituents. In addition, RKT increases reduced food intake even when administered 24 h after cisplatin administration (Yakabi, Sadakane, et al., 2010). While food intake is significantly reduced in this period, plasma ghrelin levels have already returned to normal levels. Ghrelin secretion from the hypothalamus during this time is reduced by administration of cisplatin alone and significantly increased by RKT administration. RKT mitigates cisplatin-induced anorexia by promoting peripheral and central acyl ghrelin secretion in cases where these have been reduced by cisplatin. However, RKT-induced augmentation is not reported to have an enhancing effect on endogenous ghrelin secretion, resulting in blood ghrelin levels above those of normal rats. Recently, an extremely interesting effect of RKT on ghrelin signaling has been found using COS cells in which ghrelin receptors have been overexpressed. Combined treatment with RKT and ghrelin causes sustained influx of Ca^{2+}, when compared to ghrelin treatment alone during *in vitro* tests with ghrelin binding-induced intracellular Ca^{2+} levels as indicator (Fujitsuka et al., 2011). The RKT-induced ghrelin signaling enhancing effect is due to enhanced binding between acyl ghrelin and GHSR1a. This allosteric effect of RKT on ghrelin receptors has been found in the RKT component atractylodin. These results strongly suggest the potential usefulness of RKT on cisplatin-induced dyspepsia through mitigation of reduced plasma ghrelin secretion and ghrelin signaling.

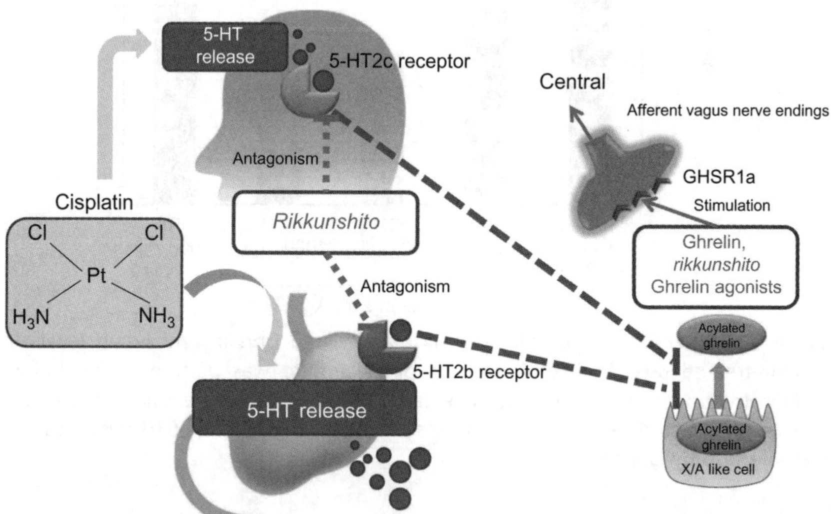

Figure 12.6 The mechanism for cisplatin-induced anorexia. *In vivo* administration of cisplatin releases serotonin present in large quantities in the enterochromaffin granule cells of the gastrointestinal tract. A portion of this binds with 5-HT2b receptors in smooth muscle of the stomach and the rest activates 5-HT2c receptors via blood or the afferent vagus nerve. These receptors reduce appetite, either directly or by controlling acyl ghrelin secretion from the stomach. Anorexia can be mitigated by supplementing insufficient ghrelin with exogenous acyl ghrelin or a ghrelin agonist. In addition, the ghrelin signaling enhancer RKT may mitigate anorexia by controlling reduced endogenous acyl ghrelin and sustaining ghrelin signaling. (See Color Insert.)

5. CONCLUSION

Cisplatin-induced anorexia is caused by peripheral and central ghrelin secretion via 5-HT2b or 5-HT2c receptor activation (Fig. 12.6). Ghrelin enhancer as like RKT may improve the anorexia in the clinical fields.

REFERENCES

Akamizu, T., Iwakura, H., Ariyasu, H., & Kangawa, K. (2010). Ghrelin and functional dyspepsia. *The International Journal of Peptide, 2010*, Pill 548457.

Akamizu, T., & Kangawa, K. (2011). Therapeutic applications of ghrelin to cachexia utilizing its appetite-stimulating effect. *Peptide*, *32*(11), 2295–2300.

Chaney, S. G., Campbell, S. I., Bassertt, E., & Wu, Y. (2005). Recognition and processing of cisplatin-and oxaliplatin-DNA adducts. *Critical Reviews in Oncology/Hematology*, *53*(1), 3–11.

Choi, D. S., & Maroteaux, L. (1996). Immunohistochemical localization of the serotonin 5-HT2B receptor in mouse gut, cardiovascular system, and brain. *FEBS Letters*, *5* (391), 45–51.

Cox, D. A., & Cohen, M. L. (1996). 5-HT2B receptor signaling in the rat stomach fundus: Dependence on calcium influx, calcium release and protein kinase C. *Behavioural Brain Research*, *73*(1–2), 289–292.

Date, Y., Murakami, N., Toshinai, K., Matsukura, S., Niijima, A., Matsuo, H., et al. (2002). The role of the gastric afferent vagal nerve in ghrelin-induced feeding and growth hormone secretion in rats. *Gastroenterology*, *123*(4), 1120–1128.

Date, Y., Shimbara, T., Koda, S., Toshinai, K., Ida, T., Murakami, N., et al. (2006). Peripheral ghrelin transmits orexigenic signals through the noradrenergic pathway from the hindbrain to the hypothalamus. *Cell Metabolism*, *4*(4), 323–331.

De Vry, J., & Schreiber, R. (2000). Effects of selected 5-HT1 and 2 receptor agonists on feeding behavior: Possible mechanisms of action. *Neuroscience and Biobehavioral Reviews*, *24*(3), 341–353.

Fujitsuka, N., Asakawa, A., Hayashi, M., Sameshima, M., Amitani, H., Kojima, S., et al. (2009). Selective serotonin reuptake inhibitors modify physiological gastrointestinal motor activities via 5-HT2c receptor and acyl ghrelin. *Biological Psychiatry*, *65*, 748–759.

Fujitsuka, N., Asakawa, A., Uezono, Y., Minami, K., Yamaguchi, T., Niijima, A., et al. (2011). Potentiation of ghrelin signaling attenuates cancer anorexia-cachexia and prolongs survival. *Translational Psychiatry*, *2011*, 1:e23.

Garcia, J. M., Cata, J. P., Dougherty, P. M., & Smith, R. G. (2008). Ghrelin prevents cisplatin-induced mechanical hyperalgesia and cachexia. *Endocrinology*, *149*(2), 455–460.

Halford, J. C., Harrold, J. A., Boyland, E. J., Lawton, C. L., & Blundell, J. E. (2007). Serotonergic drugs: Effects on appetite expression and use for the treatment of obesity. *Drugs*, *67*(1), 27–55.

Hattori, T. (2010). A new strategy using Rikkunshito (Liu-Jun-Zi-Tang), a Japanese traditional medicine, to treat gastrointestinal disease. In H. Satoh (Ed.), *Basic of evidences-based herbal medicine* (pp. 149–160). Kerala, India: Research Signpost.

Hiura, Y., Takiguchi, S., Yamamoto, K., Kurosawa, Y., Yamasaki, M., Nakajima, K., et al. (2011). Fall in plasma ghrelin concentration after cisplatin-based chemotherapy in esophageal cancer patients. *International Journal of Clinical Oncology*, *17*, 316–323. http://dx.doi.org/10.1007/s10147-011-0289-0.

Hong, Y. S., Lee, H. R., Park, S., Lee, S. C., Hwang, I. G., Park, B. B., et al. (2006). Three-week schedule of irinotecan plus cisplatin in patients with previously untreated extensive-stage small-cell lung cancer. *British Journal of Cancer, 95*(12), 1648–1652 (Epub 2006 November 28).

Kojima, M., Hosoda, H., Date, Y., Nakazato, M., Matsumoto, H., & Kangawa, K. (1999). Ghrelin is a growth-hormone-releasing acylated peptide from stomach. *Nature, 402*, 656–660.

Liu, Y., Hamaue, N., Endo, T., Hirafuji, M., & Minami, M. (2003). 5-Hydroxytryptamine (5-HT) concentrations in the hippocampus, the hypothalamus and the medulla oblongata related to cisplatin-induced PICA of rats. *Research Communication in Molecular Pathologyand Pharmacology, 113–114*, 97–113.

Malik, N. M., Moore, G. B. T., Kaur, R., Liu, Y. L., Wood, S. L., Morrow, R. W., et al. (2008). Adaptive upregulation of gastric and hypothalamic ghrelin receptors and increased plasma ghrelin in a model of cancer chemotherapy-induced dyspepsia. *Regulatory Peptides, 148*, 33–38.

Matsumura, T., Arai, M., Yonemitsu, Y., Maruoka, D., Tanaka, T., Suzuki, T., et al. (2010). The traditional Japanese medicine Rikkunshito increases the plasma level of ghrelin in humans and mice. *Journal of Gastroenterology, 45*, 300–307.

Minami, M., Endo, T., Hamaue, N., & Sertonin, M. (2004). Anticancer drug-induced emesis. *Yakugaku Zasshi, 124*(8), 491–507.

Nonogaki, K. (2008). Ghrelin and feedback systems. *Vitamins and Hormones*, 77, 149–170.

Nonogaki, K., Stack, A. M., Dallman, M. F., & Tecott, L. H. (1998). Leptin-independent hyperphagia and type 2 diabetes in mice with a mutated serotonin 5-HT(2C) receptor gene. *Nature Medicine, 4*, 1152–1156.

Ohno, T., Yanai, M., Ando, H., Toyomatsu, Y., Ogawa, A., Morita, H., et al. (2011). Rikkunshito, a traditional Japanese medicine, suppresses cisplatin-induced anorexia in humans. *Clinical and Experimental Gastroenterology, 4*, 291–296.

Roila, F., & Fatigoni, S. (2006). New antiemetic drugs. *Annals of Oncology, 17*(Suppl. 2), ii96–ii100.

Rudd, J. A., Ngan, M. P., Wai, M. K., King, A. G., Witherington, J., Andrews, P. L., et al. (2006). Anti-emetic activity of ghrelin in ferrets exposed to the cytotoxic anti-cancer agent. *Neuroscience Letters, 392*, 79–83.

Saegusa, Y., Takeda, H., Muto, S., Nakagawa, K., Ohnishi, S., Sadakane, C., et al. (2011). Decreased plasma ghrelin contributes to anorexia following novelty stress. *American Journal of Physiology. Endocrinology and Metabolism, 301*, E685–E696.

Sawchenko, P. E., & Swanson, L. W. (1981). Central noradrenergic pathways for the integration of hypothalamic neuroendocrine and autonomic responses. *Science, 214*(4521), 685–687.

Tack, J., & Janssen, P. (2011). Emerging drugs for functional dyspepsia. *Expert Opinion on Emerging Drugs, 16*(2), 283–292. Med. 4 (10)1152–1156.

Takeda, H., Sadakane, C., Hattori, T., Katsurada, T., Ohkawara, T., Nagai, K., et al. (2008). Rikkunshito, an herbal medicine, suppresses cisplatin-induced anorexia in rats via 5-HT2 receptor antagonism. *Gastroenterology, 134*(7), 2004–2013.

Tecott, L. H. (2007). Serotonin and the orchestration of energy balance. *Cell Metabolism, 6*(5), 352–361.

Winton, T., Livingston, R., Johnson, D., Rigas, J., Johnston, M., Butts, C., et al. (2005). Vinorelbine plus cisplatin vs. observation in resected non-small-cell lung cancer. *The New England Journal of Medicine, 352*(25), 2589–2597.

Xu, Y., Jones, J. E., Kohno, D., Williams, K. W., Lee, C. E., Choi, M. J., et al. (2008). 5-HT2cRS expressed by pro-opiomelanocortin neurons regulate energy homeostasis. *Neuron, 26*(609), 582–589.

Yakabi, K., Kurosawa, S., Tamai, M., Yuzurihara, M., Nahata, M., Ohno, S., et al. (2010). Rikkunshito and 5-HT2C receptor antagonist improve cisplatin-induced anorexia via hypothalamic ghrelin interaction. *Regulatory Peptides*, *161*, 97–105.

Yakabi, K., Noguchi, M., Ohno, S., Ro, S., Onouchi, T., Ochiai, M., et al. (2011). Urocortin 1 reduces food intake and ghrelin secretion via CRF2 receptors. *American Journal of Physiology—Encocrinology and Metabolism*, *301*, E72–E82.

Yakabi, K., Sadakane, C., Noguchi, M., Ohno, S., Ro, S., Chinen, K., et al. (2010). Reduced ghrelin secretion in the hypothalamus of rats due to cisplatin-induced anorexia. *Endocrinology*, *151*, 3773–3782.

Zdraveski, Z. Z., Mello, J. A., Farinelli, C. K., Essigmann, J. M., & Marinus, M. G. (2002). MutS preferentially recognized cisplatin—Over oxaliplatin-modified DNA. *Journal of Biological Chemistry*, *277*(2), 1255–1260.

CHAPTER THIRTEEN

Anorexia of Aging

Zbigniew Kmieć*[,1], Erika Pétervári†, Márta Balaskó†, Miklós Székely†
*Department of Histology, Medical University of Gdansk, Gdansk, Poland
†Department of Pathophysiology and Gerontology, Medical School, University of Pécs, Pécs, Hungary
[1]Corresponding author: e-mail address: zkmiec@gumed.edu.pl

Contents

1. Introduction 320
2. Animal Studies 322
   2.1 Spontaneous food intake in rodents of various ages 323
   2.2 Short summary of the central regulatory mechanisms of food intake 324
   2.3 Age-related differences in the expression and activity of orexigenic and anorexigenic neuropeptides involved in the control of food intake 327
   2.4 Age-related differences in the serum levels and activity of hormones involved in the control of food intake 327
3. Human Studies 335
   3.1 Involvement of neuropeptides and peripheral nervous signals in the impairments of food intake by the elderly 335
   3.2 Age-related physiologic alterations of the GI tract that affect anorexia of aging 336
   3.3 Role of leptin and insulin 340
4. Anorexia of Aging May Result from the Imbalance of Catabolism and Anabolism: Convergence of Animal and Human Studies 341
   4.1 Regulation of energy balance: Changes with aging 342
   4.2 BW/composition changes during human aging: Sarcopenia, sarcopenic obesity, and cachexia 343
5. Therapeutic Approaches to Overcome the Anorexia of Aging and Its Deleterious Effects on Body Functions 345
6. Conclusions and Perspectives 346
Acknowledgments 347
References 347

Abstract

Anorexia of aging is a physiologic decrease in food intake, which gradually leads to weight loss accompanied by age-related changes in body composition. Animal experiments have revealed that advanced age is associated with altered regulation of food intake and energy homeostasis: suppression of orexigenic mechanisms mediated by neuropeptide Y, orexins, and ghrelin, and by increased activity of the major anorexigenic neuropeptide, α-MSH. In the elderly, a reduced sense of smell and taste may contribute

Vitamins and Hormones, Volume 92
ISSN 0083-6729
http://dx.doi.org/10.1016/B978-0-12-410473-0.00013-1

to the loss of appetite, and in old humans, increased serum cholecystokinin concentration may delay gastric emptying resulting in a prolonged feeling of satiety. Although leptin and insulin play a major role in the control of energy homeostasis, their role in the loss of body weight in healthy elderly persons remains to be established. In some of the elderly, loss of body mass may result in malnutrition or even cachexia. Anorexia of aging plays some role in sarcopenia, involuntary loss of muscle mass and strength; however, there are intrinsic age-related changes in skeletal muscle, which underlie this health-endangering condition. Currently, there is no efficient pharmacological treatment for the anorexia of aging; however, it may be partially prevented by improved processing and presenting of food, physical training, and an appropriate social environment.

1. INTRODUCTION

Aging in humans and other mammals is associated with failure to maintain homeostasis in response to physiologic and environmental challenges. Disturbances in fuel and energy homeostasis occur during aging in three major forms: glucose intolerance and type 2 diabetes, increased accumulation of fat leading to obesity, and, paradoxically, at later stages, decreased food intake, called "anorexia of aging" (Kalra et al., 1999; Morley & Silver, 1988). The simple description of the anorexia of aging, which occurs in up to 20% of the elderly, defines it as an age-related decrease in calorie intake, which gradually leads to a lower body mass. Although such anorexia results in a dangerous deterioration of health status in the elderly, its causes are not well understood and, therefore, the methods to counteract it are limited.

There is an overwhelming consensus based on large epidemiologic observations such as NAHNES (National Health and Nutrition Examination Survey) that during normal human aging, a gradual decline in food consumption as well as significant weight loss takes place (Briefel et al., 1995). Since these processes can occur in otherwise healthy elderly persons, it has been proposed that they may represent a physiological response to advanced age, observed in a significant part of the human population (Morley, 1997). Longitudinal studies of healthy individuals demonstrated that after the age of 65 years, a continuous decrease in body mass in the range of ca. 0.5% of the total body weight (BW) occurs per year (Hallfrisch, Muller, Drinkwater, Tobin, & Andres, 1990). The age-related decline in food intake, also observed in laboratory animals (Wolden-Hanson, 2006), can be regarded as a normal reaction to the diminished energy expenditure observed in the elderly, and thus can be termed as a *physiologic anorexia of aging*. However, in the case of a proportional decline in energy expenditure and calorie intake, the BW should not change very much. In contrast to this, many authors have shown that there is a subgroup of the elderly who suffer much higher involuntary weight loss, which may lead to malnutrition and a life-threatening state of cachexia. Therefore, a term *pathologic anorexia of aging* seems to be more appropriate to characterize this group of elderly (Morley, 1997). Since, as will be shown later, there are multifactorial causes of the physiologic anorexia of aging, it may be assumed that pathologic anorexia of the elderly is a consequence of additional factors, which aggravate the physiologic age-associated anorexia.

The increasing life span of human populations, especially in well-developed countries, substantiates division of the elderly period into at least two phases: early aging, starting at the age of 65 years, and advanced aging, after the age of 80 years (Olshansky, Carnes, & Cassel, 1990). This distinction appears to be useful in discussing the course and consequences of both physiologic and pathologic aging.

The age-related slow decrease in body mass is accompanied by prominent changes in the body composition reflected by a gradual decrease in muscle mass (decline in lean body mass) and by an increase in fat content, although without any significant immediate change in total body mass. The first process is often described as sarcopenia (Hallfrisch et al., 1990), which is progressive and may eventually lead to serious deterioration of body functions in the presence of very high fat mass (sarcopenic obesity). Interestingly, with advancing age, the amount of body fat (and total BW) also starts declining (Hubbard, Lang, Llewellyn, & Rockwood, 2010). There are convincing epidemiologic data that show that after the age of 75 years, reduction in body fat (and BW) was accompanied by an increased mortality rate (McTigue, Hess, & Ziouras, 2006). Other epidemiologic studies demonstrated that the optimal body mass index is higher in the elderly than in young persons (Stevens, 2000; Stevens et al., 1998), emphasizing the importance of weight preservation in the elderly.

Maintenance of weight and composition of the body depends on an equilibrium between anabolic and catabolic mechanisms that involve orexigenic and anorexigenic factors (e.g., monoamines, peptides), respectively. Naturally, in various phases of life, the balance is not standard. In developing juvenile subjects, the orexigenic tone surpasses the anorexigenic one, and it may be difficult to suppress a healthy juvenile appetite. A well-balanced state between the orexigenic and anorexigenic activities may be reached by young adulthood, but later on the balance may change further: a positive balance leads to obesity (e.g., age-related obesity), while still later at old age, the balance is usually negative and the anorexic tone (anorexia of aging) causes a fall in BW. The pattern is similar in humans and other mammals, which suggests a regulatory background. This provides an opportunity to use experimental approaches on animals when investigating this balance.

Various types of experiments on aging animals have shown that anorexia of aging, which results in reduction in body mass by the end of life, is probably caused by the age-related impairment of the nervous, hormonal, and probably metabolic mechanisms, which control food intake and energy homeostasis. The object of this review is to present the currently available evidence related to the mechanisms of age-related reduction in body mass. Although the anorexia of aging presents an important health problem, the elucidation of its causes comes partly from animal experiments as obvious ethical issues exclude human experiments except for dietary and nutritional interventions. Therefore, in this review, animal studies related to the mechanisms of the anorexia of aging are briefly summarized, and this is followed by the description of more circumstantial human data. It is hoped that understanding the causes of the age-related decrease in food intake may lead to the development of therapeutic approaches that could counteract aging-associated disintegration of energy homeostasis, which results in the loss of body mass, sarcopenia, and frailty.

2. ANIMAL STUDIES

Although the age-related decline in appetite has been known for many years, there is still little understanding of its physiological basis, especially with respect to the central regulation of ingestive behavior. Because experimental verification of the central mechanisms of disturbed food intake cannot be performed in humans, answers to this problem were sought in animal experiments in which aged rats represented the most commonly used species. However, as in humans, so in rodents, the genetic interindividual and interstrain differences seem to have a big influence on the control of energy homeostasis and body mass during aging. Generally, one can distinguish two types of rat strains with respect to the changes in body mass (weight) during their life span. In the first group, represented by Wistar and Brown Norway (BN) rats, animals increase their weight only modestly after reaching maturity (Fig. 13.1A), whereas in the second group, which includes Sprague–Dawley (SD) and Fischer 344 (F344) rats, the increase in BW occurs more or less constantly throughout life. Nevertheless, it is usually accepted that the general patterns of age-related regulatory changes may have many basic similarities, including that at very old age, the BW decreases in all strains (Li, Matheny, Nicolson, Tümer, & Scarpace, 1997; Székely,

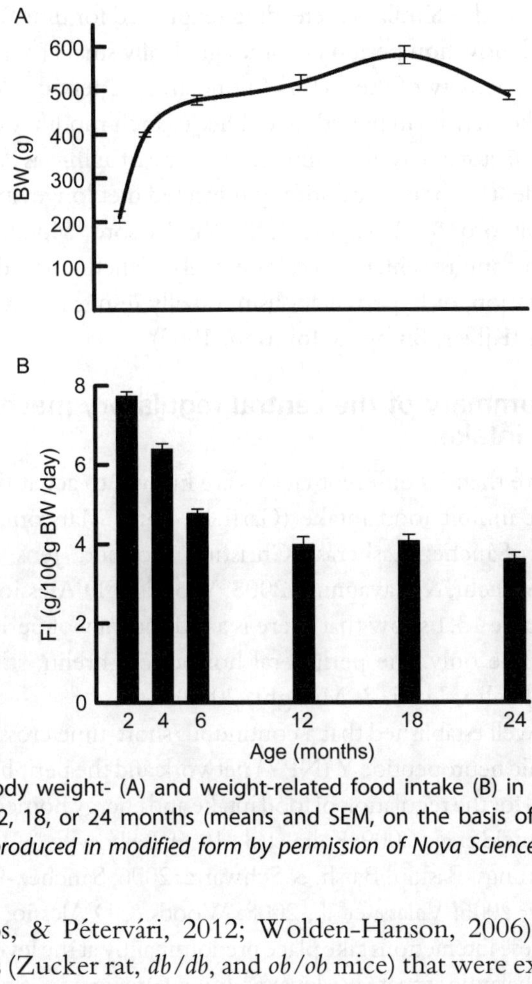

Figure 13.1 Body weight- (A) and weight-related food intake (B) in male Wistar rats aged 2, 4, 6, 12, 18, or 24 months (means and SEM, on the basis of data in Szekely et al., 2012; *reproduced in modified form by permission of Nova Science Publishers).*

Balaskó, Soós, & Pétervári, 2012; Wolden-Hanson, 2006). Some rat or mouse strains (Zucker rat, *db/db*, and *ob/ob* mice) that were extensively used in the studies of energy homeostasis cannot be regarded as valid models for aging research since they show mutant phenotypes, which may severely affect the aging process (Kmiec, 2010). In contrast to genetically modified strains, rodents maintained on a modified diet (short-/long-term calorie restriction, diet-induced obesity, etc.) may be important in the study of age-related regulatory changes.

2.1. Spontaneous food intake in rodents of various ages

The daily food intake is hardly more in adult than in juvenile rats of much smaller BW, that is, food intake expressed for unit BW decreases with age (Fig. 13.1B), suggesting that the feeding drive or spontaneous endogenous orexigenic tone is also attenuated in older animals. Very old rats eat even less than the young adults. Similarly, refeeding (expressed for unit BW) following a certain food deprivation period becomes gradually smaller with aging. This suggests that the activity of the factors (monoamines, peptides, etc.) that regulate food intake may change with age. Diet (which modifies the activity of such regulatory factors) may also influence the rate of aging: as compared with controls, in rodents kept on a calorically restricted diet longevity is known to increase (Yu, Masoro, & McMahan, 1985; Yu, Masoro, Murata, Bertrand, & Lynd, 1982). In contrast, enhanced calorie intake, whether it is due to high fat diet, cold adaptation, or hypermetabolism, usually results in faster aging and a shorter lifespan (Kibler, Silsby, & Johnson, 1963).

2.2. Short summary of the central regulatory mechanisms of food intake

Currently, more than 50 different factors are known to act at the CNS level to stimulate or inhibit food intake (Garfield, Lam, Marston, Przydzial, & Heisler, 2009; Sánchez-Lasheras, Christine Könner, Jens, & Brüning, 2010; Valassi, Scacchi, & Cavagnini, 2008; Woods & D'Alessio, 2008). Data presented in Table 13.1 show that there is a redundancy of peripheral signals that inhibit, while only one peripheral hormone, ghrelin, stimulates food intake (Ferrini, Salio, Lossi, & Merighi, 2009).

It has been well established that a continuous short-time cross talk between the hypothalamic neuropeptide Y (NPY) network and the peripheral hormone leptin is essential for the regulation of food intake and energy homeostasis (Ferrini et al., 2009; Garfield et al., 2009; Kalra et al., 1999; Leibowitz & Wortley, 2004; Morton, Cummings, Baskin, Barsh, & Schwartz, 2006; Sánchez-Lasheras et al., 2010; Schwartz, 2006; Valassi et al., 2008; Woods & D'Alessio, 2008; Zhang et al., 1994). These interactions take place predominantly at the level of two types of ARC (hypothalamic arcuate nucleus) neurons. Orexigenic "first order" neurons coexpress NPY and AgRP (agouti-related protein), whereas anorexigenic "first order" neurons coexpress the key anorexigenic peptide of the melanocortin system (α-MSH, α-melanocyte-stimulating hormone and its precursor propeptide, proopiomelanocortin, POMC). The majority of the POMC/α-MSH neurons also express another anorexigenic peptide, CART (cocaine and amphetamine-regulated transcript). The main area of NPY production is the arcuate nucleus and the release of NPY and coexpressed neurotransmitters in other hypothalamic areas, including the PVN (paraventricular nucleus), DMH (dorsomedial hypothalamic nucleus), VMH (ventromedial hypothalamic nucleus), and LHA (lateral hypothalamic area) evoke appetite.

The neurons that express POMC, precursor propeptide for many active molecules including α-MSH, are restricted to the arcuate nucleus and the

Table 13.1 Neuropeptides and hormones that control food intake

Centrally released factors that stimulate food intake	**CNS factors that suppress food intake**
AgRP	α-MSH (POMC derivative)
NPY	CART
Orexin A and B	CRH (*corticotropin-releasing hormone*) and urocortins
MCH (*melanin-concentrating hormone*)	TRH (*thyrotropin-releasing hormone*)
Galanin	BDNF (*brain-derived neurotrophic factor*)
GHRH	GALP (*galanin-like peptide*)
β-Endorphin	Oxytocin
Dynorphin	GLP-1 (*glucagon-like peptide 1*)
GABA	Prolactin
Noradrenalin	Serotonin
Dopamine (acting in VMH)	Dopamine (acting in ARC and LHA)
Endogenous cannabinoids	Neurotensin and neuromedins
	Nesfatin-1
Peripheral orexigen	**Peripheral anorexigenic signals**
Ghrelin	Leptin, adiponectin
	Insulin and amylin
	Enterostatin
	Bombesin and GRP (*gastrin-releasing peptide*)
	Oxyntomodulin
	CCK (*cholecystokinin*), PYY_{3-36} (*peptide YY*)
	GLP-1, GLP-2, GIP (*gastric inhibitory peptide*)
	Estrogens
	Cytokines (IL-1, IL-6, IL-8, TNF, IFN)

Summary of data reviewed by Kalra et al. (1999), Woods and A'Allessio (2008), Valassi et al. (2008), and Sánchez-Lasheras et al. (2010).

nucleus of the solitary tract (NTS) in the brainstem. The anorexigenic α-MSH reduces food intake and increases energy expenditure in both animals and humans. This peptide is an endogenous agonist for five melanocortin receptor types of which the melanocortin-3 receptor and melanocortin-4 receptor (MC4R) are highly expressed in the brain areas involved in the regulation of energy homeostasis (hypothalamic ARC, LHA, VMH, DMH, and NTS). The melanocortin system appears to be the dominant anorexigenic system and an important regulator of food intake and BW (Garfield et al., 2009).

Since AgRP is an endogenous inverse agonist of the melanocortin receptors, the release of NPY and AgRP in the ARC–PVN axis restrains melanocortin signaling, thus counteracting the anorexic actions of α-MSH. The NPY/AgRP and POMC/α-MSH neurons not only project to other hypothalamic and CNS nuclei involved in the control of food intake and feeding behavior but also reciprocally inhibit their own activities depending on the kind of central or peripheral signals interacting with their respective receptors. Initiation of a meal induces release of short-acting satiety signals involved in an anorexigenic feedback mediated by peripheral hormones and nutrients to two CNS centers, the hypothalamus and the NTS in the brainstem (Morton et al., 2006).

Leptin, insulin, glucose, and cholecystokinin (CCK) belong to the major peripheral signals released in the body in response to food ingestion, while ghrelin levels increase in response to fasting. These agents are transported into the hypothalamus through the blood–brain barrier, which is less tight in ARC than in other brain areas (Kastin & Pan, 2000). Leptin and insulin inhibit NPY expression by binding to their receptors on NPY/AgRP neurons, while stimulating POMC/α-MSH neurons in the ARC, which results in the termination of food intake. Ghrelin exerts opposite action since it activates NPY/AgRP neurons, thus stimulating orexigenic behavior. However, it has to be mentioned that this very simplistic description of the major regulatory pathways which control food intake, and, ultimately body mass, does not include the variety of interrelated neurocircuits involved in the regulation of one of the most complicated and most important aspects of body homeostasis. For example, in a recent report, the parabrachial nucleus has been identified in the mouse as a hub that integrates signals from several brain regions including glutamatergic neurons in the NTS and caudal serotonergic neurons to bidirectionally modulate feeding and BW (Wu, Clark, & Palmiter, 2012).

Other signals reach the brain not directly at the arcuate nucleus, but by vagus-mediated mechanisms. Afferent fibers of the abdominal vagus have receptors for leptin, CCK, ghrelin, GLP-1 (glucagon-like peptide-1), and some other gastrointestinal (GI) peptides that are involved in regulation of satiety/hunger, feeding patterns, and food intake in general (Bray, 2000). These fibers convey information about the GI stretch, and the amount/concentration of nutrients and metabolites. They project mainly to neurons of the NTS; directly or indirectly also stimulate neurons of the medulla, lower brainstem, hypothalamus, and forebrain; and induce alterations in the balance of neurotransmitter/modulator (monoamine, peptide, etc.) activities. Leptin, insulin, glucose, and some nutrients/metabolites may also act at the area postrema.

2.3. Age-related differences in the expression and activity of orexigenic and anorexigenic neuropeptides involved in the control of food intake

The data obtained in animal studies on the regulation of food intake in aging summarized in Table 13.2, suggest that, generally, there are two CNS components that may be responsible for the reduced food intake in aging animals. First, aging is associated with reduced number, sensitivity, and effectiveness of the appetite-stimulating neurons of the hypothalamus (Table 13.2). In addition, a series of experiments performed on aging Wistar rats by one of our research groups (Pétervári, Garami, Soós, Székely, & Balaskó, 2009, 2010; Pétervári, Soós, Székely, &Balaskó, 2011) strongly suggests that—in contrast to middle-aged animals—in the late phase of aging, excessive α-MSH tone and increased catabolic activity of α-MSH may participate in the reduction in food intake and BW (Fig. 13.2).

Thus, animal studies have clearly shown that the age-related decline in the reactivity of hypothalamic neurons to endogenously released orexigenic signals (e.g., during fasting) or to centrally (mostly intracerebroventricularly, ICV) administered exogenous agents, as well as the enhanced anorexigenic tone of α-MSH, represents age-dependent alterations in the central regulatory mechanisms of food intake and ingestive behavior, which are, at least partially, responsible for the anorexia of aging (Székely et al., 2012). However, it is still not known, although probable, if these age-related alterations of regulatory mechanisms participate in the involuntary weight loss observed in the elderly.

2.4. Age-related differences in the serum levels and activity of hormones involved in the control of food intake

In the short-term control of food intake, each meal is stopped by the satiety reflex via vagus nerve afferents activated by stomach distension and the gut hormone CCK, whereas in the long-term, the satiety threshold depends on fat mass stores that signal to the brain, mainly via the adipocyte hormone

Table 13.2 Effect of aging on hypothalamic peptide expression or feeding response

Neuropeptide/ hormone	Species	Effect of aging on hypothalamic peptide expression or on feeding response	References
Orexigenic peptides			
Neuropeptide Y (NPY)	BN and Wistar rat	Hypothalamic NPY mRNA levels several times lower than in young animals (ISH)	Wolden-Hanson, Marck, and Matsumoto (2004), Sohn, Wolden-Hanson, and Matsumoto (2002), Gruenewald, Marck, and Matsumoto (1996), Peralta, Carrascosa, Gallardo, Ros, and Arribas (2002), and Kaneda, Makino, Nishiyama, Asaba, and Hashimoto (2001)
NPY	F344xBN rat	No change in hypothalamic NPY content with aging	Kalra, Bagnasco, Otukonyoung, Dube, and Kalra (2003)
NPY: ICV[a] administration		No feeding response in senescent rats, high in young ones—the response gradually decreases with age	Blanton et al. (2001, 2006), Wolden-Hanson (2006), and Akimoto-Takano et al. (2005)
NPY receptors	F344 rat	Decreased mRNA levels of Y1 and Y2 NPY receptors in the PVN of rats, compared to young ones.	Coppola, Horwitz, Hamilton, and McDonald (2004)
AgRP	BN rat	Hypothalamic expression of AgRP suppressed in old rats	Wolden-Hanson et al. (2004)
AgRP: ICV[a] administration		No change in food intake in senescent rats in spite of increased serum leptin levels	Sohn et al. (2002)
Orexin A: ICV[a] administration		Lack of increase in food intake in old rats in contrast to young ones	Gruenewald et al. (1996), Akimoto-Takano et al. (2005), and Kotz, Mullett, and Wang (2005)

Orexin-type 1 receptor (OX-IR)	Rat Mouse	Reduced number of OX-IR in hypothalamus of old rats Decreased type 2 orexin receptor mRNA levels in hypothalamus of old mice	Kotz et al. (2005) and Terao, Apte-Deshpande, Morairty, Freund, and Kilduff (2002)
Orexin neurons	Rhesus macaque	The number and distribution pattern of OX-immunoreactive neurons did not change with age (age range 1–32 years)	Downs et al. (2007)
Anorexigenic peptides			
POMC, precursor of α-MSH	Rat	Hypothalamic expression of POMC was similar in young and old rats	Wolden-Hanson et al. (2004) and Kappeler, Zizzari, Alliot, Epelbaum, and Bluet-Pajot (2004)
POMC: effect of fasting	Rat	In old animals, fasting induced a smaller decrease of POMC mRNA than in young rats	Sohn et al. (2002)
α-MSH: ICV[a] administration	Wistar rat	Suppression of food intake higher in 18 and 24-month-old animals than in 6- and 12-month-old ones	Pétervári et al. (2009)
CART	Rat	In ARC of middle-aged and old rats, level of CART mRNA was higher, and in PVN, similar as in young ones	Wolden-Hanson et al. (2004)
CART	Rat	In the PVN of old rats, CART mRNA level was lower than in young animals	Sohn et al. (2002)

[a]ICV, intracerebroventricular.

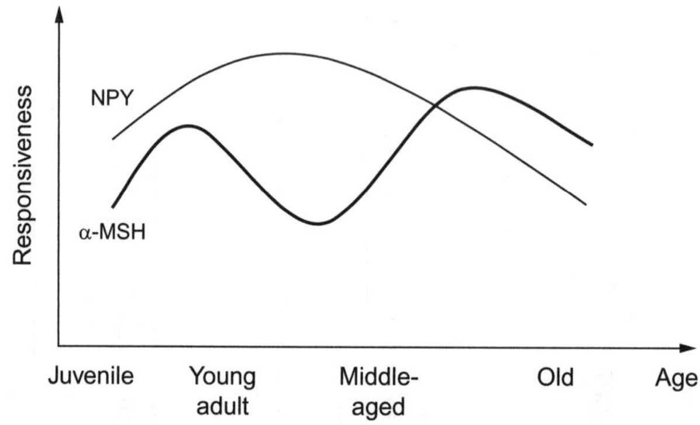

Figure 13.2 Schematic presentation of changes in the orexigenic responsiveness to NPY and anorexigenic responsiveness to α-MSH (both peptides administered intracerebroventricularly) during the life span of male Wistar rats. The age-related relationship between opposite effects of both neuropeptides on food intake may explain the age-related obesity of the middle-aged and the anorexia of aging of senescent rat groups. *Reproduced from Pétervári, Soós, et al. (2011) by permission of Bentham Science Publishers.*

leptin. On the other hand, during fasting, the secretion of the other peripheral hormone, ghrelin, increases and stimulates the activity of the orexigenic hypothalamic NPY/AgRP neurons. Thus, the measurements of the serum concentrations of the GI hormones and assessment of their activities during fasting and feeding may provide valid information about control of food intake in the course of aging.

2.4.1 Ghrelin

Ghrelin, a 28-amino acid peptide synthesized primarily in the stomach (Kojima et al., 1999), and in smaller amounts in other organs, including some neurons in the dorsal portion of the ARC and outside of the hypothalamus (Ferrini et al., 2009; Kojima et al., 1999), was discovered as an endogenous ligand of the growth hormone secretagogue receptor. Ghrelin stimulates growth hormone (GH) release and food intake when administered intravenously to rodents and humans or by an ICV route in animals (Akimoto-Takano et al., 2005), and it is suggested to inhibit brown fat metabolism (Ma et al., 2011). Ghrelin stimulates food intake primarily by direct activation of NPY/AgRP neurons in the ARC (Ferrini et al., 2009) and by inhibition of the POMC neurons. Ghrelin also activates orexin-expressing neurons in the paraventricular and lateral hypothalamic areas (Solomon, De Fanti, & Martinez, 2007). Since ghrelin is the only orexigenic peripheral agent that counteracts the satiety signal of leptin, its contribution to the control of food intake in the elderly was investigated soon after its discovery. Serum ghrelin concentrations were lower in old rats than in young ones (Porkka-Heiskanen, Alanko, Kalinchuk, Heiskanen, & Stenberg, 2004) and did not change with age in C57BL/6J male mice (Ariyasu et al., 2008). Plasma ghrelin levels are regulated by acute feeding states. They rise during fasting and are rapidly suppressed after feeding. Apparently, aging is accompanied by disturbed regulation of the secretory and sensory function of ghrelin-producing neuroendocrine "A–X"-like cells of the oxyntic glands of the stomach. This is evidenced by a blunted response of serum ghrelin concentration to 3-day fasting in old BN rats, whereas starvation nearly doubled ghrelin levels in young animals (Kotz et al., 2005). The orexigenic effect of ghrelin becomes significantly suppressed during aging. The increase in food intake after ICV ghrelin administration was significantly lower in old Wistar rats compared with young and middle-aged animals (Akimoto-Takano et al., 2005). Similarly, 2 h after intravenous ghrelin administration, food consumption in 27-month-old Long Evans rats was by ca. 30% lower than in 3-, 12-, and 24-month-old animals (Toshinai et al., 2007).

2.4.2 Leptin and central leptin resistance during aging

The key role of leptin in the long-term regulation of BW has been clearly established. Therefore, the effect of aging on serum leptin concentration, the presence of its receptors in the hypothalamus and other brain structures, and signaling in the CNS were investigated by many authors. In various strains of aging rodents, either increased (F344xBN (Morley, 2003) and Wistar (Escrivá et al., 2007; Kaneda et al., 2001; Kappeler et al., 2004) rats) or unchanged (F344 (Blanton et al., 2006) and Wistar (Ishii, Shibasaki, Murakami, Shima, & Wakabayashi, 2000; Kmiec et al., 2005; Nogalska & Swierczynski, 2001) rats) serum leptin concentrations were reported, and the variations seemed to be related to genetic differences between rat strains, as discussed by Kmiec et al. (2005).

After a decade of research, it became evident that in rodents aging is associated with central (and peripheral) leptin resistance. This age-related defect of leptin action at the level of the hypothalamus was demonstrated by the use of various experimental techniques. For example, in young SDxBN rats, hyperleptinemia induced by subcutaneous leptin infusion for 7 days caused a 50% reduction in food consumption and hypothalamic NPY levels. In old animals, however, food consumption was reduced by only 20% and hypothalamic NPY concentration was unaffected (Scarpace, Matheny, Moore, & Tümer, 2000).

In a similar experimental set-up, the resistance of peripheral tissues to leptin action was demonstrated in old SD rats (Gabriely, Ma, Yang, Atzmon, et al., 2002; Gabriely, Ma, Yang, Rossetti, & Barzilai, 2002).

The mechanism of central leptin resistance during aging may be caused by several factors. One possibility that has not been investigated in the aging studies could be decreased local production of leptin, since leptin mRNA was found in ARC, and its expression was regulated by fasting and refeeding (Wilkinson, Brown, Imrash, & Ur, 2007). Another cause of the age-related central leptin resistance may be impaired transport of leptin across the blood–brain barrier, since it is widely believed that leptin may cross the blood–brain barrier by binding to the longest variant of leptin receptors, LRb (formerly denoted as Ob-Rb) in a vessel's wall using a partially saturable transport system (Kastin & Pan, 2000). Indeed, a decreased leptin uptake in hypothalamic nuclei, which was partially caused by the diminished hypothalamic expression of the Ob-Rb receptors, was demonstrated in old Wistar rats (Fernandez-Galaz et al., 2001). However, the same group showed that adiposity plays a key role in the development of aging-associated leptin resistance, since food restriction for 1 month caused a 25% fall in BW of already obese 20–21-month-old rats who recovered leptin responsiveness and increased expression of leptin receptors in the hypothalamus by the age of 23–24 months (Fernández-Galaz et al., 2002). The importance of obesity is also demonstrated by data showing that diet-induced obesity (by reducing litter size) caused leptin resistance already at the age of 8 weeks (Stofkova et al., 2009). In contrast, other authors demonstrated that in 20-month-old rats maintained on a low-calorie diet throughout their lives preventing weight gain between age 3 and 20 months, the anorexigenic effect of leptin was still reduced, suggesting the role of age itself in the development of leptin resistance (Gabriely, Ma, Yang, Atzmon, et al., 2002; Gabriely, Ma, Yang, Rossetti, et al., 2002). However, the decreased anorexigenic effect of leptin in such fasting animals is possibly virtual, since it may be due to a chronically increased orexigenic tone (e.g., high NPY-sensitivity) concealing the presence of active leptin. Indeed, experiments on 6-month-old Wistar rats showed that in the calorie-restricted group, ICV leptin infusion elicited no anorexia but caused an extremely pronounced hypermetabolic response, while in the diet-induced obese group, a weak anorexigenic response (as compared to normally fed rats) and practically no hypermetabolism was observed (Soos, Balasko, Jech-Mihalffy, Szekely, & Petervari, 2010). A full scale of leptin effects will have to be analyzed in old rats in order to finalize the opinion about leptin resistance in old age.

Aging-associated suppression of leptin action at the CNS level may also be caused by changes in the signal transduction pathway(s) in the hypothalamic neurons as has been recently discussed by Kmiec (2011).

2.4.3 Central insulin action is decreased in aging

Thirty years ago, Woods, Lotter, McKay, and Porte (1979) demonstrated that chronic ICV infusion of insulin reduced food intake and BW of baboons. Since then many reports that demonstrated expression of insulin receptors and different elements of the insulin signal transduction pathway in hypothalamic nuclei, or reported on activation of insulin signaling in hypothalamic neurons and described the effects of central insulin administration on food intake and BW in different animal models, have convincingly supported insulin's role in the regulation of fuel homeostasis also at the central level (Woods & D'Alessio, 2008). Insulin shares some of the hypothalamic targets of leptin. Together with leptin, insulin is increasingly often regarded as an adiposity signal. However, the effects of leptin at the CNS level on food intake and energy balance seem to be more efficient than those of insulin. Using ICV insulin administration, García-San Frutos et al. (2007) showed that insulin signaling was clearly impaired in old Wistar rats at the level of insulin receptor and IRS-2 (insulin receptor substrate 2) as well as downstream of the PI3K (phosphoinositide-3-kinase) pathway, a pathway also used by leptin (Figlewicz & Benoit, 2009; Metlakunta, Sahu, & Sahu, 2008; Yang et al., 2010). Interestingly, food restriction improved both insulin responsiveness and insulin signaling (García-San Frutos et al., 2007). These data suggest that during aging, Wistar rats develop hypothalamic insulin resistance, which is probably caused by the alterations in the signal transduction pathway(s). The central insulin resistance is accompanied by the age-dependent decrease in insulin sensitivity of peripheral tissues (with unchanged serum insulin concentrations in young, adult, and old rats) that has been related mainly to the increased content of retroperitoneal fat in old animals (Escrivá et al., 2007). Removal of visceral fat in 20-month-old Zucker diabetic fatty rats improved the insulin sensitivity and glucose tolerance (Gabriely, Ma, Yang, Atzmon, et al., 2002; Gabriely, Ma, Yang, Rossetti, et al., 2002).

2.4.4 Changes of gut hormone levels and activity during aging

Ingestion of food gives rise to mechanical and chemical stimulation of the GI tract and results in the activation of afferent sensory nerves and secretion of a variety of GI hormones. These events activate vagal afferent neurons, which project to and stimulate neurons located in the medulla (particularly in the

NTS), pons, hypothalamus, and forebrain (Suzuki, Simpson, Minnion, Shillito, & Bloom, 2010). The CNS circuits mediate the food intake-inhibitory action of GI signals and control of various aspects of food intake such as initiation of meal, its size, duration, and frequency. Unfortunately, despite the recognition of the importance of the brain–gut axis for the regulation of food intake in aging, only few reports have dealt with this subject.

2.4.4.1 Cholecystokinin

CCK, released in the proximal small intestine in response to nutrients in gut lumen, particularly to fat and protein, stimulates pancreatic enzyme secretion, induces gallbladder contraction, reduces gastric emptying, and stimulates postprandial satiety, acting as an anorexigenic hormone (Moran & Kinzig, 2004). When administered to either rodents or humans, CCK decreases food intake, meal size, and meal duration by binding to mainly peripheral CCK1 and central CCK2 receptors. These effects result mainly from CCK-mediated stimulation of vagal afferent neurons in the nodose ganglion, although CCK receptors are widely distributed in the brain including the brainstem and hypothalamus (Dockray, 2009). Despite the recognized role for CCK in the regulation of food intake, there are relatively few reports on CCK status during aging. The intestinal CCK concentration was higher in old than in young guinea pigs (Poston, Singh, Draviam, Upp, & Thompson, 1988). The CCK release in brain samples was found to be smaller in old than young rats, although the CCK content rather increased (Ohta, Tanaka, Masuda, Miyasaka, & Funakoshi, 1995). Recent experiments (Balaskó et al., 2012) have shown that the strong anorexigenic effect of intraperitoneal CCK-octapeptide (CCK-8) (acting mainly on CCK-1 receptors of the afferent vagus) that was characteristic for young adult rats was minimal in middle-aged, but again very pronounced in old Wistar rats. Other studies also demonstrated that, irrespective of the basal plasma levels, the efficacy of some peptides may also be different in various age groups of rodents: the satiety-inducing effect of peripherally applied CCK was more pronounced in old than in young animals (Silver, Flood, & Morley, 1988; Voigt, Huston, Voits, & Fink, 1996). Miyasaka et al. (1995) and Dockray (2009) found that ICV administration of CCK-8 (acting on CCK-2 receptors of the brain) inhibited food intake to a higher degree in old versus young Wistar rats while the CCK plasma concentrations were similar. In rats, the hypothalamic (Miyasaka et al., 1995) and substantia nigra (Schuligoi, Fernandez, Heavens, & Sirinathsinghji, 1993) CCK mRNA levels and the plasma concentration of CCK-8 (Miyasaka et al., 1995) did not change with aging, although in humans the plasma level of CCK increased with age (Chapman, MacIntosh, Morley, & Horowitz, 2002; Di Francesco et al., 2005; MacIntosh et al., 1999, 2001; Sturm et al., 2003).

3. HUMAN STUDIES

The animal studies of both central and peripheral mechanisms of the anorexia of aging are being performed in standardized ways (genetic homogeneity of rodent strains, control of the quality and quantity of consumed food, constant light/dark cycling, peripheral or central administration of neuropeptides and hormones, measurements of the metabolic parameters and observations of ingestive behavior, etc.). On the contrary, human studies of the physiologic and pathologic aging-related anorexia are hampered by many biases which are difficult to overcome. Apart from obvious ethical limitations, other typically human factors such as psychological, lifestyle, social, and economic issues have to be considered when investigating anorexia of the elderly. Due to the complexity of the problem, we limit our considerations to the biologically oriented approach.

3.1. Involvement of neuropeptides and peripheral nervous signals in the impairments of food intake by the elderly

In contrast to the animal studies, the evidence for the age-related changes in neuropeptides involved in the control of food intake in humans is scarce. In a study of 75 nonobese Polish centenarians (mean age 101 years), 26 elderly (mean age 67 years), and 47 young women (mean age 26 years), serum concentration of NPY was almost two times lower in the centenarians compared to the elderly; however, the serum level of NPY was much lower in the young women compared to the other groups. This finding suggests a possible resistance to the orexigenic action of NPY in old women, since similar BMI values were reported for all compared groups. Unfortunately, food intake was not measured in this study (Baranowska et al., 2006). It has been assumed that in humans, the major sources of the circulating NPY were hypothalamic neurons; however, NPY can also be released at the periphery from NPY-ergic neurons. In studies of aging animals, a decreased NPY level in the hypothalamus and its reduced orexigenic effectiveness were found (Table 13.2). Other authors reported (Escobar, Krajewski, Sandoval-Guzmán, Voytko, & Rance, 2004) an enhanced NPY gene expression in the hypothalami of elderly women, due possibly to the negative energy balance or to decreased suppression by leptin. Indeed, in patients with senile anorexia, high serum and CSF NPY levels were demonstrated (Martinez et al., 1993). In contrast to these high levels, in animal experiments, the efficacy of NPY was shown to decrease with aging (Akimoto-Takano et al., 2005; Blanton et al., 2001).

In humans, the number of CRH-containing neurons in the paraventricular nucleus was reported to increase with age in men (Bao & Swaab, 2007). However, the hypothalamo–pituitary–adrenal axis usually becomes activated during stress, and thus, possible changes in the level of food intake-suppressing CRH might not be primary controller of food intake in the long-term.

3.2. Age-related physiologic alterations of the GI tract that affect anorexia of aging

For the short-term regulation of ingestive behavior, factors that initiate and end food intake are of importance, and they may become impaired during aging. Normally, meals follow shorter or longer fasting periods, and feeling of hunger is the driving force which initiates feeding. However, in many elderly, loss of appetite occurs in the course of aging. This may be caused by impaired central neurohormonal mechanisms (which is difficult to prove in humans, though being well established in animals), as well as by decreased sensory input from taste and smell receptors and that from the gut wall. The feeling of satiety that determines the end of feeding is driven mainly by GI mechanisms. When food leaves the stomach and enters the small intestine, mechano- and chemoreceptors send signals to the hypothalamus and the brainstem, which results in cessation of food intake. These signals are provided by both GI hormones (CCK, GLP-1, and PYY; cf. Table 13.1) acting on the hypothalamus and afferent nerves providing information mainly to the NTS in the brainstem.

3.2.1 Sensation of smell and taste

Human aging is associated with altered smell perception. It was found that 62.5% of 80–97-year olds had an olfactory impairment (Schubert, Cruickshanks, Klein, Klein, & Nondahl, 2011) and that the elderly also lose the ability to discriminate between smells (Boyce & Shone, 2006; Rolls & McDermott, 1991), probably due to the altered function of ion channels and receptors (Wilson, Yu, & Bennett, 2011). These physiologic alterations may, to some extent, disrupt the appetite drive and represent one of the causes of the involuntary weight loss in the elderly (Bhutto & Morley, 2008).

3.2.2 *Delayed gastric emptying results in earlier feeling of fullness and satiety*

Aging is associated with slower gastric emptying, observed especially for large solid meals (Brogna et al., 2006), which may prolong postprandial satiety and reduce bile output from the gallbladder (Di Francesco et al., 2007). It was found that old subjects were less hungry and more satiated after a test meal than young ones, and this was inversely related to the rate of gastric emptying (Clarkston et al., 1997). However, in older adults, appetite control was influenced by food form and portion size (Leidy, Apolzan, Mattes, & Campbell, 2010). The delayed gastric emptying in older people may result from the enhanced release of intestinal hormones, such as CCK, which also suppresses the feeling of hunger at the level of the hypothalamus (Di Francesco et al., 2005). Moreover, in healthy elderly, meals with a high fat content increased the satiety signal from GLP-1 and lowered the acylated to des-acylated ghrelin ratio, that is, decreased the level of active ghrelin, consequently decreasing hunger (Di Francesco et al., 2010).

It has been suggested that age-related alterations in gut anatomy and histology may affect function of the GI tract (Chapman, 2007). Interestingly, there are only subtle changes in the microscopic structure of the stomach and gut in aging animals and humans (Bhutto & Morley, 2008; Majumdar, 2003; Majumdar, Jaszewski, & Dubick, 1997). Also, gut motor function and whole gut transit time seem to be little affected by aging (Chapman, 2007; Madsen & Graff, 2004), although many textbooks describe slow transit and obstipation in the elderly (probably resulting from low-fiber diet).

3.2.3 *Age-related changes of serum levels and activity of gut hormones involved in the regulation of food intake*

Enteroendocrine cells present in the epithelium of the stomach and intestines secrete more than 50 different peptides which generally affect the secretory and motor function of the gut. Some of these hormones, such as CCK, ghrelin, PYY, and GLP-1, are generally regarded as important factors that affect the short-term regulation of food intake, acting both at the CNS level and locally.

3.2.3.1 Cholecystokinin

In healthy elderly subjects, the plasma CCK concentrations were higher (Chapman et al., 2002; Di Francesco et al., 2005; MacIntosh et al., 1999, 2001; Sturm et al., 2003) or similar (Serra-Prat, Palomera, Clave, & Puig-Domingo, 2009) compared with young adults, while the number of

CCK-immunoreactive cells in the duodenum did not change significantly with age (Sandström & El-Salhy, 1999). In contrast to the high basic CCK level, the postprandial rise of CCK was found to be smaller in old subjects than in young ones (Serra-Prat et al., 2007). Because CCK is an anorectic signal for the hypothalamus and also delays gastric emptying, in this way prolonging the feeling of satiety, the endogenous age-related increase in plasma CCK levels may be an important mediator of the anorexia of aging. Agonists of CCK may cause more severe and more progressive fall of BW in old than in young patients (Berna, Tapia, Sancho, & Jensen, 2007). The observation that the sensitivity to the satiating effect of exogenous CCK was retained or increased in healthy older adults (MacIntosh et al., 2001) suggests that CCK antagonists might be used to increase energy intake in undernourished older people. However, CCK1 receptor antagonists showed only a moderate positive effect on food intake, which was similar in young and old subjects (Roy et al., 2005).

3.2.3.2 Peptide YY and glucagon-like peptide 1

PYY and GLP-1 belong to the group of enteric peptides released from the distal small intestine that are involved in GI motility and inhibit food intake by both decreasing the meal size and increasing the satiating potency of consumed nutrients (Suzuki et al., 2010). In one study, no differences were found in the PYY plasma level of old subjects over 2 h after a test meal (MacIntosh et al., 1999); however, other authors showed a higher rise of PYY during the late postprandial period in the elderly compared with young subjects (Di Francesco et al., 2005). Similar to CCK, abnormally high postprandial PYY levels may delay the search for a second meal, thus leading to longer fasting intervals.

GLP-1, a strong anorexigen, is produced in the small intestine after food ingestion (Suzuki et al., 2010). In contrast to CCK and PYY, both basal and stimulated (by introduodenal lipid or glucose infusion) plasma concentrations of GLP-1 were similar in the elderly and young subjects (MacIntosh et al., 1999, 2001).

3.2.3.3 Ghrelin

In contrast to the aging-related increase (or no change) of gut peripheral anorexigens (CCK, PYY, GLP-1), data on the plasma levels of the only one peripheral orexigen, ghrelin, are not consistent. Although some authors reported a decline in serum ghrelin levels in old humans (Rigamonti et al., 2002; Sturm et al., 2003), a recent study did not confirm these findings

(Bauer et al., 2010). The plasma concentration of ghrelin in a group of centenarian women was lower by 33% and in a group of elderly (mean age 66 years) by 25% than in young subjects (Baranowska et al., 2006). However, the number of investigated subjects was in all studies too small to allow for definite conclusions. Ghrelin secretion depends also on the composition of the diet (Ferrini et al., 2009), which was different in the studied populations. The low secretion of ghrelin in the elderly may result from impaired sensitivity of ghrelin-secreting cells since after a carbohydrate-rich test meal their serum ghrelin level did not change postprandially, whereas the decline was substantial in middle-aged individuals (Ariyasu et al., 2008).

It was found that GH responses to ghrelin administration in the elderly were lower than those seen in young people (Broglio et al., 2003). If the orexigenic response of the NPY/AgRP neurons to ghrelin decreases similarly in the elderly, it may be concluded that decreased serum ghrelin levels and an inadequate orexigenic response to ghrelin (Akimoto-Takano et al., 2005) may contribute to the age-related impairment of food intake and anorexia of aging.

Ghrelin administration to old patients with heart failure or chronic obstructive pulmonary disease improved food intake, BW, functional capacities, and attenuated muscle wasting (Depoortere, 2009; Nagaya et al., 2005, 2004). Moreover, it was also useful in elderly patients when applied prior to hip replacement (Akamizu et al., 2008).

The presented data that demonstrated the effects of aging on the secretion or efficacy of the anorexigenic enteric peptides involved in the control of food intake have to be regarded with caution since the results were subjected to several biases. The obvious ones were gender, the small number of participating old subjects, and the different body mass and health status of the elderly ("healthy," "frail," or "undernourished"). In some of the studies, the basic blood levels of hormones were measured after an overnight fast (Leidy et al., 2010), whereas other authors performed measurements before and after a test meal not reporting on the time elapsed since the previous meal. In all studies, the sensation of hunger, fullness, and satiation were measured by similar methods; however, the types of test meals were different in respect to their caloric content, proportions of fat and carbohydrates, food form, and portion size. For example, Leidy et al. (2010) showed in a study of 25 elderly persons that postprandial hunger and ghrelin concentration were greater following a beverage versus a solid meal, whereas no effects were observed for CCK or GLP-1 (Leidy et al., 2010). Fatty meals (40% vs. 20% fat) increased the serum concentration of GLP-1 and lowered the level of active ghrelin more in the elderly than in young subjects (Di Francesco et al., 2010). Thus, the consumption of fat-rich meals in the elderly increases the satiety signal from the gut, and this condition may lead to a reduction in calorie intake.

3.3. Role of leptin and insulin

The two hormones, insulin secreted by the endocrine pancreas and leptin produced primarily by adipocytes, circulate in levels proportional to body fat and are considered the main endocrine adiposity signals in mammals that communicate current energy availability to the brain. Within the brain, and in particular, the hypothalamus, leptin and insulin signaling are integrated with other signals such as neurotransmitters and nutrients. The hypothalamus, in turn, orchestrates nutrient partitioning and appetite (Schwartz & Porte, 2005). The prevailing paradigm of insulin's and leptin's role in the regulation of energy homeostasis at the CNS level is that they act synergistically. Both hormones suppress food intake via signaling in the hypothalamus (Schwartz & Porte, 2005); however, it has to be noted that the anorectic effects of insulin in the brain have been challenged recently (Jessen, Clegg, & Bouman, 2010).

Almost 20 years after the discovery of leptin, there is a general consensus that this hormone plays an important role in the long-term regulation of body mass and energy metabolism. Its role in the suppression of feeding drive has been shortly described in the previous chapter. However, it is very difficult to assess the role of leptin in the anorexia of aging in humans. Generally, leptin levels positively correlated with BMI and percent body fat (Sinha & Caro, 1998). The elderly represent a heterogeneous group regarding the amount of white adipose tissue, which is the main source of leptin and can affect blood leptin concentration. Comparison of young and elderly nonobese women revealed a tendency to slightly higher serum leptin levels in the elderly group (Baranowska et al., 2006). It was repeatedly demonstrated that plasma concentration of leptin was much higher in all age groups of women than in men (Andreasson, Undén, Elofsson, & Brismar, 2012; Hickey et al., 1996). This may be caused by different size and/or distribution of fat tissue depots influenced by sex hormones since estrogens stimulate, whereas testosterone inhibits leptin secretion. Many clinical studies on the adipokine's serum levels were performed in nonhealthy elderly who suffered from type 2 diabetes, obesity, or frailty. However, we are not aware of studies in which serum leptin levels were evaluated in apparently healthy humans experiencing age-related involuntary weight loss. In definitely frail old patients, the serum leptin level was low in contrast to high levels of inflammatory cytokines (Hubbard, O'Mahony, Calver, & Woodhouse, 2008).

The role of insulin as a long-term modulator of energy homeostasis has been well established (Woods et al., 1979). In contrast to many animal studies, there were no human studies of healthy elderly directed specifically at serum insulin levels. It appears that it is not age *per se* but rather the BMI, adipose tissue, skeletal muscle mass, and physical activity that are major determinants of serum insulin levels (McDonald & Ruhe, 2010).

Since pathologic anorexia of aging affects humans who have rather low or normal BMI, it seems unlikely that altered serum concentrations of insulin and leptin may be causative factors for this condition, assuming unaltered actions of these peripheral hormones at the level of hypothalamus (although in animal studies resistance was suggested). These peptides certainly have a role in abnormalities of the earlier stages of aging, but after the onset of aging anorexia, negative energy balance, and decrease in BW or in manifest cachexia, other mechanisms (e.g., inflammatory substances (Engineer & Garcia, 2012)) may play more important roles.

4. ANOREXIA OF AGING MAY RESULT FROM THE IMBALANCE OF CATABOLISM AND ANABOLISM: CONVERGENCE OF ANIMAL AND HUMAN STUDIES

The decreased feeding drive in old humans might be partially caused by impairments in the action of peripheral feedback signals such as the feeling of early satiety and fullness, delayed gastric emptying, enhanced serum concentration of CCK, a strong anorexigen, and decreased serum level of ghrelin, the only peripheral orexigen. Reduced sensory input from olfactory receptors could also play some role. In animals, such abnormalities of hunger/satiety are shown by reduced duration and/or number of feeding bouts (meal size vs. feeding frequency).

Indirect observations suggest that human aging, similar to animal aging, is associated with the impairment of homeostatic mechanisms at the CNS level, which regulate food intake, body mass, and energy preservation/expenditure. In accordance with these changes, experimental data (Wolden-Hanson, 2006) have proven that—in contrast to young rats—after a 72-h food deprivation in old rats, the food intake did not increase adequately and the old animals failed to regain the fasting-induced loss of BW. Moriguti et al. (2000) showed that old men and women who had volunteered to a 6-week-long period of underfeeding, lost considerably more weight than younger individuals and, in contrast to young subjects, they were unable to regain their weight during the next 6 months of normal feeding. Studies on the control of food intake in older men (Roberts et al., 1994) have shown that, unlike in their young counterparts, neither a 3-week-long calorie-restricted diet, nor an excessive calorie-containing diet of the same length was readily compensated following the dietary period—they named this phenomenon as "dysorexia" of the elderly. Decrease in BW in such cases is usually accompanied by a pronounced fall in fat-free mass, while in the case of weight gain, it is due mainly to fat accumulation (Newman et al., 2005). In everyday practice, overfeeding periods are rare in the elderly, while the multitude of events causing a decrease in food intake (sensory deficits, depression, acute/chronic illness, surgeries, social environment, etc.) may remain uncompensated and may cause lasting anorexia, making recovery extremely difficult. In fact, apart from the general observations in humans (and in all mammals) that aging is often coupled with anorexia and fall in BW, it is also known that weight recovery following an acute illness or operation is more difficult in old patients compared with young ones.

Apparently, although its mechanism has not been clearly clarified, decreased involuntary loss of lean body mass seems to be a physiologic marker of normal human aging. Extensive research over the last 10 years in the field of the regulation of energy homeostasis clearly suggests that during the second part of the animal or human life span, a change in the set point for the homeostatic control of body mass takes place. From the thermodynamic point of view, loss of BW results from the prevalence of the catabolic over the anabolic processes, which, presenting in part as the anorexia of aging, may lead to a severe deterioration of health in older individuals.

The next sections of this review deal with the physiologic and pathologic implications of the anorexia of aging and the emerging ways of their therapeutic interventions.

4.1. Regulation of energy balance: Changes with aging

The overall energy balance (calorie intake, metabolic rate, energy expenditure) is determined as a balance between the anabolic and catabolic factors. The anabolic factors are orexigenic, enhance food intake and also suppress energy expenditure, whereas the catabolic ones act in the opposite way. In the case of thermal stability, the long-term balance affects mainly the BW and body composition. It changes continuously with age: in the period of growth and development, a positive balance is needed, while in adults, a positive balance affects BW and increases mainly adiposity, and a negative balance causes a fall in BW with a decrease in fat mass and, in more severe cases, in the fat-free mass as well.

The expression and activity/effect of catabolic and anabolic peptides change with age, but the age-related changes are not necessarily linear. Figure 13.2 shows that the pronounced anorexic effect of α-MSH in young adult rats is followed by a decreased effect at age 12 months and an extremely strong effect in the oldest group. Although the hypermetabolic effects of α-MSH do not follow this pattern (Pétervári, Szabad, et al., 2011), together with the age-related changes in NPY effects (pronounced in young and early middle-aged adults, but gradually decreasing with age), the age-related obesity may be explained, just as well as the weight loss in old animals.

Altered responsiveness of the central integrative circuitry to peripheral metabolic cues, altered expression of central neurotransmitters/modulators or altered effectiveness to them is presumed to be responsible for the age-related changes (Wernette, White, & Zizza, 2011). Apparently, old animals—like aged humans—seem to be more sensitive to the catabolic factors and less to the anabolic ones. Although resistance to leptin and insulin is characteristic at old age, the sensitivity to catabolic peptides (e.g., α-MSH, CART, CRH) of the ARC and other hypothalamic or brainstem nuclei becomes enhanced, while the sensitivity to the anabolic peptides (e.g., NPY, orexin) is attenuated. Similarly, the activity of the main peripheral catabolic peptide, CCK, increases, but the activity of the peripheral orexigenic ghrelin becomes smaller at old age.

4.2. BW/composition changes during human aging: Sarcopenia, sarcopenic obesity, and cachexia

The term "sarcopenia" refers to loss of muscle. Although muscle can be lost even at a young age in the course of various disease states (Puthucheary, Montgomery, Moxham, Harridge, & Hart, 2010) (e.g., chronic inflammatory processes, tumors, etc.), sarcopenia is characteristic of both animal (Fig. 13.3) and human aging, which implies a common biological basis for this process. It may be defined as a progressive loss of skeletal muscle mass (loss of lean body mass) (Muscaritoli et al., 2010), which is often accompanied by a relative or an absolute increase in fat mass. In fact—similar to peak bone mass—there is a maximum level (depending mainly on physical activity) for lean body mass in young adults or early middle-aged subjects, which gradually decreases after the age of 35–40 years. The rate of muscle loss is variable, depending on intrinsic age-related changes in muscle tissue, significant loss of spinal motoneurons after the age of 60 years, physical activity, and hormonal and nutritional status (Narici & Maffulli, 2010). In the late phase of aging, loss of muscle tissue becomes faster and manifest sarcopenia develops, with all of its functional consequences.

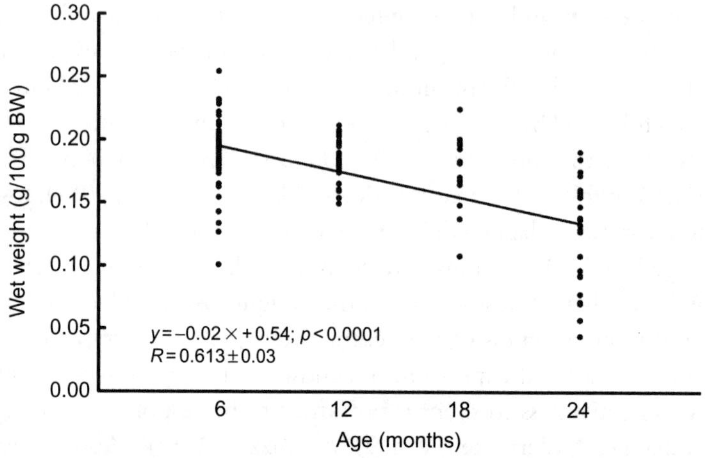

Figure 13.3 Beyond the age of 6 months, the weight of anterior tibialis muscle (expressed as the percentage of total body weight) steadily decreases. This age-related dependency is particularly pronounced in the oldest group, although in this group, the total body mass also starts decreasing (on the basis of unpublished data of Pétervári et al.).

Loss of skeletal muscle results in a gradual decrease of muscle strength which manifests in aging humans as weaker grip force, slower walking (gait) speed, and the general decrease of motor activity. With severe sarcopenia, any change of position (climbing stairs, rising from a chair, changing position in bed, bathroom activities, etc.) becomes difficult, and there is often impairment of movement coordination. The gait is altered (e.g., wider base, rigid upper extremities), and turning around is slow and takes the whole body. In brief, there are two basic consequences of sarcopenia for the elderly: (1) increasingly compromised mobility (which makes sarcopenia even more severe in a vicious circle of decreasing muscle use), (2) development of frailty (age-related state of vulnerable health) and functional deterioration of the elderly, observed for example, as increase in the frequency and severity of falls, life-threatening forms of disability, or even depression and cognitive decline.

During the earlier stages of aging, the loss of lean body mass is compensated for, or often overcompensated by an increase in the body's fat mass. Thereby, the total BW does not change; rather, it increases despite the loss of muscle mass, concealing the progressively developing sarcopenia. In effect, in old subjects, fat accumulates at the expense of skeletal muscle, and also within muscle tissue and muscle fibers (intra- and intermuscular fat deposits). Thus, in many elderly, obesity and sarcopenia coexist (a condition termed sarcopenic obesity), and their additive results lead to higher health risks than each condition alone.

In advanced aging, the amount of fat and total BW also decrease: while loss of the remaining lean body mass continues, the fat mass also disappears gradually, resulting, in some subjects, in cachexia, a complex shrinkage of the whole body. Anorexia is the main factor in the development of cachexia (Evans et al., 2008): both α-MSH (administered by ICV route, Pétervári et al., 2010) and peripherally administered CCK (Balaskó et al., 2012) show extremely strong anorectic action in old animals. In addition, the efficacy of several orexigenic mechanisms becomes insufficient during aging (Akimoto-Takano et al., 2005). In advanced aging, changes at the CNS level may promote anorexia and an overall negative energy balance, as in starvation. Still, anorexia may not be the only factor in inducing cachexia since enhanced energy loss due to increased catabolism may contribute to the loss of BW. Although in animal experiments the resting metabolism was similar in old and young rats, the α-MSH-induced hypermetabolism was most pronounced at later ages (Pétervári, Szabad, et al., 2011).

Cachexia means loss of both fat and protein content, and the increased demand for gluconeogenesis in a condition of relative starvation or undernutrition exaggerates and accelerates the so far moderate/slow protein loss. At this stage, serum leptin levels may be already decreased (Hubbard et al., 2008) and with the possible persistence of the age-related leptin resistance, at the later stages of cachexia, inflammatory signals may replace the anti-anabolic action of leptin at the level of the hypothalamus (Engineer & Garcia, 2012). Proinflammatory cytokines, which were shown to exhibit increased levels in many elderly persons (a process termed inflamm-aging (Cannizzo, Clement, Sahu, Follo, & Santambrogio, 2011; Giunta, 2008)) can enhance proteolysis of muscle proteins (Plata-Salamán, 2001) and contribute to the late phase of the anorexia–cachexia.

5. THERAPEUTIC APPROACHES TO OVERCOME THE ANOREXIA OF AGING AND ITS DELETERIOUS EFFECTS ON BODY FUNCTIONS

Since there are no data suggesting defective absorption of nutrients, normal diet should be sufficient, there is no need to recommend the healthy elderly to apply higher intake of protein or other nutrients (with a possible exception of vitamin D). However, the taste of food, its seasoning, preparation, and presentation may be important factors that influence appetite. In a case of underfeeding or cachexia, enhanced total calorie intake may be necessary: a high-energy high-protein diet is advised (Yaxley & Miller, 2011).

However, caloric support *per se* usually does not reverse cachexia (Tisdale, 2002); it should be treated by means of special diets (e.g., rich in certain branched chain amino acids).

Because various changes in peptidergic regulation have been suggested to contribute to the aging anorexia, intervention at this level is believed to be useful, for example, administration of ghrelin (Akamizu et al., 2008; Depoortere, 2009; Nagaya et al., 2005, 2004), CCK antagonists (Roy et al., 2005), or MC4R antagonist (Foster & Chen, 2007). Unfortunately, such therapeutic approaches have only limited use, partly because there is not enough clinicopharmacological experience, including long-term safety. Recent trials deal with substances capable of blocking protein catabolism (Eley, Russell, Baxter, Mukerji, & Tisdale, 2007).

Physical activity is usually regarded as beneficial for decreasing obesity, but it may also be an important method to fight sarcopenia. A 7-year-long study of 70–79-year-old subjects demonstrated that at the start the less fit persons had a higher weight, a higher fat mass and a lower fat-free mass than the fit ones, but by the end of the training period, they had lost more weight, more fat and also more fat-free mass (Koster et al., 2010). Others reported that elderly persons with leisure-time physical activity lost muscle mass and total body potassium in a 3-year period, while those with higher level of physical activity maintained muscle mass and had less total and truncal fat (Raguso et al., 2006). Still others found that over a 20-year period, the training level did not influence the change in body composition, but the muscle function was better in those with higher activity (Westerterp & Meijer, 2001). Apart from influencing skeletal muscles directly, physical activity also decreases the isolation and the concurrent tendency for depression, it improves cognitive functions and improves appetite in the frail elderly.

6. CONCLUSIONS AND PERSPECTIVES

Aging is accompanied by characteristic changes in energy homeostasis manifested by alterations in BW and composition. Starting from middle age, an intrinsic gradual decrease in muscle mass occurs, which is counterbalanced in many subjects by an increase in fat mass. The decline in metabolically active muscle tissue corresponds to the decrease in food intake, termed "physiologic anorexia," which probably results from the altered age-related integration of peripheral and central signaling at the level of the hypothalamus and brainstem. During the early phase of aging in many elderly persons, the body fat mass increases at a faster rate than the accompanying loss of muscle mass, a condition termed sarcopenic obesity. However, in the later phases of aging, the body's fat mass also decreases so that anorexia of aging results in the decline of the total body mass. In these old subjects, severe sarcopenia and the developing cachexia become major causes of frailty with substantially worsened quality of life and shortening of life expectancy. These aging-related changes develop on the basis of altered energy balance regulation: the anabolic mechanisms become attenuated with a simultaneous enhancement of the catabolic ones.

Anorexia of aging appears to be basically a physiological process; however, at later stages, it turns pathological with serious consequences. Maintenance of normal BW and body composition at the earlier stages of life (and prevention of an early increase in serum levels of proinflammatory cytokines) may be important. Although at present no safe pharmacological intervention seems to be applicable, and there are no reliable and simple methods to alter the homeostatic regulatory mechanisms that lie in the background, other methods are important to prevent or at least to slow down the progression of the anorexia of aging. They include preparation and presentation of food, social environment, physical activity, and probably lifestyle, as well as maintenance of normal BW and body composition from the early to the late stages of life. Since severe sarcopenia is the most serious health-threatening factor of the complex age-related changes of body mass and composition, further investigations are necessary to find methods of preventing or slowing down the age-dependent loss of muscle tissue.

ACKNOWLEDGMENTS

The expert secretarial assistance of Mrs. Iwona Pakulska is highly appreciated. The authors' studies mentioned earlier have been supported by Grant ST-12 from the Medical University of Gdansk, Poland, by a grant from the Hungarian Agency for Scientific Grants OTKA PD-84241, and other grants from the University of Pécs (SROP-4.2.1.B-10/2/KONV-2010-0002, SROP-4.2.2/B-10/1-2010-0029, 34039/KA-OTKA/13-02), Hungary.

REFERENCES

Akamizu, T., Iwakura, H., Ariyasu, H., Murayama, T., Sumi, E., Teramukai, S., et al. (2008). Osteoarthritis-total hip replacement clinical study team: Effects of ghrelin treatment on patients undergoing total hip replacement for osteoarthritis: Different outcomes from studies in patients with cardiac and pulmonary cachexia. *Journal of the American Geriatrics Society*, *56*(12), 2363–2365.

Akimoto-Takano, S., Sakurai, C., Kanai, S., Hosoya, H., Ohta, M., & Miyasaka, K. (2005). Differences in the appetite-stimulating effect of orexin, neuropeptide Y and ghrelin among young, adult and old rats. *Neuroendocrinology*, *82*(5–6), 256–263.

Andreasson, A. N., Undén, A. L., Elofsson, S., & Brismar, K. (2012). Leptin and adiponectin: Distribution and associations with cardiovascular risk factors in men and women of the

general population. *American Journal of Human Biology*, *24*(5), 595–601. http://dx.doi.org/10.1002/ajhb.22279.
Ariyasu, H., Iwakura, H., Yamada, G., Nakao, K., Kangawa, K., & Akamizu, T. (2008). Efficacy of ghrelin as a therapeutic approach for age-related physiological changes. *Endocrinology*, *149*(7), 3722–3728.
Balaskó, M., Soós, S., Párniczky, A., Koncsecskó-Gáspár, M., Székely, M., & Pétervári, E. (2012). Anorexigenic effect of peripheral cholecystokinin (CCK) varies with age and body composition. *Acta Physiologica Hungarica*, *99*(2), 166–172.
Bao, A. M., & Swaab, D. F. (2007). Gender difference in age-related number of corticotrophin-releasing hormone-expressing neurons in the human hypothalamic paraventricular nucleus and the role of sex hormones. *Neuroendocrinology*, *85*, 27–36.
Baranowska, B., Bik, W., Baranowska-Bik, A., Wolinska-Witort, E., Szybinska, A., Martynska, I., et al. (2006). Neuroendocrine control of metabolic homeostasis in Polish centenarians. *Journal of Physiology and Pharmacology*, *57*, 55–61.
Bauer, J. M., Haack, A., Winning, K., Wirth, R., Fischer, B., Uter, W., et al. (2010). Impaired postprandial response of active ghrelin and prolonged suppression of hunger sensation in the elderly. *The Journals of Gerontology. Series A, Biological Sciences and Medical Sciences*, *65*(3), 307–311.
Berna, M. J., Tapia, J. A., Sancho, V., & Jensen, R. T. (2007). Progress in developing cholecystokinin (CCK)/gastrin receptor ligands that have therapeutic potentials. *Current Opinion in Pharmacology*, 7(6), 583–592.
Bhutto, A., & Morley, J. E. (2008). The clinical significance of gastrointestinal changes with aging. *Current Opinion in Clinical Nutrition and Metabolic Care*, *11*(5), 651–660.
Blanton, C. A., Horwitz, B. A., Blevins, J. E., Hamilton, J. S., Hernandez, E. J., & Mc Donald, R. B. (2001). Reduced feeding response to neuropeptide Y in senescent Fischer 344 rats. *American Journal of Physiology. Regulatory, Integrative and Comparative Physiology*, *280*(4), 1052–1060.
Blanton, C. A., Horwitz, B. A., Murtagh-Mark, C., Gietzen, D. W., Griffey, S. M., & McDonald, R. B. (2006). Meal patterns associated with the age-related decline in food intake in the Fischer 344 rat. *The American Journal of Physiology*, *275*(5 Pt. 2), 1494–1502.
Boyce, J. M., & Shone, G. R. (2006). Effects of ageing on smell and taste. *Postgraduate Medical Journal*, *82*, 239–241.
Bray, G. A. (2000). Afferent signals regulating food intake. *The Proceedings of the Nutrition Society*, *59*(3), 373–384.
Briefel, R. R., McDowell, M. A., Alaimo, K., Caughman, C. R., Bischof, A. L., Carroll, M. D., et al. (1995). Total energy intake of the US population: The third National Health and Nutrition Examination Survey, 1988–1991. *The American Journal of Clinical Nutrition*, *62*(Suppl. 5), 1072S–1080S.
Broglio, F., Benso, A., Castiglioni, C., Gottero, C., Prodam, F., Destefanis, S., et al. (2003). The endocrine response to ghrelin as a function of gender in humans in young and elderly subjects. *The Journal of Clinical Endocrinology and Metabolism*, *88*(4), 1537–1542.
Brogna, A., Loreno, M., Catalano, F., Bucceri, A. M., Malaguarnera, M., Muratore, L. A., et al. (2006). Radioisotopic assessment of gastric emptying of solids in elderly subjects. *Aging Clinical and Experimental Research*, *18*, 493–496.
Cannizzo, E. S., Clement, C. C., Sahu, R., Follo, C., & Santambrogio, L. (2011). Oxidative stress, inflamm-aging and immunosenescence. *Journal of Proteomics*, *74*(11), 2313–2323.
Chapman, I. M. (2007). The anorexia of aging. *Clinics in Geriatric Medicine*, *23*, 735–756.
Chapman, I. M., MacIntosh, C. G., Morley, J. E., & Horowitz, M. (2002). The anorexia of ageing. *Biogerontology*, *3*(1–2), 67–71.
Clarkston, W. K., Pantano, M. M., Morley, J. E., Horowitz, M., Littlefield, J. M., & Burton, F. R. (1997). Evidence for the anorexia of aging: Gastrointestinal transit and hunger in healthy elderly vs. young adults. *The American Journal of Physiology*, *272*(1 Pt. 2), R243–R248.

Coppola, J. D., Horwitz, B. A., Hamilton, J., & McDonald, R. B. (2004). Expression of NPY Yl and Y5 receptors in the hypothalamic paraventricular nucleus of aged Fischer 344 rats. *American Journal of Physiology. Regulatory, Integrative and Comparative Physiology, 287*(1), 69–75.

Depoortere, I. (2009). Targeting the ghrelin receptor to regulate food intake. *Regulatory Peptides, 156*(1–3), 13–23.

Di Francesco, V., Barazzoni, R., Bissoli, L., Fantin, F., Rizzotti, P., Residori, L., et al. (2010). The quantity of meal fat influences the profile of postprandial hormones as well as hunger sensation in healthy elderly people. *Journal of the American Medical Directors Association, 11*(3), 188–193.

Di Francesco, V., Fantin, F., Omizzolo, F., Residori, L., Bissoli, L., Bosello, O., et al. (2007). The anorexia of aging. *Digestive Diseases, 25*(2), 129–137.

Di Francesco, V., Zamboni, M., Dioli, A., Zoico, E., Mazzali, G., Omizzolo, F., et al. (2005). Delayed postprandial gastric emptying and impaired gallbladder contraction together with elevated cholecystokinin and peptide YY serum levels sustain satiety and inhibit hunger in healthy elderly persons. *The Journals of Gerontology. Series A, Biological Sciences and Medical Sciences, 60*(12), 1581–1585.

Dockray, G. J. (2009). Cholecystokinin and gut-brain signalling. *Regulatory Peptides, 155* (1–3), 6–10.

Downs, J. L., Dunn, M. R., Borok, E., Shanabrough, M., Horvath, T. L., Kohama, S. G., et al. (2007). Orexin neuronal changes in the locus coeruleus of the aging rhesus macaque. *Neurobiology of Aging, 28*(8), 1286–1295.

Eley, H. L., Russell, S. T., Baxter, J. H., Mukerji, P., & Tisdale, M. J. (2007). Signaling pathways initiated by beta-hydroxy-beta-methylbutyrate to attenuate the depression of protein synthesis in skeletal muscle in responses to cahectic stimuli. *American Journal of Physiology. Endocrinology and Metabolism, 293*(4), E923–E931.

Engineer, D. R., & Garcia, J. M. (2012). Leptin anorexia and cachexia syndrome. *International Journal of Peptides, 2012*, 1–13. http://dx.doi.org/10.1155/2012/287457. Article ID 287457.

Escobar, C. M., Krajewski, S. J., Sandoval-Guzmán, T., Voytko, M. L., & Rance, N. E. (2004). Neuropeptide Y expression is increased in the hypothalamus of older women. *The Journal of Clinical Endocrinology and Metabolism, 89*(5), 2338–2343.

Escrivá, F., Gavete, M. L., Fermín, Y., Pérez, C., Gallardo, N., Alvarez, C., et al. (2007). Effect of age and moderate food restriction on insulin sensitivity in Wistar rats: Role of adiposity. *The Journal of Endocrinology, 194*(1), 131–141.

Evans, W. J., Morley, J. E., Argilés, J., Bales, C., Baracos, V., Guttridge, D., et al. (2008). Cachexia: A new definition. *Clinical Nutrition, 27*(6), 793–799.

Fernandez-Galaz, C., Fernandez-Agullo, T., Campoy, F., Arribas, C., Gallardo, N., Andres, A., et al. (2001). Decreased leptin uptake in hypothalamic nuclei with ageing in Wistar rats. *The Journal of Endocrinology, 171*(1), 23–32.

Fernández-Galaz, C., Fernández-Agulló, T., Pérez, C., Peralta, S., Arribas, C., Andrés, A., et al. (2002). Long-term food restriction prevents aging associated central leptin resistance in Wistar rats. *Diabetologia, 45*(7), 997–1003.

Ferrini, F., Salio, C., Lossi, L., & Merighi, A. (2009). Ghrelin in central neurons. *Current Neuropharmacology*, 7(1), 37–49.

Figlewicz, D. P., & Benoit, S. C. (2009). Insulin, leptin, and food reward: Update 2008. *American Journal of Physiology. Regulatory, Integrative and Comparative Physiology, 296*(1), R9–R19.

Foster, A. C., & Chen, C. (2007). Melanocortin-4 receptor antagonists as potential therapeutics in the treatment of cachexia. *Current Topics in Medicinal Chemistry*, 7(11), 1131–1136.

Gabriely, I., Ma, X. H., Yang, X. M., Atzmon, G., Rajala, M. W., Berg, A. H., et al. (2002). Removal of visceral fat prevents insulin resistance and glucose intolerance of aging. *Diabetes, 51*(10), 2951–2958.

Gabriely, I., Ma, X. H., Yang, X. M., Rossetti, L., & Barzilai, N. (2002). Leptin resistance during aging is independent of fat mass. *Diabetes*, *51*(4), 1016–1021.

García-San Frutos, M., Fernández-Agulló, T., De Solís, A. J., Andrés, A., Arribas, C., Carrascosa, J. M., et al. (2007). Impaired central insulin response in aged Wistar rats: Role of adiposity. *Endocrinology*, *148*(11), 5238–5247.

Garfield, A. S., Lam, D. D., Marston, O. J., Przydzial, M. J., & Heisler, L. K. (2009). Role of central melanocortin pathways in energy homeostasis. *Trends in Endocrinology and Metabolism*, *20*(5), 203–215.

Giunta, S. (2008). Exploring the complex relations between inflammation and aging (inflamm-aging): Anti-inflamm-aging remodelling of inflamm-aging, from robustness to frailty. *Inflammation Research*, *57*(12), 558–563.

Gruenewald, D. A., Marck, B. T., & Matsumoto, A. M. (1996). Fasting-induced increases in food intake and neuropeptide Y gene expression are attenuated in aging male Brown Norway rats. *Endocrinology*, *137*(10), 4460–4467.

Hallfrisch, J., Muller, D., Drinkwater, D., Tobin, J., & Andres, R. (1990). Continuing diet trends in men: The Baltimore Longitudinal Study of Aging (1961–1987). *Journal of Gerontology*, *45*, M186–M191.

Hickey, M. S., Israel, R. G., Gardiner, S. N., Considine, R. V., McCammon, M. R., Tyndall, G. L., et al. (1996). Gender differences in serum leptin levels in humans. *Biochemical and Molecular Medicine*, *59*, 1–6.

Hubbard, R. E., Lang, I. A., Llewellyn, D. J., & Rockwood, K. (2010). Frailty, body mass index, and abdominal obesity in older people. *The Journals of Gerontology. Series A, Biological Sciences and Medical Sciences*, *65*, 377–381.

Hubbard, R. E., O'Mahony, M. S., Calver, B. L., & Woodhouse, K. W. (2008). Nutrition, inflammation, and leptin levels in aging and frailty. *Journal of the American Geriatrics Society*, *56*(2), 279–284.

Ishii, S., Shibasaki, T., Murakami, T., Shima, K., & Wakabayashi, I. (2000). Response of leptin mRNA to 24-h food deprivation and refeeding is influenced by age in rats. *Regulatory Peptides*, *92*(1–3), 45–50.

Jessen, L., Clegg, D. J., & Bouman, S. D. (2010). Evaluation of the lack of anorectic effect of intracerebroventricular insulin in rats. *American Journal of Physiology. Regulatory, Integrative and Comparative Physiology*, *298*(1), R43–R50.

Kalra, S. P., Bagnasco, M., Otukonyoung, E. E., Dube, M. G., & Kalra, P. S. (2003). Rhythmic, reciprocal ghrelin and leptin signaling: New insight in the development of obesity. *Regulatory Peptides*, *111*(1–3), 1–11.

Kalra, S. P., Dube, M. G., Pu, S., Xu, B., Horvath, T. L., & Kalra, P. S. (1999). Interacting appetite-regulating pathways in the hypothalamic regulation of body weight. *Endocrine Reviews*, *20*(1), 68–100.

Kaneda, T., Makino, S., Nishiyama, M., Asaba, K., & Hashimoto, K. (2001). Differential neuropeptide responses to starvation with ageing. *Journal of Neuroendocrinology*, *13*(12), 1066–1075.

Kappeler, L., Zizzari, P., Alliot, J., Epelbaum, J., & Bluet-Pajot, M. T. (2004). Delayed age-associated decrease in growth hormone pulsatile secretion and increased orexigenic peptide expression in the Lou C/JaLL rat. *Neuroendocrinology*, *80*(5), 273–283.

Kastin, A. J., & Pan, W. (2000). Dynamic regulation of leptin entry into brain by the blood-brain barrier. *Regulatory Peptides*, *92*(1–3), 37–43.

Kibler, H. H., Silsby, H. D., & Johnson, H. D. (1963). Metabolic trends and life span of rats living at 9 C and 28 C. *Journal of Gerontology*, *18*(7), 235–239.

Kmiec, Z. (2010). Central control of food intake in aging. *Interdisciplinary Topics in Gerontology*, *37*, 37–50.

Kmiec, Z. (2011). Aging and peptide control of food intake. *Current Protein & Peptide Science*, *12*, 271–279.

Kmiec, Z., Pokrywka, L., Kotlarz, G., Kubasik, J., Szutowicz, A., & Mysliwski, A. (2005). The effects of fasting and refeeding on serum leptin, adiponectin and free fatty acids concentrations in young and old male rats. *Gerontology*, *51*(6), 357–362.

Kojima, M., Hosoda, H., Date, Y., Nakazato, M., Matsuo, H., & Kangawa, K. (1999). Ghrelin is a growth hormone-releasing acylated peptide from stomach. *Nature*, *402* (6762), 656–660.

Koster, A., Visser, M., Simonsick, E. M., Yu, B., Allison, D. B., Newman, A. B., et al. (2010). Health, Aging and Body Composition Study: Association of fitness with changes in body composition and muscle strength. *Journal of the American Geriatrics Society*, *58*(2), 219–226.

Kotz, C. M., Mullett, M. A., & Wang, C. F. (2005). Diminished feeding responsiveness to orexin A (hypocretin 1) in aged rats is accompanied by decreased neuronal activation. *American Journal of Physiology. Regulatory, Integrative and Comparative Physiology*, *289*(2), 359–366.

Leibowitz, S. F., & Wortley, K. E. (2004). Hypothalamic control of energy balance: Different peptides, different functions. *Peptides*, *25*(3), 473–504.

Leidy, H. J., Apolzan, J. W., Mattes, R. D., & Campbell, W. W. (2010). Food form and portion size affect postprandial appetite sensations and hormonal responses in healthy, nonobese, older adults. *Obesity*, *18*(2), 293–299.

Li, H., Matheny, M., Nicolson, M., Tümer, N., & Scarpace, P. J. (1997). Leptin gene expression increases with age independent of adiposity in rats. *Diabetes*, *46*(12), 2035–2039.

Ma, X., Lin, L., Qin, G., Lu, X., Fiorotto, M., Dixit, V. D., et al. (2011). Ablations of ghrelin and ghrelin receptor exhibit differential metabolic phenotypes and thermogenic capacity during aging. *PLoS One*, *6*, e16391.

MacIntosh, C. G., Andrews, J. M., Jones, K. L., Wishart, J. M., Morris, H. A., Jansen, J. B., et al. (1999). Effects of age on concentrations of plasma cholecystokinin, glucagon-like peptide 1, and peptide YY and their relation to appetite and pyloric motility. *The American Journal of Clinical Nutrition*, *69*(5), 999–1006.

MacIntosh, C. G., Morley, J. E., Wishart, J., Morris, H., Jansen, J. B., Horowitz, M., et al. (2001). Effects of exogenous cholecystokinin (CCK-8) on food intake, plasma CCK, leptin and insulin concentrations in older and young adults: Evidence for increased CCK activity as a cause of the anorexia of aging. *The Journal of Clinical Endocrinology and Metabolism*, *86*(12), 5830–5837.

Madsen, J. L., & Graff, J. (2004). Effects of ageing on gastrointestinal motor function. *Age and Ageing*, *33*, 154–159.

Majumdar, A. P. (2003). Regulation of gastrointestinal mucosal growth during aging. *Journal of Physiology and Pharmacology*, *54*(Suppl. 4), 143–154.

Majumdar, A. P., Jaszewski, R., & Dubick, M. A. (1997). Effect of aging on the gastrointestinal tract and the pancreas. *Proceedings of the Society for Experimental Biology and Medicine*, *215*(2), 134–144.

Martinez, M., Hernanz, A., Gómez-Cerezo, J., Pena, J. M., Vazquez, J. J., & Arnalich, F. (1993). Alterations in plasma and cerebrospinal fluid levels of neuropeptides in idiopathic senile anorexia. *Regulatory Peptides*, *49*(2), 109–117.

McDonald, R. B., & Ruhe, R. C. (2010). Changes in food intake and its relationship to weight loss during advanced age. *Interdisciplinary Topics in Gerontology*, *37*, 51–63.

McTigue, K. M., Hess, R., & Ziouras, J. (2006). Obesity in older adults: A systematic review of the evidence for diagnosis and treatment. *Obesity (Silver Spring)*, *14*(9), 1485–1497.

Metlakunta, A. S., Sahu, M., & Sahu, A. (2008). Hypothalamic phosphatidylinositol 3-kinase pathway of leptin signaling is impaired during the development of diet-induced obesity in FVB/N mice. *Endocrinology*, *149*(3), 1121–1128.

Miyasaka, K., Kanai, S., Masuda, M., Ohta, M., Kawanami, T., Matsumoto, M., et al. (1995). Gene expressions of cholecystokinin (CCK) and CCK receptors, and its satiety effect in young and old male rats. *Archives of Gerontology and Geriatrics*, *21*(2), 147–155.

Moran, T. H., & Kinzig, K. P. (2004). Gastrointestinal satiety signals II: Cholecystokinin. *American Journal of Physiology. Gastrointestinal and Liver Physiology*, *286*(2), 183–188.

Moriguti, J. C., Das, S. K., Saltzman, E., Corrales, A., McCrory, M. A., Greenberg, A. S., et al. (2000). Effects of a 6-week hypocaloric diet on changes in body composition, hunger, and subsequent weight regain in healthy young and older adults. *The Journals of Gerontology. Series A, Biological Sciences and Medical Sciences*, *55*(12), B580–B587.

Morley, J. E. (1997). Anorexia of aging: Physiologic and pathologic. *The American Journal of Clinical Nutrition*, *66*, 760–773.

Morley, J. E. (2003). Anorexia and weight loss in older persons. *The Journals of Gerontology. Series A, Biological Sciences and Medical Sciences*, *58*(2), 131–137.

Morley, J. E., & Silver, A. J. (1988). Anorexia in the elderly. *Neurobiology of Aging*, *9*(1), 9–16.

Morton, G. J., Cummings, D. E., Baskin, D. G., Barsh, G. S., & Schwartz, M. W. (2006). Central nervous system control of food intake and body weight. *Nature*, *443*(7109), 289–295.

Muscaritoli, M., Anker, S. D., Argilés, J., Aversa, Z., Bauer, J. M., Biolo, G., et al. (2010). Consensus definition of sarcopenia, cachexia and pre-cachexia: Joint document elaborated by Special Interest Groups (SIG) "cachexia-anorexia in chronic wasting diseases" and "nutrition in geriatrics". *Clinical Nutrition*, *29*(2), 154–159.

Nagaya, N., Itoh, T., Murakami, S., Oya, H., Uematsu, M., Miyatake, K., et al. (2005). Treatment of cachexia with ghrelin in patients with COPD. *Chest*, *128*(3), 1187–1193.

Nagaya, N., Moriya, J., Yasumura, Y., Uematsu, M., Ono, F., Shimizu, W., et al. (2004). Effects of ghrelin administration on left ventricular function, exercise capacity, and muscle wasting in patients with chronic heart failure. *Circulation*, *110*(24), 3674–3679.

Narici, M. V., & Maffulli, N. (2010). Sarcopenia: Characteristics, mechanisms and functional significance. *British Medical Bulletin*, *95*, 139–159.

Newman, A. B., Lee, J. S., Visser, M., Goodpaster, B. H., Kritchevsky, S. B., Tylavsky, F. A., et al. (2005). Weight change and the conservation of lean mass in old age: The Health, Aging and Body Composition Study. *The American Journal of Clinical Nutrition*, *82*(4), 872–878.

Nogalska, A., & Swierczynski, J. (2001). The age-related differences in obese and fatty acid synthase gene expression in white adipose tissue of rat. *Biochimica et Biophysica Acta*, *1533* (1), 73–80.

Ohta, M., Tanaka, Y., Masuda, M., Miyasaka, K., & Funakoshi, A. (1995). Impaired release of cholecystokinin (CCK) from synaptosomes in old rats. *Neuroscience Letters*, *198*(3), 161–164.

Olshansky, S. J., Carnes, B. A., & Cassel, C. (1990). In search of Methuselah: Estimating the upper limits to human longevity. *Science*, *250*, 634–640.

Peralta, S., Carrascosa, J. M., Gallardo, N., Ros, M., & Arribas, C. (2002). Ageing increases SOCS-3 expression in rat hypothalamus: Effects of food restriction. *Biochemical and Biophysical Research Communications*, *296*(2), 425–428.

Pétervári, E., Garami, A., Soós, Sz., Székely, M., & Balaskó, M. (2009). Suppression of food intake by intracerebroventricular injection of alpha-MSH varies with age in rats. *Acta Physiologica Hungarica*, *96*(4), 483–487.

Pétervári, E., Garami, A., Soós, S., Székely, M., & Balaskó, M. (2010). Age dependence of alpha-MSH-induced anorexia. *Neuropeptides*, *44*, 315–322.

Pétervári, E., Soós, S., Székely, M., & Balaskó, M. (2011). Alterations in the peptidergic regulation of energy balance in the course of aging. *Current Protein and Peptide Science*, *12*, 316–324.

Pétervári, E., Szabad, Á. O., Soós, S., Garami, A., Székely, M., & Balaskó, M. (2011). Central alpha-MSH infusion in rats: Disparate anorexic vs. metabolic changes with aging. *Regulatory Peptides*, *166*(1–3), 105–111.

Plata-Salamán, C. R. (2001). Cytokines and feeding. *International Journal of Obesity and Related Metabolic Disorders, 25*(S5), S48–S52.
Porkka-Heiskanen, T., Alanko, L., Kalinchuk, A., Heiskanen, S., & Stenberg, D. (2004). The effect of age on prepro-orexin gene expression and contents of orexin A and B in the rat brain. *Neurobiology of Aging, 25*(2), 231–238.
Poston, G. J., Singh, P., Draviam, E. J., Upp, J. R., & Thompson, J. C. (1988). Development and age-related changes in pancreatic cholecystokinin receptors and duodenal cholecystokinin in guinea pigs. *Mechanisms of Aging and Development, 46*(1–3), 59–66.
Puthucheary, Z., Montgomery, H., Moxham, J., Harridge, S., & Hart, N. (2010). Structure to function: Muscle failure in critically ill patients. *The Journal of Physiology, 588*(23), 4641–4648.
Raguso, C. A., Kyle, U., Kossovsky, M. P., Roynette, C., Paolini-Giacobino, A., Hans, D., et al. (2006). A 3-year longitudinal study on body composition changes in the elderly: Role of physical exercise. *Clinical Nutrition, 25*(4), 573–580.
Rigamonti, A. E., Pincelli, A. I., Corra, B., Viarengo, R., Bonomo, S. M., Galimberti, D., et al. (2002). Plasma ghrelin concentrations in elderly subjects: Comparison with anorexic and obese patients. *The Journal of Endocrinology, 175*(1), 1–5.
Roberts, S. B., Fuss, P., Heyman, M. B., Evans, W. J., Tsay, R., Rasmussen, H., et al. (1994). Control of food intake in older men. *JAMA: The Journal of the American Medical Association, 272*(20), 1601–1606.
Rolls, B. J., & McDermott, T. M. (1991). Effects of age on sensory-specific satiety. *The American Journal of Clinical Nutrition, 54*(6), 988–996.
Roy, P., Wangsa, J., Patel, A., Nolting, A., Persiani, S., Abramowitz, W., et al. (2005). The singe-dose pharmacokinetics of the novel CCK1 receptor antagonist, dexloxiglumide, are not influenced by age and gender. *International Journal of Clinical Pharmacology and Therapeutics, 43*(9), 444–451.
Sánchez-Lasheras, C., Christine Könner, A. C., Jens, C., & Brüning, J. C. (2010). Integrative neurobiology of energy homeostasis-neurocircuits, signals and mediators. *Frontiers in Neuroendocrinology, 31*(1), 4–15.
Sandström, O., & El-Salhy, M. (1999). Aging and endocrine cells of human duodenum. *Mechanisms of Ageing and Development, 108*(1), 39–48.
Scarpace, P. J., Matheny, M., Moore, R. L., & Tümer, N. (2000). Impaired leptin responsiveness in aged rats. *Diabetes, 49*(3), 431–435.
Schubert, C. R., Cruickshanks, K. J., Klein, B. E., Klein, R., & Nondahl, D. M. (2011). Olfactory impairment in older adults: Five-year incidence and risk factors. *The Laryngoscope, 121*(4), 873–878.
Schuligoi, R., Fernandez, J., Heavens, R. P., & Sirinathsinghji, D. J. (1993). Decreased tyrosine hydroxylase mRNA but not cholecystokinin mRNA in the pars compacta of the substantia nigra and ventral tegmental area of aged rats. *Brain Research. Molecular Brain Research, 19*(4), 333–338.
Schwartz, M. W. (2006). Central nervous system regulation of food intake. *Obesity, 14*, 1–8.
Schwartz, M. W., & Porte, D., Jr. (2005). Diabetes, obesity, and the brain. *Science, 307*(5708), 375–379.
Serra-Prat, M., Fernández, X., Burdoy, E., Mussoll, J., Casamitjana, R., & Puig-Domingo, M. (2007). The role of ghrelin in the energy homeostasis of elderly people: A population-based study. *Journal of Endocrinological Investigation, 30*, 484–490.
Serra-Prat, M., Palomera, E., Clave, P., & Puig-Domingo, M. (2009). Effect of age and frailty on ghrelin and cholecystokinin responses to a meal test. *The American Journal of Clinical Nutrition, 89*(5), 1410–1417.
Silver, A. J., Flood, J. F., & Morley, J. E. (1988). Effect of gastrointestinal peptides on ingestion in old and young mice. *Peptides, 9*(2), 221–225.
Sinha, M. K., & Caro, J. F. (1998). Clinical aspects of leptin. *Vitamins and Hormones, 54*, 1–30.

Sohn, E. H., Wolden-Hanson, T., & Matsumoto, A. M. (2002). Testosterone (T)-induced changes in arcuate nucleus cocaine-amphetamine-regulated transcript and NPY mRNA are attenuated in old compared to young male Brown Norway rats: Contribution of T to age-related changes in cocaineamphetamine-regulated transcript and NPY gene expression. *Endocrinology, 143*(3), 954–963.

Solomon, A., De Fanti, B. A., & Martinez, J. A. (2007). Peripheral ghrelin interacts with orexin neurons in glucostatic signaling. *Regulatory Peptides, 144*, 17–24.

Soos, S., Balasko, M., Jech-Mihalffy, A., Szekely, M., & Petervari, E. (2010). Anorexic vs. metabolic effects of central leptin infusion in rats of various ages and nutritional states. *Journal of Molecular Neuroscience, 41*(1), 97–110.

Stevens, J. (2000). Impact of age on associations between weight and mortality. *Nutrition Reviews, 58*(11), 129–137.

Stevens, J., Cai, J., Pamuk, E. R., Williamson, D. F., Thun, M. J., & Wood, J. L. (1998). The effect of age on the association between body-mass index and mortality. *The New England Journal of Medicine, 338*(1), 1–7.

Stofkova, A., Skurlova, M., Kiss, A., Zelezna, B., Zorad, S., & Jurcovicova, J. (2009). Activation of hypothalamic NPY, AgRP, MC4R, and IL-6 mRNA levels in young Lewis rats with early diet-induced obesity. *Endocrine Regulations, 43*(3), 99–106.

Sturm, K., MacIntosh, C. G., Parker, B. A., Wishart, J., Horowitz, M., & Chapman, I. M. (2003). Appetite, food intake, and plasma concentrations of cholecystokinin, ghrelin, and other gastrointestinal hormones in undernourished older women and well-nourished young and older women. *The Journal of Clinical Endocrinology and Metabolism, 88*(8), 3747–3755.

Suzuki, K., Simpson, K. A., Minnion, J. S., Shillito, J. C., & Bloom, S. R. (2010). The role of gut hormones and the hypothalamus in appetite regulation. *Endocrine Journal, 57*(5), 359–372.

Székely, M., Balaskó, M., Soós, S., & Pétervári, E. (2012). *Peptidergic regulation of food intake: Changes related to age and body composition. In J. L. Morrison (Ed.), Food intake: Regulation, assessing and controlling* (pp. 83–104). Hauppauge, New York: Nova Science Publishers, Inc. Chapter 4. https://www.novapublishers.com/catalog/product_info.php?products_id=19499.

Terao, A., Apte-Deshpande, A., Morairty, S., Freund, Y. R., & Kilduff, T. S. (2002). Age-related decline in hypocretin (orexin) receptor 2 messenger RNA levels in the mouse brain. *Neuroscience Letters, 332*(3), 190–194.

Tisdale, M. J. (2002). Cachexia in cancer patients. *Nature Reviews. Cancer, 2*(11), 862–871.

Toshinai, K., Mondal, M. S., Shimbara, T., Yamaguchi, H., Date, Y., Kangawa, K., et al. (2007). Ghrelin stimulates growth hormone secretion and food intake in aged rats. *Mechanisms of Aging and Development, 128*(2), 182–186.

Valassi, E., Scacchi, M., & Cavagnini, F. (2008). Neuroendocrine control of food intake. *Nutrition, Metabolism, and Cardiovascular Diseases, 18*(2), 158–168.

Voigt, J. P., Huston, J. P., Voits, M., & Fink, H. (1996). Effects of cholecystokinin octapeptide (CCK-8) on food intake in adult and aged rats under different feeding conditions. *Peptides, 17*(8), 1313–1315.

Wernette, C. M., White, D., & Zizza, C. A. (2011). Signaling proteins that influence energy intake may affect unintentional weight loss in elderly persons. *Journal of the American Dietetic Association, 111*(6), 864–873.

Westerterp, K. R., & Meijer, E. P. (2001). Physical activity and parameters of aging: A physiological perspective. *The Journals of Gerontology. Series A, Biological Sciences and Medical Sciences, 56*(S2), 7–12.

Wilkinson, M., Brown, R., Imrash, S. A., & Ur, E. (2007). Adipokine gene expression in brain and pituitary gland. *Neuroendocrinology, 86*(3), 191–209.

Wilson, R. S., Yu, L., & Bennett, D. A. (2011). Odor identification and mortality in old age. *Chemical Senses, 36*, 63–67.

Wolden-Hanson, T. (2006). Mechanisms of the anorexia of aging in the Brown Norway rat. *Physiology & Behavior, 88*(3), 267–276.

Wolden-Hanson, T., Marck, B. T., & Matsumoto, A. M. (2004). Blunted hypothalamic neuropeptide Y gene expression in response to fasting, but preservation of feeding responses to AgRP in aging male Brown Norway rats. *American Journal of Physiology. Regulatory, Integrative and Comparative Physiology, 287*(1), 138–146.

Woods, S. C., & D'Alessio, D. A. (2008). Central control of body weight and appetite. *The Journal of Clinical Endocrinology and Metabolism, 93*(11), 37–50.

Woods, S. C., Lotter, E. C., McKay, L. D., & Porte, D., Jr. (1979). Chronic intracerebroventricular infusion of insulin reduces food intake and body weight of baboons. *Nature, 282*(5738), 503–505.

Wu, Q., Clark, M. S., & Palmiter, R. D. (2012). Deciphering a neuronal circuit that mediates appetite. *Nature, 483*(7391), 594–597.

Yang, M.-J., Wang, F., Wang, J.-H., Wu, W.-N., Hu, Z.-L., Cheng, J., et al. (2010). PI3K integrates the effects of insulin and leptin on large-conductance Ca^{2+}-activated K^{+} channels in neuropeptide Y neurons of the hypothalamic arcuate nucleus. *American Journal of Physiology. Endocrinology and Metabolism, 298*(2), E193–E201.

Yaxley, A., & Miller, M. D. (2011). The challenge of appropriate identification and treatment of starvation, sarcopenia, and cachexia: A survey of Australian dietitians. *Journal of Nutrition and Metabolism, 2011*, 1–6. http://dx.doi.org/10.1155/2011/603161. Article ID 603161.

Yu, B. P., Masoro, E. J., & McMahan, C. A. (1985). Nutritional influences on aging of Fischer 344 rats. I. Physical, metabolic and longevity characteristics. *Journal of Gerontology, 40*(6), 657–670.

Yu, B. P., Masoro, E. J., Murata, I., Bertrand, H. A., & Lynd, F. T. (1982). Life span study of SPF Fischer 344 male rats fed ad libitum or restricted diets: Longevity, growth, lean body mass and disease. *Journal of Gerontology, 37*(2), 130–141.

Zhang, Y., Proenca, R., Maffei, M., Barone, M., Leopold, L., & Friedman, J. M. (1994). Positional cloning of the mouse obese gene and its human homologue. *Nature, 372*(6505), 425–432.

INDEX

Note: Page numbers followed by "*f*" indicate figures, and "*t*" indicate tables.

A

ACTH. *See* Adrenocorticotropic hormone (ACTH)
Adipose triglyceride lipase (ATGL), 277–278, 279
Adrenocorticotropic hormone (ACTH)
  secretion, 128
  in steroidogenesis, 127–128
  stimulation, 127–128
Advanced glycation end-products (AGE), 276
AGE. *See* Advanced glycation end-products (AGE)
Agouti gene-related protein (AGRP)
  anx/anx mouse, 43
  immunofluorescence micrographs, 35–36, 36*f*
  NPY projections
    brain, 29
    IHC, 33–34
    ISH, 34
    POMC/CART neurons, 30, 31*f*
Agouti-related peptide (AgRP)
  central melanocortin system, 4, 5*f*
  and NPY/AgRP neurons, 4
AGRP. *See* Agouti gene-related protein (AGRP)
AgRP. *See* Agouti-related peptide (AgRP)
AIDS-associated cachexia, 90–91
α-Melanocyte-stimulating hormone (α-MSH)
  anorexigenic, 324–326
  central melanocortin system, 4, 5*f*
  dendritic and axonal release, 7, 17
  enhanced anorexigenic tone, 327
  expression, *NUCB2* gene, 12
  nesfatin-1 colocalization, 13
  POMC-CRH-OT feeding circuit, 17, 18*f*
Amenorrhea
  adolescents and young adult women, 255–256
  chronic, 244
  estrogen therapies, 246
  HRT, 248, 249*t*
AN. *See* Anorexia nervosa (AN)
Anorexia
  caloric intake, 199
  cancer patients, 274
  chronic diseases, 275
  CKD, 219
  food intake, patients, 274
  ghrelin, 206
  lipopolysaccharide (LPS) injection, 205
  proinflammatory cytokines, 274–275
Anorexia and hypothalamic degeneration
  anx/anx mouse (*see Anx/anx* mouse)
  cachexia, 28
  children, 29
  food intake, 29–30
  neurodegeneration and mitochondrial dysfunction, 48–49
  opioid receptor gene, 28–29
  weight disturbances, 42–48
Anorexia nervosa (AN)
  adipokine, bone anomalies, 266
  adolescents, 244, 260–261
  amenorrhea, 244
  Arg51Gln and Leu72Met SNP, 112–113
  BDNF gene, 144–145
  biological variables and bone parameters, 264–265, 264*t*
  bivariate analysis, 264–265, 264*t*
  BMD (*see* Bone mineral density (BMD))
  BMI, 263
  body weight, 266
  bone mineral density, 142
  caloric restriction, 111
  clinical characteristics, 263, 263*t*
  data collection, 255
  definition, 62
  denial, 126
  DSM-IV, 143
  endocrine manifestations, 125–126
  estrogen therapy (*see* Estrogen therapy)

Anorexia nervosa (AN) (*Continued*)
etiology, 144–145
genetic factors, 111–112
and ghrelin
ANRT, 85
laboratory examinations, 85–87
onetime ghrelin infusion, 85–87
orexigenic effects, 87
GHRL polymorphisms, 113–115
GHSR polymorphisms, 115
GH values, 260–261
GOAT polymorphisms, 115
hormonal axes, 266–267
hypothalamic degeneration (*see* Anorexia and hypothalamic degeneration)
implications, 252–256
Leu72Met polymorphism, 113–115, 114*t*
materials and methods
biochemical assessment, 262
experimental protocol, 261–262
patients selection, 261
statistical analysis, 262–263
menstrual function, 244
mortality rates, 142
nutritional and hormonal parameters, 263–264, 264*t*
osteoporosis, 265
plasma levels, 110–111
prevalence, 143–144
psychiatric disorder, treatment, 267
refeeding, 136–137
steroid excretion, 130–136
steroid metabolism, 129–130
therapies, 144
women's skeletal integrity, 265–266
Anorexia nervosa restrictive type (ANRT)
caloric restriction, 85
ghrelin levels, 85
onetime ghrelin infusion, 85–87
therapy, 87
Anorexia of aging
animal studies
body weight, 322–323, 323*f*
food intake (*see* Food intake)
body fat mass, 346–347
body weight (BW), 320–321
catabolism and anabolism
animal/human life span, 342
BW/composition, 343–345
energy balance, 342–343
food intake, 341–342
homeostatic mechanisms, 341–342
olfactory receptors, 341
definition, 320
epidemiologic observations, 320–321
health problem, 322
human studies
gastric emptying, 337
leptin and insulin, 340–341
neuropeptides and peripheral nervous signals, 335–336
physiology and pathology, 335
serum levels and activity, gut hormones, 337–340
smell and taste sensation, 336
orexigenic and anorexigenic activities, 321–322
sarcopenia, 321
severe sarcopenia, 347
therapeutic approaches, 345–346
AN-OTP *vs.* non-OTP patients
clinical characteristics, 263, 263*t*
nutritional and hormonal parameters, 263–264, 264*t*
Anx/anx mouse
cell death/degeneration, 38–39
microglia (*see* Microglia)
mitochondrial complex I dysfunction, 39
Ndufaf1 gene, 40–41
neurochemical aberrances (*see* Neurochemical aberrances)
neuronal expression, 37–38
phenotype, 30–32
ATGL. *See* Adipose triglyceride lipase (ATGL)

B

BCAAs. *See* Branched -chain amino acids (BCAAs)
BMD. *See* Bone mineral density (BMD)
BMI. *See* Body mass index (BMI)
BN. *See* Bulimia nervosa (BN)
Body mass index (BMI)
and BMD, 266
calculation, 261
Caucasian women, 261

imped anciometer, 262
osteoporosis, patients, 263
Body weight
AGRP gene, 153–154
amenorrhea, 143–144
and food intake, 147
KO mice, ER alpha/beta, 148
Bone mineral density (BMD)
biological variables and bone parameters, AN patients, 264–265, 264*t*
and BMI, 260–261, 266
and HRT, 248–251
IGF-1 and estrogen, 251–252
oral contraceptives, 247
T-score at LS, 262
Branched -chain amino acids (BCAAs), 282
Bulimia nervosa (BN)
Arg51Gln and Leu72Met SNP, 112–113
basal ghrelin concentrations, 111
GHRL SNPs, 113–115
GHSR polymorphisms, 115
Leu72Met polymorphism, 113–115, 114*t*

C

Cachexia
aging, 224
AMPK, 289
anabolic and catabolic side, 287
anorexia, 274–275
anti-inflammatory strategies, 283–284
appetite regulation, 198–199
body and tissue wasting, 273–274
burn/thermal injury, 220–223
cancer, 209–215
cancer treatment-induced cachexia, 225
cardiac, 215–218
C26 colon carcinoma, 288–289
chronic pathologies, 272
colitis, 223
cytokine production, 284–285
cytokine-receptor interaction, 285–286
definition, 272
derangements, protein and lipid metabolism, 286–287
description, 198
ERK inhibition, 288–289
HIV/AIDS, 223–224
hypoanabolism/hypercatabolism, 279–281
inflammation, 275–278
inhibitors, lipolysis, 290
insulin/IGF-1 pathway, 287
"latent" to "overt" condition, 272, 290
metabolic perturbations, 290
MKK2/p38, 287–288
molecular mediators (*see* Mediators, cachexia)
nutritional interventions, 281–282
parameters, 272
peripheral and central appetite regulation (*see* Central melanocortin system)
proteasome inhibitors, 289
protein turnover modulations, 289
renal, 219–220
skeletal muscle, 287
symptoms, 198
therapeutic strategies, 281
tumor-bearing mice, 289–290
Cancer cachexia
anti-inflammatory treatment, 210–211
appetite regulation, 210
definition, 62
and ghrelin
animal models, 73–74, 75*t*
BMIs, 74–77
ghrelin mimetics, 82–83
human studies, 78–82, 79*t*
proinflammatory cytokines, 73–74
therapy, 78–82
leptin and ghrelin levels, 209–210
MC4-R antagonism and ghrelin administration, 211–215, 212*t*
megestrol acetate (MA), 210–211
Cancer treatment-induced cachexia
AgRP, 225
in animals, ghrelin, 225
cisplatin administration, 225
Cannabinoid (CB) receptors
AEA and 2-AG, 169
characterisation, 168
CNS and peripheral organs, 170–171
type 1 (CB1)
CCK and AEA signaling systems, 181–182

Cannabinoid (CB) receptors (*Continued*)
control of feeding and energy homeostasis, 172
expression, 168–169
hypothalamus, 173
type 2 (CB2)
endocannabinoid system, 172
expression, 168–169
glucose homeostasis, 172
Cardiac cachexia
causes, 215
classification, 215
infliximab, 216
MC4-R antagonism and ghrelin administration, 216, 217*t*
proinflammatory cytokines, 215–216
CART. *See* Cocaine- and amphetamine-regulated transcript (CART)
CCK. *See* Cholecystokinin (CCK)
Cell death-inducing DNA fragmentation factor-[alpha]-like effector A (CIDEA), 279
Central melanocortin system
activation model, 202–203, 202*f*
anorexic signal, 203–204
cytokines, 207
description, 201–202
expression, NPY and AgRP, 204
ghrelin, 206–207
leptin, 208
LIF, 207–208
MC4R antagonism, 205
MC3R modulation, 205
α-MSH, 203–204
receptor-ligand interactions, 202–203
serotonin, 209
stimulation, MC4R, 204–205
Central nervous system (CNS)
ghrelin-mediated orexigenic mechanisms, 311
ghrelin production, 310
5-HT1b/5-HT2c receptors, 304
5-HT receptors, 303
Central POMC-CRH-OT feeding circuit
alpha-MSH, 17
CRF receptor antagonist, 17
functional central melanocortin receptors, 16
intracerebroventricular administration, 17
nesfatin-1, food intake, 16
nutritional status information, 17, 18*f*
CHF. *See* Congestive heart failure (CHF)
Cholecystokinin (CCK). *See also* Feeding
affinity, 177–178
bioactive forms, 176
CCK1 receptors, 177
CCK2 receptors, 177
central CCK and feeding
meal completion, 180
opiod, dopaminergic, and melanocortin systems, 180–181
satiety effects, 180
description, 175–176
and endocannabinoid receptors, 181–183
gut hormone levels and activity, aging, 334–335, 337–338
leptin, 326–327
peripheral CCK and feeding
adaptive responses, 179
body weight regulation, 179
feeding modulation, 178
and ghrelin, 179
vagal afferent neurons, 178–179
receptors, 176
synthesis, 176
Chronic heart failure (CHF). *See* Cardiac cachexia
Chronic kidney disease (CKD)
characterisation, 219
clinical trials and application, 219–220
MC4-R antagonism and ghrelin administration, 220, 221*t*
proinflammatory cytokines, 219
Chronic obstructive pulmonary disease (COPD)
cachexia, 62
caloric deficiency, 83–84
and ghrelin
animal models, 83–84
chronic smoke exposure, 83–84
immune modulatory function, 84–85
non-GH-dependent mechanisms, 84–85
normal weight (NW) controls, 84–85

CIDEA. *See* Cell death-inducing DNA fragmentation factor-[alpha]-like effector A (CIDEA)
Ciliary neurotrophic factor (CNTF), 47, 48
Cisplatin-induced anorexia and ghrelin
  chemical structure, 302, 302*f*
  chemotherapy-induced nausea and vomiting, 302–303
  GHSR, 303
  5-HT (*see* 5-hydroxytryptamine (5-HT))
  mechanisms, 302, 314*f*, 315
  neurotransmitter abnormalities, 302–303
  treatment
    anti-dyspepsia effects, 311–312
    RKT (*see* Rikkunshito (RKT))
    therapeutic agent, 311
CNS. *See* Central nervous system (CNS)
CNTF. *See* Ciliary neurotrophic factor (CNTF)
Cocaine- and amphetamine-regulated transcript (CART)
  and AGRP/NPY, 31*f*, 37
  and IHC, 34
  and NPY, 34–35
  and POMC cells synthesize, 30
Congestive heart failure (CHF)
  anorexia, 62
  cachectic rat model, 68–69
  epidemiologic studies, 87–88
  and ghrelin
    anabolic/catabolic imbalance, 87–88
    GHRP treatment, 88
    in humans, 88–89
    in rat models, 88
  sympathetic nerve outflow, 89
COPD. *See* Chronic obstructive pulmonary disease (COPD)
Corticotropin-releasing hormone (CRH)-producing neurons
  central melanocortin system, 13
  CRH1R/CRH2R antagonist, 12–13
  hypothalamus, 12–13
  and POMC-OT (*see* Central POMC-CRH-OT feeding circuit)
Cytokine production
  atractylenolide I, 285
  body weight and mid-arm muscle, 285
  phospho diesterase inhibitors, 284–285
  proinflammatory cytokines, 285
  TACE, 285
  teratogenicity, 284
  thalidomide, 284
Cytokine-receptor interaction, 286–290
Cytokines, cachexia treatment
  IGF-1, 201
  LIF, 207–208
  melanocortin system, 203*t*, 207
  TNF-α, 200

D

DHA. *See* Docosahexaenoic acids (DHA)
Diagnostic and Statistical Manual of Mental Disorders (DSM-IV), 143, 261
Diet-induced obesity (DIO), 47
DIO. *See* Diet-induced obesity (DIO)
DMH. *See* Dorsomedial hypothalamic nucleus (DMH)
Docosahexaenoic acids (DHA), 282, 283
Dorsomedial hypothalamic nucleus (DMH), 33–34, 33*f*

E

Eating disorder (EDs)
  AN (*see* Anorexia nervosa (AN))
  BN (*see* Bulimia nervosa (BN))
  genetic factors, 108
  and ghrelin (*see* Ghrelin)
  multifactorial psychiatric diseases, 142–143
Eating disorders not otherwise specified (EDNOS), 142–143
ECLIA. *See* Electrochemiluminescence immuno assay (ECLIA)
Eicosapentaenoic (EPA)
  malnourished patients, 283
  patients with head and neck cancer, 283
  tumor-bearing animals treatment, 283
Electrochemiluminescence immuno assay (ECLIA), 262
Endocannabinoids. *See also* Feeding
  AEA and 2-AG, 169
  CB1 and CB2 receptors, 168–169
  and CCK, 181–183
  central endocannabinoids and feeding
    functional levels, 172–173
    hypothalamus, 173

Endocannabinoids (*Continued*)
mesolimbic dopaminergic system, 174–175
progressive ratio schedules, 174–175
sensory pleasure/hedonic feelings, 173–174
taste reactivity test, 173–174
THC administration, 173
complex network, 169–170
description, 168
FAAH, 170
G-protein-coupled receptor, 169
medical effects, 168
peripheral mechanisms and feeding
AEA levels, 171
CB1 and CB2 receptors, 170–171
humeral and nervous pathways, 171–172
in obesity and eating disorders, 172
receptors, 168
End-stage renal disease (ESRD)
anorexia, 62
ghrelin
and CKD, 89–90
in human trials, 90
in rats, 90
Energy homeostasis
aging, 320, 322–323
and body mass, 322–323
characteristic changes, 346–347
regulation, 324–326, 340, 342
EPA. *See* Eicosapentaenoic (EPA)
ESRD. *See* End-stage renal disease (ESRD)
Estrogen
in AN
animal models, 147–148
and food intake, brain, 148–149
human genetics (*see* Genetics, estrogen pathway)
hypoestrogenism, 150–151
sexual hormones, 150
cytochrome P450 members, 145
description, 145
ERs (*see* Estrogen receptors (ERs))
growth factors, 146
replacement, 146
Estrogen receptors (ERs)
activation, 149
alpha
ESR1 and *ESR2*, 151–152
expression, 146–147
gene encoding, KO mice, 148
ligand binding domain, 152–153
beta
ESR1 and *ESR2*, 151–152
expression, 146–147
gene encoding, KO mice, 148
feeding regulation, 146
isoforms, 145–146
transcription, 153–154
Estrogen therapy
bone mass, 245
clinical disadvantages, 246

F

FAAH. *See* Fatty acid amide hydrolase (FAAH)
Fatty acid amide hydrolase (FAAH), 170
Feeding
and CCK, 175–181
and endocannabinoids, 168–175
"fat sensor", 167
lumen, 167
peptidic signals, 166–167
peripheral signaling, 166
vagal afferent pathways, 166
Food intake
adipocytes, 2
central melanocortin system, 4–6
central oxytocin system, 6–8
central POMC-CRH-OT feeding circuit, 16–17
central regulatory mechanisms, 324–327
gut hormones
cholecystokinin, 337–338
ghrelin, 338–340
peptide YY and glucagon-like peptide 1, 338
hypothalamic neurogenesis, 46–48
hypothalamic regulation, 29–30
nesfatin-1 (*see* Nesfatin-1)
neural control, appetite, 2–4
neurodegeneration/hypothalamic inflammation
experimental and selective ablation, 46
HFD, 45

Ubb-dependent protein degradation, 45
neuronostatin (*see* Neuronostatin)
neuropeptides, 2
neuropeptides and peripheral nervous signals, 335–336
orexigenic and anorexigenic neuropeptides, 327, 328*t*
oxytocinergic and nonoxytocinergic-mediated anorexia, 18–19
physiologic alterations, gastrointestinal tract
gastric emptying, 337
smell and taste, 336
rodents, 323–324
serum levels and activity, hormones (*see* Hormones, control food intake)

G

GABA. *See* Gamma-aminobutyric acid (GABA)
Gamma-aminobutyric acid (GABA), 31*f*, 46
Gas chromatography (GC), 130–131, 131*f*
Genetics, estrogen pathway
AGRP gene, 153–154
BDNF gene, 153–154
candidate genes, 151–152
CYP19 gene, 153–154
ESR1 gene, 152–153
ESR2 gene, 152
GH. *See* Growth hormone (GH)
Ghrelin
anthropometry and eating pathology, 116
appetite and body weight regulation, 110
cachexia treatment
administration, 206
in aging, 224
anti-inflammatory properties, 206–207
in cancer cachexia, 211–215, 212*t*
in cardiac cachexia, 216, 217*t*
in colitis, 223
description, 206
in HIV/AIDS, 224
orexigenic action, 203*t*, 206
in renal cachexia, 220, 221*t*
in thermally injured rats, 223
description, 108
discovery, 62–64
and eating disorders
genes, 111–112
genome-wide association analysis, 116
polymorphisms, 112–115, 117
GHS-R1a, 64–65, 66
GOAT, 64–65
growth hormone secretion, 110
human and mouse ghrelin gene, 64–65
mechanisms of action, 66–72
regulation, 108
secretion, 64–65
signaling system, 108–110
UAG and AG, 64–65
Ghrelin *O*-acyl transferase (GOAT)
description, 109–110
genetic variation, 85
knockout mice, 64–65
polymorphisms, 115
Ghrelin/obestatin prepropeptide gene (GHRL)
anthropometry measures, 116
exons, 108–109
nonsynonymous polymorphisms, 112, 113
Ghrelin signaling system
des-acyl ghrelin, 109
GHSR, 109
GOAT, 109–110
N-terminal and C-terminal peptide, 108–109
GHRL. *See* Ghrelin/obestatin prepropeptide gene (GHRL)
GHS. *See* Growth hormone secretagogues (GHS)
GHSR. *See* Growth hormone secretagogue receptor (GHSR)
GHS-R1a. *See* Growth hormone secretagogue receptor (GHS-R1a)
GOAT. *See* Ghrelin *O*-acyl transferase (GOAT)
G protein-coupled receptors (GPCR), 8, 9, 12–13, 15–16
Growth hormone (GH)
description, 66–67
GHS (*see* Growth hormone secretagogues (GHS))
GHS-R1a (*see* Growth hormone secretagogue receptor (GHS-R1a))

Growth hormone (GH) (*Continued*)
and IGF (*see* Insulin-like growth factor-1 (IGF-1))
and IGF-1, 260–261
secretion, 64–65
on skeletal muscle, 67–68
Growth hormone secretagogue receptor (GHS-R1a)
AGRP and NPY, 69
discovery, 63–64
GH secretion, 64–65
knockout mice, 66
Growth hormone secretagogue receptor (GHSR)
cisplatin administration, 310–311
description, 109
gene and types, 109
gene expression, 310–311
ghrelin, 307–308
polymorphisms, 115
in stomach, 310–311
Growth hormone secretagogues (GHS)
cancer cachexia and ghrelin
animal models, 73–74, 75*t*
human studies, 78–82, 79*t*
discovery, 63–64
GHRP-6, 63–64
GHS-R1a (*see* Growth hormone secretagogue receptor (GHS-R1a))
on immune system, 71–72
in setting of cancer, 82–83

H

Heat shock protein 27 (HSP27)
cytoplasmic Akt complex, 287–288
hyperexpression, 287–288
phosphorylation, 287–288
HFD. *See* High-fat diet (HFD)
High-fat diet (HFD), 45
Hormone replacement therapy (HRT), 248–251, 249*t*
Hormones, control food intake
central insulin action, 333
ghrelin, 330–331
gut hormone levels and activity, 333–335
leptin and central leptin resistance, 331–333
serum concentrations, 327–330
Hormone-sensitive lipase (HSL), 277–278, 279
HRT. *See* Hormone replacement therapy (HRT)
HSL. *See* Hormone-sensitive lipase (HSL)
HSP27. *See* Heat shock protein 27 (HSP27)
5-Hydroxytryptamine (5-HT) receptor
cisplatin-induced ghrelin regulation
chemotherapy, 308
clinical approach, 308
feeding behavior, 307–308
GHSR mRNA expression, 310–311
5-HT2c receptor, 310
intraperitoneal administration, 309–310
plasma acyl ghrelin levels, 308–309
secretion, 307–308, 310
structure, acylated ghrelin, 307–308, 307*f*
cisplatin-induced overproduction
delayed gastric emptying/decreased food intake, 305*f*
enterochromaffin cells, 303
food intake, 304
5-HT1b, 5-HT2b and 5-HT2c activation, 304, 306*f*
metabolite 5-hydroxyindole-acetic acid, 303
POMC neuron, 306–307
vomiting and nausea, 303–304
Hypoanabolism/hypercatabolism
adipogenesis, cachexia, 279
adipose tissue and skeletal muscle, 279
anabolic signals, 279–280
CIDEA, 279
FoxO family, 280
lipid mobilization, 279
PI3K/Akt/mTOR pathway, 279–280
protein metabolism, 279–280
"side effect", 281
tumor-bearing mice, 279
Hypoestrogenism, 150–151
Hypothalamic peptide expression/feeding response, 327, 328*t*
Hypothalamus
AGRP gene, 153–154
ESR1 gene expression, 152–153
homeostatic functions, 149

I

ICV. *See* Intracerebroventricular (ICV)
IGF-1. *See* Insulin-like growth factor-1 (IGF-1)
Immunohistochemistry (IHC), 32–34
Inflammation and ghrelin, 71–72
In situ hybridization (ISH), 32–33, 34
Insulin-like growth factor-1 (IGF-1)
 catabolism and anabolism, 67
 downstream mediators, IGF-1 pathway, 68–69
 estrogen, 251–252
 family, 66–67
 and GH, 260–261
 GH/IGF-1 axis, 66–67
 ghrelin administration, 84–85
 nutritional and hormonal parameters, AN patients, 263–264, 264*t*
 serum levels, 262
 skeletal muscle protein synthesis, 67–68
Intracerebroventricular (ICV)
 chronic, 333
 ghrelin administration, 330–331
 hypothalamic peptide expression/feeding response, 328*t*
 insulin administration, 333
 leptin infusion, 332
ISH. *See In situ* hybridization (ISH)

L

Lateral hypothalamic area (LHA), 324, 325*t*
Leukemia inhibitory factor (LIF), 207–208

M

Major histocompatibility complex I (MHC I)
 microglial expression, 36–37
 neuronal expression, 37–38
Mammalian target of rapamycin (mTOR)
 AMPK, 289
 PI3K/Akt pathway, 279–280, 287–288
MAPK. *See* Mitogen-activated protein kinase (MAPK)
MAPK-kinase 2 (MKK2), 287–288
Mechanisms of action, ghrelin
 appetite regulation, 69
 inflammation, 71–72
 lipid metabolism
  activation of lipogenic pathways, 69–70
  brown adipose tissue (BAT), 70–71
  des-acyl ghrelin, 70–71
  ghrelin administration, rats, 69–70
 muscle and GH-IGF-1 axis
  catabolism and anabolism, 67
  description, 66
  downstream mediators, 68–69
  growth hormone (GH), 66–67
  skeletal muscle protein synthesis, 67–68
Mediators, cachexia
 albumin and prealbumin, 201
 catecholamines, 200
 IGF-1, 201
 proinflammatory cytokines, 201
 suppression of food intake, 199
 TNF-α, 199–200
Melanocortin
 central system (*see* Central melanocortin system)
 colitis, 223
 cytokines, 207
 leptin, 208
 ligand-receptor interaction, 202–203, 203*t*
 MC3R, 205
 MC4R (*see* Melanocortin 4 receptor (MC4R))
Melanocortin 4 receptor (MC4R)
 in cancer cachexia, 211, 212*t*
 in cardiac cachexia, 216, 217*t*
 intracerebroventricular injection, α-MSH, 204–205
 KO mice, 204–205
 ligand-receptor interaction, 202–203, 203*t*
 in renal cachexia, 220, 221*t*
MHC I. *See* Major histocompatibility complex I (MHC I)
Microglia
 activation, 35–36
 expression, MHC class I, 36–37
Mitogen-activated protein kinase (MAPK)
 ERK inhibition, 288–289
 MKK2, 287–288
 muscle wasting, 287–288

MKK2. *See* MAPK-kinase 2 (MKK2)
mTOR. *See* Mammalian target of rapamycin (mTOR)

N

National Health and Nutrition Examination Survey (NAHNES), 320–321
Nesfatin-1
 brain, 11–12
 Brunner's glands, 11–12
 Edinger-Westphal nucleus, 11–12
 endocrine cells, 11–12
 humans, 11–12
 induced anorexia
  autonomic activity and fluid intake, 14–15
  central circuits mediating, 12–13
  food intake and metabolism, 13–14
  physiological relevance, 15–16
 periphery, 11–12
Neurochemical aberrances
 anx/anx mouse brain, 32–33
 NPY/AGRP system, 33–34
 POMC/CART system, 34–35
 serotonergic systems, 35
Neurodegeneration
 hypothalamic inflammation
  experimental and selective ablation, 46
  HFD, 45
  Ubb-dependent protein degradation, 45
 mitochondrial deficiencies
  anx/anx mouse, 42–43
  ATP sensitive K^+ channels, 43–44
  Kir 6.2/SUR1 expression, 44–45
  NPY/AGRP system, 43
Neuronostatin
 bioinformatic analyses, 8
 GPCRs, 9
 induced anorexia
  and autonomic function, 10
  central circuits, 9–10
  physiological relevance, 10–11
 production, 8
 somatostatin, 8
Neuropeptide Y (NPY)
 and AgRP, 4, 326
 and AGRP neurons (*see* Agouti gene-related protein (AGRP))
 central melanocortin system, 4
 coexpressed neurotransmitters, 324
 hypothalamic peptide expression/feeding response, 328*t*
 hypothalamus, 335–336
 serum concentration, 335–336
Non-small cell lung cancer (NSCLC), 278, 283, 286
NPY. *See* Neuropeptide Y (NPY)
NSCLC. *See* Non-small cell lung cancer (NSCLC)
NUCB2. *See* Nucleobindin 2 (NUCB2)
Nucleobindin 2 (NUCB2)
 alpha-MSH expression, 12
 mRNA/immunoreactivity, 11–12
 and *NEFA* gene, 14
 and NEFA precursor protein, 11–12

O

Osteoporosis
 AN women, 263, 265–266
 densitometric criteria, 262–263
 diagnosis, 262
 osteopenia, 260–261, 265
 risk factor, 265
Oxidative phosphorylation system (OXPHOS)
 dysfunction, 42–43
 microarray and subsequent pathway, 39
 mitochondrial inner membrane, 39
 ROS, 39
OXPHOS. *See* Oxidative phosphorylation system (OXPHOS)

P

Paraventricular nuclei (PVN)
 and AgRP, 326
 central oxytocin system, 6–7, 6*f*
 POMC-CRH-OT feeding circuit, 17, 18*f*
Phosphoinositide-3-kinase (PI3K), 279–280, 287–288
PI3K. *See* Phosphoinositide-3-kinase (PI3K)
ω-3 Polyunsaturated fatty acids (PUFAs)
 anorexia, 282
 beneficial effects, 283
 chronic inflammation, cachexia, 283

POMC. *See* Pro-opiomelanocortin (POMC)
POMC-producing neurons
  AgRP, NPY/AgRP neurons, 4
  brain nuclei, 3–4
  brainstem nuclei, 4
  central melanocortin system, 4, 5*f*
  and CRH-OT (*see* Central POMC-CRH-OT feeding circuit)
Pro-opiomelanocortin (POMC)
  and CART (*see* Cocaine- and amphetamine-regulated transcript (CART))
  hypothalamic peptide expression/feeding response, 328*t*
  α-MSH neurons, 324, 326
Psychiatric disorder. *See* Anorexia nervosa (AN)
PVN. *See* Paraventricular nuclei (PVN)

R

RA. *See* Rheumatoid arthritis (RA)
Randomized controlled trials (RCT) and cohort studies
  HRT, 248, 249*t*
  quality, 252, 253*t*
RBP. *See* Retinol binding protein (RBP)
Refeeding
  fat gain, 136
  in men, obesity, 136–137
  11-OH/11-oxo ratio, 137
  20-OH/20-oxo ratio, 137
  steroid metabolites, 131–133, 134*t*
Renal cachexia. *See* Chronic kidney disease (CKD)
Retinol binding protein (RBP)
  measurement, 262
  nutritional and hormonal parameters, AN patients, 263–264, 264*t*
  and SHBG, 263–264
Rheumatoid arthritis (RA)
  anorexia, 62
  description, 91
  ghrelin infusion/GHS, 93
  ghrelin role, 91–92
  in humans, 92–93
  mechanisms of cachexia, 91
  in rat adjuvant arthritis (AA), 91–92
Rikkunshito (RKT)
  cisplatin-induced anorexia and dyspepsia, 312–314
  dysmotility-type functional dyspepsia symptoms, 312
  and flavonoids, 312–314
  induced ghrelin signal, 312–314
  plasma acylated ghrelin and leptin levels, 312, 313*f*
  plasma ghrelin secretion, rats, 312
  treatment, 312–314
RKT. *See* Rikkunshito (RKT)

S

Sarcopenia
  BW/composition, human aging, 343–345
  definition, 62
  and ghrelin, 72–73
Sexual hormone-binding globulin (SHBG)
  measurement, 262
  nutritional and hormonal parameters, AN patients, 263–264, 264*t*
  and RBP, 263–264
SHBG. *See* Sexual hormone-binding globulin (SHBG)
Single-nucleotide polymorphism (SNP)
  Arg51Gln, 112–113
  3056C allele, 116
  GHSR, 115
  Gln90Leu, 112–113
  GOAT, 115
  Leu72Met, 112–113
SNP. *See* Single-nucleotide polymorphism (SNP)
SON. *See* Supraoptic nuclei (SON)
Steroids
  ACTH, 127–128
  cholesterol, 127–128
  cyclopentanoperhydrophenanthrene structure, 127, 127*f*
  excretion, AN (*see* Urinary steroid profiling)
  glucocorticoids, 126–127
  metabolism, AN, 129–130
  mineralocorticoids, 126–127
  regulation, 128
  synthesis, 126

Sulfonylurea receptor (SUR)
arcuate and substantia nigra neurons, 44–45
K^+ channels, 43–44
Supraoptic nuclei (SON), 6–7, 6*f*
SUR. *See* Sulfonylurea receptor (SUR)

T

Terminal dUTP nick end labeling (TUNEL), 39
Thermal injury, cachexia, 220–223
TNF α-converting enzyme (TACE), 285

U

Urinary steroid profiling
biosynthesis and origin, 131, 132*f*
capillary GC, 130–131
chromatogram, 131, 133*f*
concentration of steroid, 130–131
enhanced androgen and cortisol metabolite excretion, 135
hydroxysteroid dehydrogenase (HSD), 133–135
metabolites of cortisol, 131, 131*f*
20-OH/20-oxo, 136
purification step, 130–131
starvation and after refeeding, AN patients, 131–133, 134*t*
weight-reducing diets, 135

V

Ventromedialhypothalamic nucleus (VMH), 324–326, 325*t*
VMH. *See* Ventromedialhypothalamic nucleus (VMH)

W

Weight disturbances
food intake (*see* Food intake)
mitochondrial deficiencies (*see* Neurodegeneration)

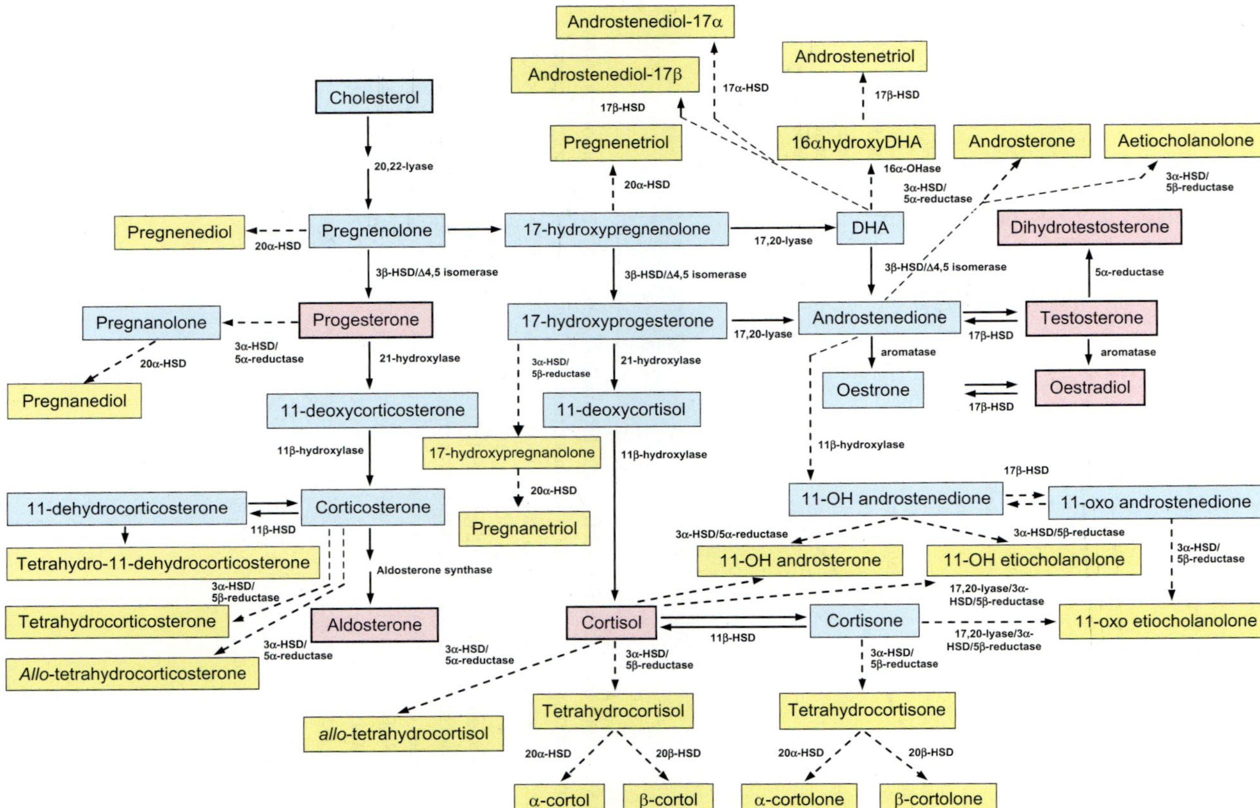

Wassif Samuel Wassif and Andrew Rashad Ross, Figure 5.3 Biosynthesis and origin of urinary steroid metabolites. Anabolic pathways are represented by a solid arrow (⟶); catabolic pathways (- - →); major hormonal steroids ▢; major urinary metabolites ▢; intermediates ▢. DHA represents dehydroepiandrosterone; HSD, hydroxy dehydrogenase (courtesy of Dr. N. Taylor).

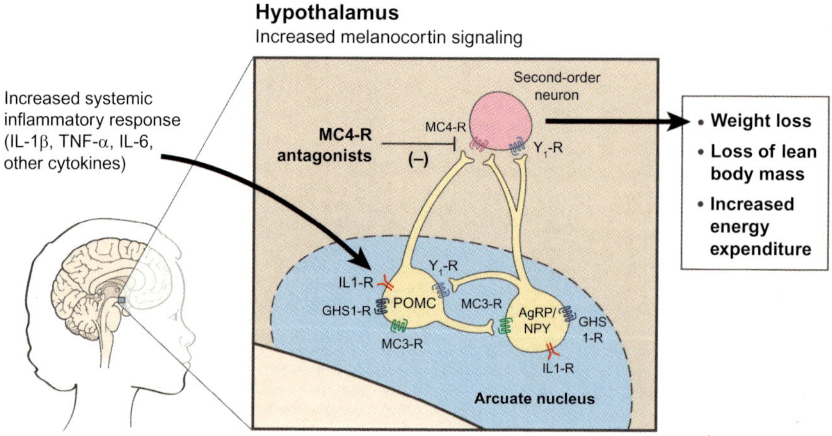

Jeremy Steinman and Mark Daniel DeBoer, Figure 8.1 Model for activation of the central melanocortin system in the hypothalamus during cachexia. The melanocortin system comprises two sets of neurons, ones expressing either POMC or AgRP and NPY. Each set of these expresses receptors to IL-1β, Ghrelin, and α-MSH. During cachexia, inflammatory cytokines are released; IL-1β acts on the IL-1-RI to increase the release of α-MSH from POMC neurons and decrease the release of AgRP. This causes an increase in activity at the MC4-Rs at second-order neurons and downstream events characteristic of cachexia. Blockade of this signal by AgRP/NPY neurons attenuates these downstream events. Increased production of AgRP, as is caused by the effect of ghrelin at the GHS-1R, also blocks melanocortin output. AgRP, Agouti-related protein; GHS-1R, growth hormone secretagogue receptor 1; IL1-R, interleukin-1 receptor; IL-1β, interleukin-1b; IL-6, interleukin-6; MC3-R, melanocortin-3 receptor; MC4-R, melanocortin-4 receptor; NPY, neuropeptide Y; TNF-α, tumor necrosis factor-α; Y1-R, NPY receptor-1. *Figure adapted from DeBoer (2010); used with permission.*

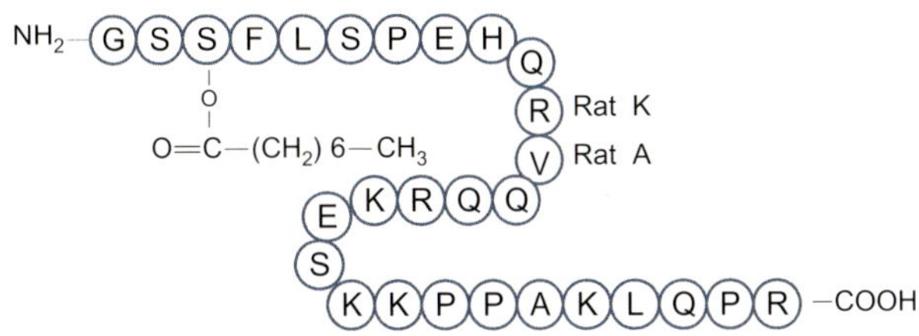

Tomohisa Hattori *et al.*, Figure 12.4 Structure of acylated ghrelin.

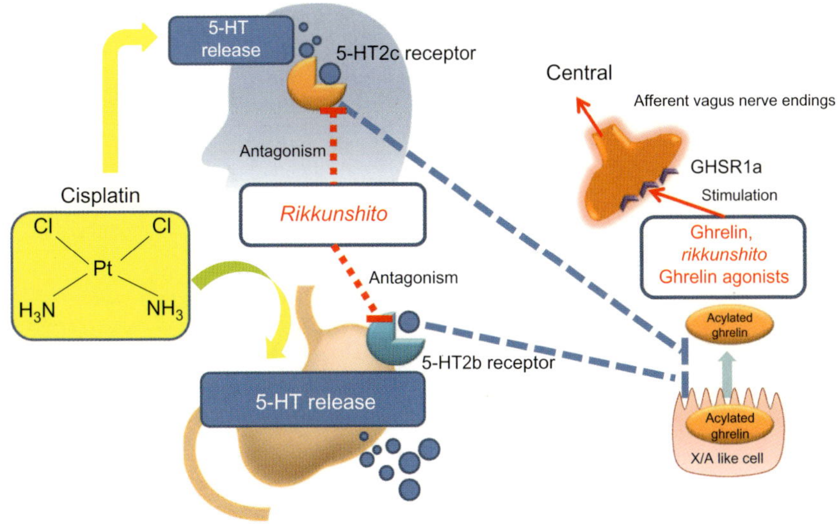

Tomohisa Hattori *et al.*, Figure 12.6 The mechanism for cisplatin-induced anorexia. *In vivo* administration of cisplatin releases serotonin present in large quantities in the enterochromaffin granule cells of the gastrointestinal tract. A portion of this binds with 5-HT2b receptors in smooth muscle of the stomach and the rest activates 5-HT2c receptors via blood or the afferent vagus nerve. These receptors reduce appetite, either directly or by controlling acyl ghrelin secretion from the stomach. Anorexia can be mitigated by supplementing insufficient ghrelin with exogenous acyl ghrelin or a ghrelin agonist. In addition, the ghrelin signaling enhancer RKT may mitigate anorexia by controlling reduced endogenous acyl ghrelin and sustaining ghrelin signaling.